PUBLIC HEALTH FOUNDATIONS

PUBLIC HEALTH FOUNDATIONS

Concepts and Practices

ELENA ANDRESEN
ERIN DEFRIES BOULDIN

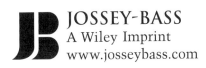

JOSSEY-BASS
A Wiley Imprint
www.josseybass.com

Library of Congress Cataloging-in-Publication Data

Public health foundations : concepts and practices / [edited by] Elena Andresen, Erin DeFries Bouldin.
    p. cm.
    Includes bibliographical references and index.
    ISBN 978-0-470-44587-7 (pbk.); ISBN 9780470890165 (ebk.); ISBN 9780470890172 (ebk.);
ISBN 9780470890189 (ebk.)
  1. Public health–United States. I. Andresen, Elena. II. Bouldin, Erin DeFries.
    RA445.P834 2010
    362.10973–dc22

                        2010036301

Printed in the United States of America

FIRST EDITION

PB Printing 10 9 8 7 6 5 4 3 2 1

To my husband.
EMA

To my husband, mom, and dad.
EDB

CONTENTS

Part 3: Behavior and Health

Part 4: Health Services and Social Determinants

Part 5: Forecasting Public Health

FIGURES AND TABLES

Figures

Tables

PUBLIC HEALTH is all around us. It is in the air we breathe, the water we drink, the homes we live in, and the behaviors in which we engage. It includes our health care systems and the agencies and services that protect our health and environment. Public health is a vital yet often overlooked component of modern life; most of us do not think about it as part of our daily lives. It may only receive public attention when a crisis occurs or when the public health system falters or fails. It may become an important personal focus when we need a specialized service, when we don't have access to a private clinic, or when we face a neighborhood environmental concern. Public health encompasses a broad range of activities and functions, but among its most important are promoting and preserving the health of populations through prevention. Prevention has several meanings or levels, as we discuss in the ensuing chapters, giving public health a breadth of purview uncommon to many disciplines. To address this breadth, the field of public health includes professionals from many backgrounds, including not only medicine and health professions but also sociology, microbiology, engineering, planning and development, marketing, and others. Public health even includes nonprofessionals; the entire public is part of the field because public health's activities and its funding are largely determined by the will and the needs of the people. This focus on populations and on the public is reflected in the cover photo for this textbook.

Audience

In recent years, multiple public health- and education-related organizations have highlighted the need to create an educated citizen as part of general undergraduate training. In 2003, the Institute of Medicine called for the educated citizen to have a basic grounding in public health and for all undergraduate students to have access to a public health education[1]. The Association of American Colleges and Universities (AAC&U) began The Educated Citizen and Public Health initiative to help integrate public health into the liberal arts education programs offered at colleges and universities across the United States[2]. Partly as a result of this movement, undergraduate public health courses are becoming more common throughout the United States and elsewhere. This book is designed to meet the needs of undergraduate instructors teaching introductory public health courses, including upper-division undergraduate courses.

This book is designed to be flexible and accommodate a variety of introductory public health courses. For a course targeting freshman or sophomore students, an instructor may choose to cover only the basics of each discipline, leaving aside the more in-depth chapters on study design, qualitative methods, and risk assessment, for example. Likewise, instructors could choose to cover the material in a different sequence than that presented here, using section headings as guides for similar content areas. The book is laid out in such a way that it follows the ten essential public health services[3], but other configurations would work equally well.

Content

In this book, we outline the history of public health, tracing the field from its roots in sanitation to its early endeavors to assure a basic level of education and services to all people. We then explore its more modern effort at quantifying health and intervening to improve the health of disadvantaged groups. Today, public health often is divided into five core disciplines: epidemiology, biostatistics, environmental health, social and behavioral sciences, and health policy and management. We have a chapter devoted to each of these broad subspecialties and also delve deeper into how public health is structured. We discuss quantitative and qualitative study designs, including a special look at pharmacoepidemiology, infectious diseases and tuberculosis, and risk management and communication. We end with a projection of where public health is likely to go in the rest of the twenty-first century as we face new challenges and continue to address ancient issues.

Features

- **Learning Objectives** Each chapter begins with a set of learning objectives to help students organize the material.

- **Introduction** Following the learning objectives, each chapter provides an overview of the content to prepare students for the information to come and to link it to previous chapters.

- **Public Health Connections** Throughout the text, more detailed explanations and case studies content of interest appear in text boxes. These features not only link to the chapter's content but also connect students to the practicality of the field of public health.

- **Summary** A summary closes each chapter, providing a recap for students and emphasizing key content and themes.

- **Key Terms** An indexed list of key terms is available in each chapter to bring students' attention to important concepts introduced and also to assist them in locating these topics within the text.

- **Review Questions** Each chapter's review questions encourage students to apply new concepts to practical applications or to recall specific details of a model or concept.

- **References** Resources used to construct each chapter are cited at the end of each chapter and provide a valuable link to both students and instructors looking for more information on a topic.

- **Glossary** Brief definitions of all key terms used in the text are included as an appendix to facilitate students' learning.

An overall goal of the textbook is to encourage the development of practical interpretation and problem-solving skills. In everyday life we must make decisions about what behaviors to engage in, what substances we are willing to ingest or inhale, and how to apply statistics and data about the relationship between various exposures and health outcomes. This book provides a framework through which to consider these decisions as well as a basic toolkit for synthesizing information and delivering it to others.

References

1. Institute of Medicine. *Who Will Keep the Public Healthy?* Washington, D.C.: National Academies Press; 2003.
2. Association of American Colleges and Universities (AAC&U). The Educated Citizen and Public Health initiative Web page. Available at: www.aacu.org/public_health/index.cfm. Accessed March 10, 2010.
3. Public Health in America. Mission statement. Available at: www.health.gov/phfunctions/public.htm. Accessed March 10, 2010.

Elena M. Andresen, PhD, is a professor in the Department of Epidemiology and Biostatistics at the University of Florida's College of Public Heath and Health Professions. Dr. Andresen received her PhD in epidemiology from the University of Washington, Seattle. She also trained in health services research and was a pre-doctoral Health Services Research and Development fellow at the Seattle VA Medical Center. Dr. Andresen has taught Introduction to Public Health and Public Health Concepts together with Erin DeFries Bouldin, MPH, to undergraduates at the University of Florida since 2006. In addition, she has many years of graduate teaching experience, including epidemiology methods courses and disability epidemiology courses, both in the United States and abroad. Her training and research interests include chronic disease epidemiology among older adults, disability epidemiology, and outcomes research in rehabilitation and disability.

Erin DeFries Bouldin, MPH, is a lecturer in the Department of Epidemiology and Biostatistics at the University of Florida's College of Public Heath and Health Professions. She received her MPH in epidemiology from the University of Florida, Gainesville. Ms. Bouldin has taught Introduction to Public Health and Public Health Concepts together with Elena Andresen, PhD, to undergraduates at the University of Florida since 2006. Ms. Bouldin's training and research interests include nutrition and maternal and child health, and her current work focuses on the health impacts of caregiving and improving the health and quality of life of Floridians with disabilities through the Florida Office on Disability and Health.

David Ashkin, MD, is the medical director and co-principal investigator of the Southeastern National Tuberculosis Center (SNTC), medical executive director at the A.G. Holley TB Hospital in Lantana, Florida, and Florida State TB health officer for the Florida Department of Health.

Alan Becker, PhD, MPH, is an assistant professor of environmental and occupational health at Florida A&M University, College of Pharmacy and Pharmaceutical Sciences, Institute of Public Health.

Lori Bilello, MBA, MHS, is a doctoral student in the Department of Health Services Research, Management and Policy at the University of Florida's College of Public Health and Health Professions.

Babette A. Brumback, PhD, is an associate professor in the Department of Epidemiology and Biostatistics at the University of Florida's College of Public Health and Health Professions.

Lisa R. Chacko, MPH, is a medical student in the School of Medicine at the University of Pennsylvania.

Sara A. Chacko, MPH, is a doctoral candidate in the Department of Epidemiology at the University of California Los Angeles.

Lisa Conti, DVM, MPH, DACVPM, CEHP, is the director of the Division of Environmental Health at the Florida Department of Health.

Barbara A. Curbow, PhD, is professor and chair of the Department of Behavioral Science and Community Health at the University of Florida's College of Public Health and Health Professions.

Amy B. Dailey, PhD, MPH, is an assistant professor in the Department of Epidemiology and Biostatistics at the University of Florida's College of Public Health and Health Professions.

Kendra Goff, PhD, is a toxicologist in the Division of Environmental Health at the Florida Department of Health.

Allyson G. Hall, PhD, MBA/MHS, is an associate professor in the Department of Health Services Research, Management and Policy at the University of Florida's College of Public Health and Health Professions.

Stephanie L. Hanson, PhD, ABPP (Rp), is the executive associate dean of the College of Public Health and Health Professions at the University of Florida.

Vito Ilacqua, PhD, is a research assistant professor in the Department of Environmental and Global Health at the University of Florida's College of Public Health and Health Professions.

JoAnne Julien, MD, is the deputy TB health officer for the Florida Department of Health, medical consultant for the Southeastern National Tuberculosis Center, and an adjunct assistant professor in the Division of Pulmonary, Critical Care and Sleep Medicine at the University of Florida.

Greg Kearney, DrPH, MPH, RS, is an epidemiologist in the National Center for Environmental Health at the Centers for Disease Control and Prevention.

Michael Lauzardo, MD, MSc, is the director of the Southeastern National Tuberculosis Center, deputy TB health officer for the Florida Department of Health, and chief of the Division of Mycobacteriology at the University of Florida.

Ellen D. S. López, MPH, PhD, is an assistant professor in the Department of Psychology and the Center for Alaska Native Health Research at the University of Alaska Fairbanks.

Cindy Prins, PhD, MPH, CIC, is an infection control practitioner at Shands Hospital at the University of Florida.

Sharleen Simpson, PhD, ARNP, is an associate professor in the Department of Women's, Children's, and Family Nursing at the University of Florida's College of Nursing.

Sandra Whitehead, MPA, is an environmental health planner in the Division of Environmental Health at the Florida Department of Health.

Almut G. Winterstein, PhD, is an associate professor and director FDA/CDER Graduate Training Program in the Department of Pharmaceutical Outcomes and Policy at the University of Florida's College of Pharmacy.

Mary Ellen Young, PhD, CRC/R, is a clinical associate professor in the Department of Behavioral Science and Community Health at the University of Florida's College of Public Health and Health Professions.

Public Health became a college discipline at the University of Florida in 2003 under the direction of the dean of the College of Public Health and Health Professions, Dr. Robert (Bob) Frank. The college was established in 1958 as the College of Health Related Services and included occupational therapy, physical therapy, and medical technology. Today, the mission of the College of Public Health and Health Professions is to preserve, promote, and improve the health and well-being of populations, communities, and individuals. It is a unique environment in which faculty and students work across a variety of levels of prevention and research, from preventing hearing loss to improving function after a spinal cord injury and from basic science research to population level interventions. The college has a number of graduate programs, including a master of public health degree, and a large bachelor of health science degree program. To raise awareness about the new discipline in the college, Dean Frank suggested that an undergraduate level public health course be implemented and offered to both the bachelor of health science students and other undergraduates across campus. We were excited by this proposal and agreed to teach Introduction to Public Health (PHC2100) to a group of thirty students in the fall of 2006.

In the summer of 2008, Andy Pasternack, senior editor at Jossey-Bass, contacted us. He had seen our course syllabus for Introduction to Public Health and wondered if we were interested in writing a textbook for the course. By that time, we had reworked the class to be an upper-level undergraduate course called Public Health Concepts (PHC4101). We had not, however, found a textbook that suited the course and were excited at the idea of crafting our own. We could not have imagined the journey on which we were embarking, but we are grateful to Andy for his vision and his request. We hope this textbook will serve the needs of many other undergraduate public health instructors who, like us, have found it challenging to identify a single textbook that covers the basics of public health, including methodology and topics of current interest. Our Public Health Concepts course is now required for all bachelor of health science students in our college, and the yearly enrollment in the class is nearly three hundred students. This book is the result of the assistance of many of our colleagues, some of whom have visited our course over the years and contributed their expertise to make the class, and now this book, a success. This book's production would not have been possible without the support, direction, and keen editorial skills of Seth Schwartz, Sandra Kiselica, Gary Kliewer, and Jane Loftus. We are also grateful to Robert E. Aronson, University of North Carolina at Greensboro; Yaw A. Nsiah, Eastern Connecticut State University; and Ashley C. Wells, University of Georgia, who served as reviewers for many of the chapters in this book.

Elena Andresen
Erin DeFries Bouldin

HISTORY, DEVELOPMENT, AND ORGANIZATION

CHAPTER 1

HISTORY AND DEVELOPMENT OF PUBLIC HEALTH

Erin D. Bouldin, MPH

LEARNING OBJECTIVES

- Define health and public health.
- Describe major historical milestones in the development of public health and identify major figures such as John Graunt, John Snow, and Lemuel Shattuck.
- Compare and contrast endemic, epidemic, and pandemic diseases.
- Identify and describe the three hallmarks of public health: philosophy of social justice, focus on prevention, and focus on populations.
- List and distinguish the five core public health disciplines.
- Understand ethics and be aware of situations in public health in which ethical concerns arise.

Public health is all around us. It is the air we breathe, the water we drink, the places we work. Public health is a broad discipline, encompassing professionals from various backgrounds: anthropology, sociology, economics, health behavior, biology, and statistics, to name a few. Perhaps because of its amorphous and expansive nature, public health is not well understood by the American public[1]. Although its functions touch our everyday lives, public health is not always identified as the source of the benefits it provides. In the absence of large-scale national or global health threats, the public may become complacent about the need for sustaining public health activities, even though it is a field that is always working to improve lives and health.

In this chapter, we will describe public health, beginning with a definition of health. We will discuss public health's mission and its core functions, which will provide a foundation for the rest of this book. We will trace public health's development over the centuries, identifying some of the major historical figures who advanced the field. We will also cover three hallmarks of public health: a philosophy of social justice, a focus on populations, and a focus on prevention. Finally, we will introduce you to some ethical considerations in public health.

What Is Public Health?

So what is public health? Let us first consider what we mean by health. The World Health Organization (WHO)[2] defines **health** as "a state of complete physical, mental, and social well-being and not merely the absence of disease or infirmity." This holistic view of health, incorporating body, mind, and community, is one consistent with the concept of public health, and it will be used as the definition of health in this text. **Public health** has been defined in different ways. In 1920, Charles Edward Amory Winslow said it is "the science and art of preventing disease, prolonging life, and promoting health and efficiency through organized community effort … to ensure everyone a standard of living adequate for the maintenance of health … ."[3, p. 10] In 1958, Geoffrey Vickers said public health consists of "successive re-defining of the unacceptable"[3, p. 10]. Both of these definitions highlight the role played by members of the community in improving health and in defining what is socially and publicly acceptable. Thus public health seeks to improve or maintain the health of a population, but does so according to the values and norms of its people.

The **mission of public health** is to "[fulfill] society's interest in assuring conditions in which people can be healthy"[4]. This mission comprises two areas that are vital to an understanding of public health. The first is *fulfilling society's interest*. As mentioned, public health is very much concerned with the needs and demands of the public. Much of the financing for public health activities comes from the federal government, and activities funded with public dollars are subject to input from the citizenry. This responsiveness to the will of the public also means public health is a fluid discipline. Although it has core functions and hallmarks, the purview and activities of public health change over time. The second part of this mission statement, *assuring conditions in which people can be healthy*, highlights the supportive role public health plays in the health of the populace. Public health does not necessarily provide medical care to individuals but rather assures conditions that support health. For example, smoking bans in restaurants and food-labeling requirements are public health efforts to prevent harmful exposures and to provide information to the public in order to promote healthful choices. This aspect of public health is one of the cornerstones of the field, namely that public health embraces a **social-ecological model** of health. This model essentially holds that health is not a result of individual factors alone but is also a result of external factors, such as those produced by family members, peers, and society as a whole. The social-ecological model will be described in more detail in later chapters of this text. One other cornerstone of public health not directly addressed in this mission statement is the focus on prevention. A complete definition of prevention, including a discussion of its three levels, appears in the next chapter.

History of Public Health

To fully understand the field of public health, it is helpful to understand how it became a discipline. For thousands of years, populations have been concerned with sanitation, housing, the provision of safe, clean food and water, and the control and treatment of disease. Public health evolved to address these concerns. These issues continue to be important today, along with the many new topics constantly added to the field. Although it was not always identified as a separate discipline, we can see examples of public health concerns in the earliest civilizations. Figure 1.1 shows some of the major historical events in the development of public health over the centuries.

Ancient Greece and Rome

The great writers, philosophers, and physicians of ancient Greece tell us of the beginnings of public health. In "Airs, Waters and Places," Hippocrates, the esteemed Greek physician, discussed the relationship between one's environment

FIGURE 1.1 Timeline of Major Developments in Public Health History

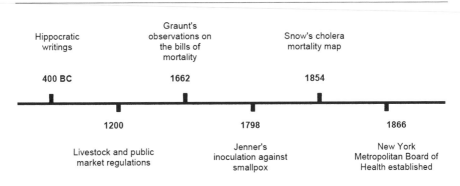

and health. He considered climate, soil, water, nutrition, and lifestyle to be important predictors of health outcomes[5]. In addition, he distinguished between endemic and epidemic diseases. **Endemic** diseases are those that occur at an expected rate in a population and **epidemic** diseases are those that occur at a rate higher than expected. These terms will be further defined and their importance to public health discussed in Chapter 4.

The Romans continued the medical inquiries of the Greeks and formalized public health administration systems[6]. The Romans constructed vast water supply and sanitation systems and established government positions dedicated to overseeing these systems. They also created offices to oversee the food supply at markets and to assess the public bathhouses. In addition, the Romans established perhaps the earliest example of a medical care system. Some physicians were associated with wealthy families, and others worked in what we would today call private practice offices. The government, however, paid other physicians to supply free medical care to citizens who could not afford to pay for it. Hospitals, including military hospitals and charity hospitals, were also created by the Romans[6]. Nonetheless, early advances in public health did not benefit all citizens equally. Slaves and citizens living in poverty often did not have access to clean water or sanitary living conditions, and Roman writers noted higher rates of disease among these lower classes of citizens. These **health disparities**, differences in the rate or severity of health outcomes between two groups of people, continue to be a focus of public health work today. Chapter 16 is devoted to describing modern health disparities.

Middle Ages

The Middle Ages began and ended with pandemics of bubonic plague: the Plague of Justinian in 543 and the Black Death in 1348. A **pandemic** is an epidemic, or unexpectedly large disease outbreak, that impacts the entire globe. The **etiology**, or cause, of bubonic plague was not understood during the Middle Ages, but poor living conditions were known to contribute to frequent epidemics. Today, we know bubonic plague is caused by infection with *Yersinia pestis*, a bacterium transmitted from rats to humans by the fleas that bite both. In the Middle Ages, overcrowded cities with unreliable municipal sanitation systems and close proximity of animals and humans allowed rat populations to flourish and bubonic plague to spread rapidly. Near the end of the Middle Ages, around 1200, European cities began passing laws to improve public health and combat epidemics. These measures included the establishment of slaughterhouses and the regulation of livestock possession[6]. Both of these improvements decreased the chances of passing disease between people and their animals. The regulation of food at public markets improved during the Middle Ages as well, with specific guidelines for the length of time specific food products could be sold and dedicated areas for waste disposal. These regulations prevented foodborne illnesses associated with eating rotten or outdated food and also prevented pests, including rats, from scavenging near the markets[6].

The long-standing practice of isolating people with leprosy was extended to those with the plague during the Middle Ages. **Isolation** is the separation from healthy individuals those people who are actively ill or who exhibit symptoms of illness. At the same time, in Venice ships entering the port were segregated to prevent the introduction of new diseases. This practice led to the term *quarantine*, which comes from the Italian *quarantenaria*, meaning forty days[6]. **Quarantine** is the separation of people who are not ill or symptomatic but who have been exposed to an illness.

Renaissance

The Renaissance (late 1300s to early 1600s) brought great strides in scientific discovery, laying the groundwork for advances in public health. During the Renaissance, two theories on the origin of epidemics prevailed. The first, taken from Hippocrates, held that *environmental factors* dictated the potential for outbreaks and that an *individual's susceptibility* determined whether he or she would fall ill. The opposing theory of contagion, championed by Giolamo Fracastoro (1478–1533), evolved into our present understanding of infection. Fracastoro believed microscopic agents were responsible for disease and that these agents could be transmitted by direct contact, through the air, or by intermediate fomites (inanimate objects such as doorknobs or drinking glasses that harbor infectious disease). He and his contemporaries did not imagine these infectious agents to be alive, however. It was not until Anton von Leeuwenhock (1632–1723) observed the first microscopic organisms that people believed this to be possible. Despite earlier conjecture by some leading scientists, the germ theory of disease did not truly take hold until the late nineteenth century[6].

As mercantilism and the conquest for wealth and power swept Europe from the sixteenth to eighteenth centuries, public health progress was part of each nation's interest. The necessity to quantify people and their health became clear. William Petty (1623–1687) coined the term *political arithmetic* and advocated the collection of data on income, education, and health conditions. (Gottfried Achenwall introduced the term *statistics* to replace *political arithmetic* in 1749.) It was John Graunt (1620–1674), however, who published one of the first statistical analyses of a population's health, noting associations between demographic variables and disease. Graunt also produced the first calculations of life expectancy. It was during this time that people began to recognize the need for state-supported programs to prevent premature (early) death[6]. Chapter 3 takes up the topic of modern data (information) systems, and Chapter 6 discusses modern biostatistics in more detail.

Enlightenment

As France led the world into the Age of Enlightenment in the eighteenth century, public health began in earnest. A humanitarian spirit and the desire for equality led to a *social* understanding of health. Infant mortality (death during the first year of life) was high on the list of concerns and disparities. The public health movement involved concerned citizens lobbying their governments to regulate alcohol and to provide for the safe conditions and fair treatment of all infants and children, regardless of their social standing[6]. Simultaneously, health education became popular, in line with the Enlightenment tenets of universal education and information dissemination. Despite earlier interest in the relationship of environment, social factors, and disease, it was in this era that health surveys were first employed[6]. Occupational health received attention as well, and the health of members of the armed services, especially sailors, and of metal workers and miners received attention. Rosen lists the various occupational ailments described during this time, including "dermatoses of shoemakers and metal workers, grocer's itch, eczema of washerwoman, and baker's itch"[6, p. 118]. John Howard (1726–1790) exposed the appalling conditions in which English prisoners lived, rousing public outcry that led to improved conditions. Mental illness, which carried a severe stigma and generally led to institutionalization, began to be viewed as a public health problem, especially after physicians demonstrated that a stable, nurturing environment produced better treatment results among the "insane" than restraints and physical punishment. Variolation (deliberate infection with smallpox), a common practice originating in China and spreading through the East over the centuries, became popular in the West in the 1700s. Although somewhat effective at preventing a serious case of disease, the practice of exposing susceptible people to smallpox could also induce severe forms of the disease and contributed to epidemics. In 1798, Edward Jenner (1749–1823) used naturally acquired and fairly benign cowpox to inoculate against smallpox. Within three years, more than one hundred thousand people were vaccinated in England alone. As early as 1800, publications heralded the impending eradication of smallpox, an event that would be officially achieved in 1980[6].

Industrial Revolution and Victorian Era

As the Industrial Revolution (between 1700 and 1900) spread from England through Europe and eventually to the United States, the health of workers quickly deteriorated, and calls for improved public health measures followed. The industrialization process widened gaps in income, causing the number of individuals receiving financial assistance from local governments to increase beyond capacity. In 1834, Edwin Chadwick (1800–1890) led the development of England's Poor Law Amendment Act, which withdrew government support from the able-bodied poor in an effort to encourage self-sufficiency. The only assistance offered was placement in workhouses. The administration of this system occurred at the national level, with a hierarchy of regional and local boards below. This market system mobilized the workforce, leading to a significant social change. Factories appeared, and the population moved toward industrial centers, creating crowded urban areas and work conditions ripe for the spread of disease. Little city planning occurred as builders rushed to provide enough housing for the influx of workers. Meanwhile, the wealthy, who could afford to travel, moved to suburban or rural areas vacated by the masses. Sanitation systems and public parks were not planned in most cities. Few toilets were available to city dwellers, and there was no infrastructure for garbage removal or sewage systems. In 1833, the passage of the Factory Act dealt with working conditions and the poor living conditions of those workers it sought to protect. Throughout the 1830s and 1840s, legislation regulating mines, factories, and child labor passed in England and Europe[6].

During an 1848 cholera (an acute diarrheal illness) outbreak in London, John Snow (1813–1858), often deemed the father of epidemiology, identified a particular public water pump as the likely source of the epidemic. Again, in 1854, he mapped reported cholera deaths during an outbreak and associated the clusters with a water supply company that drew its supply downstream from London on the Thames River, where we now know that the water was more contaminated by sewage (see the map in Chapter 4, Figure 4.6). Snow hypothesized cholera transmission was possible via water. In addition, he is generally credited with ending the 1848 outbreak by breaking the handle off the Broad Street Pump, although some historians believe the epidemic had already begun to recede by this point. It would be several decades, however, before his hypothesis was proven correct. Nonetheless, his disease investigations and the epidemiological methods he employed generated knowledge that could prevent disease without knowing the causative agent[6].

Disease outbreaks were associated with the poorest, dirtiest parts of cities, but quickly began to affect all social classes. Chadwick understood the poverty–

disease cycle and sought statistics to quantify the relationship. Surveys on sanitary conditions resulted in the *Report on and Inquiry into the Sanitary Condition of the Laboring Population of Great Britain* in 1842. The report became a standard for epidemiological investigation and community health action and formed the basis for sanitary reform[6]. Chadwick linked disease and the environment and called for city engineers, rather than physicians, to wage the war on disease outbreaks. The General Board of Health, created by the Public Health Act of 1848, was an attempt at organized government responsibility for the health of its citizens. Although disbanded after a few years, the board laid the groundwork for public health as we now know it. The explosion of vital statistics (birth and death records) and survey data collection during this period prompted the publication of several data-based health reports during the mid-1850s[6]. There were no standards for analysis, however, and few authors employed the same methods, citing the inapplicability of mathematics to health. Adolphe Quetelet (1796–1874) began the work necessary to remedy the perceived incompatibility and published a compendium of practical applications of mathematics in health, today called *biostatistics*.

In the United States, Lemuel Shattuck (1793–1859) produced *Report on the Sanitary Condition of Massachusetts* in 1850, calling for the establishment of state and local boards of health, increased attention to vital statistics collection, and improved health education. In 1866, the New York Metropolitan Health Bill created the Metropolitan Board of Health, and it reorganized four years later into what is today the New York City Health Department. This board was the foundation for the U.S. public health system[6]. In 1869, Massachusetts used Shattuck's recommendations to create the first effective state health department. Around the same time, efforts to create a national board of health failed[6]. In 1878, the authority for port quarantine was bestowed upon the surgeon general of Marine Hospital Services. As the responsibilities of the Marine Hospital Service expanded in the late nineteenth and early twentieth centuries to include infectious disease investigation, immigrant screening at Ellis Island, vital statistics collection, and the dissemination of knowledge through its journal *Public Health Reports*, the agency's name was changed first to the Public Health and Marine Hospital Service (1902) and ultimately to the United States Public Health Service (PHS; 1912)[7].

During the nineteenth century, two theories relating to communicable (contagious or infectious) disease prevailed. The first was the miasma theory, which held that disease was due to a particular state of the air or environment. The second theory was that a specific contagion was responsible for each disease. In fact, many people believed some combination of the two was the real explanation: some contagious agent, whether disease specific or not, in combination with social or environmental factors, produced disease[6]. By the end of the century, the germ theory of disease had been firmly established by Koch, Pasteur, and many others. From 1880 to 1898, the causative agents for a multitude of diseases, from malaria to tuberculosis and plague to typhoid were identified. Antiseptics became popular in medical care, which resulted in a marked decrease in **morbidity** (the existence of any form of disease, or to the degree to which the health condition affects the patient) and **mortality** (susceptibility to death). A more complete understanding of immunity was established late in the nineteenth century, and the development of vaccines proceeded nearly as rapidly as the discovery of pathogenic organisms. The United States Marine Hospital established one of the first bacteriological laboratories in the world in 1887. Although the United States was not the site of most scientific discovery in the era, it was the leader in applying new knowledge to public health[6].

Modern Public Health

Armed with increasingly more effective weapons against disease, public health's mission throughout most of the twentieth century continued to be preventing and controlling communicable or infectious disease. As you can see in Tables 1.1 and 1.2, deaths due to infectious agents occurred at a much higher rate than deaths due to noninfectious causes in the United States for much of the century.

Public health remained largely a local enterprise until social change occurred following the Depression (1929–1941), when people needed, and thus allowed, government intervention and subsidy. Throughout the 1900s, public health achievements such as water fluoridation, mass immunizations, motor vehicle safety, occupational safety, food supply safety and fortification, improved maternal and child health, family planning, prevention of heart disease and stroke, and, of course, control of infectious diseases led to substantially reduced morbidity and mortality[10]. Public health programs have been credited with a twenty-five-year increase in life span over the course of the twentieth century[10]. The establishment of agencies such as the Centers for Disease Control and Prevention (CDC) in 1946 (born out of the Office of Malaria Control as the Communicable Disease Center, part of the U.S. Public Health Service) and the World Health Organization in 1948 (the United Nations' dedicated health agency) have allowed the advancement of public health by establishing centralized agencies to which people can turn for information and assistance.

The definition of public health was established primarily during the twentieth century by individuals such as C.E.A. Winslow (mentioned above) and through groundbreaking works such as the series of Institute of Medicine (IOM) reports dedicated to the field. IOM's 1988 *The Future of Public Health* clearly

Table 1.1 Number of Deaths and Crude Mortality Rate for Leading Causes of Death in the United States in 1900

Cause of Death	Number of Deaths	Crude Mortality Rate per 100,000
Pneumonia and influenza	40,362	202.2
Tuberculosis	38,820	194.4
Diarrhea, enteritis, and other gastrointestinal problems	28,491	142.7
Heart disease	27,427	137.4
Stroke	21,353	106.9
Kidney diseases	17,699	88.6
Unintentional injuries (accidents)	14,429	72.3
Cancer	12,769	64.0
Senility	10,015	50.2
Diphtheria	8,056	40.3

Source: Reference 8.

Table 1.2 Number of Deaths and Crude Mortality Rate for Leading Causes of Death in the United States in 2000

Cause of Death	Number of Deaths	Crude Mortality Rate per 100,000
Heart disease	710,760	258.1
Cancer	553,091	200.9
Stroke	167,661	60.9
Chronic lower respiratory diseases	122,009	44.3
Unintentional injuries (accidents)	97,900	35.6
Diabetes mellitus	69,301	25.2
Influenza and pneumonia	65,313	23.7
Alzheimer's disease	49,558	18.0
Kidney diseases	37,251	13.5
Septicemia	31,224	11.3

Source: Reference 9.

defined public health's mission as "assuring conditions in which people can be healthy."[4] It also delineated steps needed to improve a fractured public health system and identified the three core functions of public health: assessment, policy development, and assurance, described in detail in the following chapter. In 2002, *Who Will Keep the Public Healthy* established requirements for the training of the public health workforce[11], and *The Future of the Public's Health in the 21st Century* translated the 1988 recommendations into practice while embracing the concept of "healthy people in healthy communities"[12].

PUBLIC HEALTH CONNECTIONS 1.1

INSTITUTE OF MEDICINE

The Institute of Medicine (IOM), founded in 1970, is a part of the nonprofit organization, the National Academy of Sciences. The IOM acts as an advisory body to the United States, generating unbiased, evidence-based reports on some of the most important health and scientific policy issues of the day. The IOM works by establishing panels of experts in the field to collaborate on topical reports.

Throughout this textbook, we will refer to three recent IOM reports on public health: *The Future of Public Health* (1988), *The Future of the Public's Health in the 21st Century* (2002), and *Who Will Keep the Public Healthy?* (2003).

Public health, and its tenets and activities, has evolved throughout time in response to shifts in societies' values and scientific knowledge. Some of the historical issues of infectious diseases, health disparities, and population assessment continue to be modern public health challenges. There are new public health challenges also: populations are more mobile than ever, heightening concerns about pandemics. The mortality of many vaccine-preventable diseases declined so dramatically over the course of the twentieth century that often there is complacency about these diseases, and immunization rates have dropped. Antibiotic resistance has also made the apparent victory over common infections less certain. Medical care and insurance in the United States continues to cost more than many people can afford, and as the population ages, the federal government will face increasing fiscal demands. Bioterrorism and natural disasters have required planning for mass immunization, prophylaxis, evacuation, and treatment. We will address these and a variety of other public health topics and challenges throughout the rest of this textbook.

Hallmarks of Public Health

Although the issues facing public health may vary over time, the underlying principles of public health remain constant. There are three hallmarks of public health that define the field and also provide a contrast to the related field of medicine. Public health and medicine often have the similar goals of reducing the impact of disease and improving health and quality of life, but there are some notable differences between the two in the methods of reaching these goals. The hallmarks of public health are a philosophy of **social justice**, a focus on **populations**, and a focus on **prevention**.

Philosophy of Social Justice

The term *social justice* has been used by various groups in different contexts. In public health, the concept of social justice connotes the idea that all individuals in a population should have access to the same programs and services, regardless of social condition or standing. This is in contrast to a concept of access to goods, services, and programs based on market forces, a concept known as *market justice*. Public health seeks to provide a basic level of health provisions, such as clean food and water, safe neighborhoods, and access to health care services, to all members of a community or population. In this vein, public health works to ensure there are no health disparities. In fact, the elimination of health disparities in the United States was one of the two overarching goals of a federal initiative called *Healthy People 2010*, the health blueprint for the nation[13]. (The other overarching goal is to increase the quality and years of healthy life[13].)

Focus on Populations

In medicine, patients typically are seen and managed individually. In public health, the focus is on groups of people or populations rather than on individuals. Public health endeavors to implement programs that benefit a group of people: water fluoridation, folic acid fortification of grain products, the development of safe walking trails throughout a city, etc. Ultimately, these public health interventions will impact individuals' health, but the needs, desires, and attributes of the population as a unit are considered when making decisions in public health, rather than what will benefit each individual person. The methods of measuring population characteristics are described in more detail in later chapters. Also, as alluded to above, some public health systems, such as local health departments, indeed provide individual-level medical care and treatment, but often these programs are established to serve subgroups in a population with limited access to these services.

Focus on Prevention

Throughout this text, you will often read about prevention and the numerous efforts to prevent people from being exposed to harmful or unhealthful substances or experiences. Indeed, public health focuses on preventing poor health outcomes or exposures that lead to these outcomes, and this focus is a hallmark of the field. As you will learn in Chapter 2, prevention has multiple levels, some of which may surprise you. Public health seeks to identify risk factors for disease and then works to learn methods for eliminating or limiting these risk factors to prevent populations from becoming ill or experiencing poor health. In addition, public health typically aims to maintain health rather than to address decrements in health after they have occurred.

In May 2009, an opinion survey of registered voters in the United States revealed that the public views prevention as an important component of health care in the country and believes that prevention efforts should receive more funding[14]. Regardless of political party affiliation, geographic region, or demographic subgroup, the majority of U.S. voters (76 percent) believe the federal and state governments should invest more strongly in prevention efforts. The survey also revealed a change in this opinion: in 1987, 45 percent of voters said the United States should put more emphasis on prevention (versus treatment), and in 2009, 59 percent said prevention should be given more emphasis than treatment. Despite the common concern in public health groups that cost savings must be demonstrated in order to gain support for prevention efforts, 72 percent of voters said that prevention is worth the investment even if it does not save money because the lives saved and quality of life improvements are worth the cost[14].

Core Public Health Disciplines

Although public health is a multidisciplinary field comprising individuals who may not have formal training in the subject, there are five core disciplines within public health in which practitioners are trained: epidemiology, biostatistics, social and behavioral sciences, environmental health, and health management and policy (Figure 1.2). **Epidemiology** is the study of the determinants and distribution of health outcomes. It encompasses describing health outcomes based on the frequency or number of events and analyzing health outcomes to identify risk factors. Epidemiology may be divided into the two broad areas of chronic disease and infectious disease epidemiology. You will learn more about epidemiology in Chapters 4 and 5. **Biostatistics** provides the tools to understand public health data. It is a branch of statistics devoted to understanding health and health outcomes and allows the analysis of complex studies. Chapter 6 discusses biostatistics in more detail. **Environmental health** is largely concerned with the impact of various exposures on health. Environment is broadly

FIGURE 1.2 Core public health disciplines

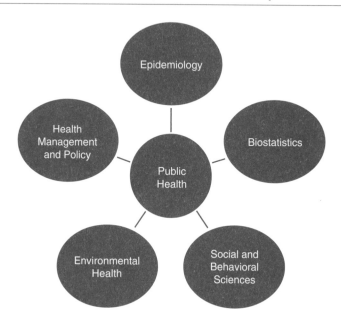

defined and may include any aspect of the physical environment and its relationship to health outcomes. Details about environmental health appear in Chapters 9 and 10. **Social and behavioral sciences** focus on individual-level factors and the impact of external factors on health, primarily the influence of the social environment. This discipline includes understanding how people respond to external messages and information and how to change behavior. Social and behavioral science is covered in more depth in Chapters 11 and 12. **Health management and policy** is the discipline most concerned with issues of health care access and the policies at various levels of an organization or government, as well as how these policies impact health outcomes. More information about health management and policy is included in Chapters 14 and 15.

Modern public health training programs typically include each of these disciplines in their master's of public health (MPH) degree program. Although each discipline has specialty skills and techniques for conducting its part of public health research and practice, public health education also includes cross-disciplinary training. This cross-training allows professionals in different disciplines to work together to solve problems that benefit from the application of more than one set of skills. For more information about how public health training programs are organized and the competencies of these disciplines, visit the Council on Education in Public Health Web site, http://CEPH.org/.

Public Health Ethics

As we have discussed in this chapter, public health seeks to understand disease and improve health at the population level. To achieve this, some individuals may be encouraged or required to take actions that may be uncomfortable or undesirable in order to prevent harm to others. Likewise, in order to understand risk factors for disease, injury, and other poor health outcomes, public health professionals must conduct research studies. Research also is required to compare the effectiveness of vaccines, drugs, interventions, and treatment options in preventing or curing disease. Many public health activities must be carefully assessed and scrutinized to ensure that the activities conform to **public health ethics**, in other words, that the actions taken maintain human rights, individual autonomy, and legal requirements.

Ethical dilemmas abound in public health as we weigh the benefit to the group against the freedoms of the individual. For example, should we compel someone with an infectious disease to take medication or to remain in isolation to prevent others from becoming ill? If we know a behavior greatly increases the risk of morbidity or mortality, should laws be enacted to prevent it? If we are trying to understand the risks associated with an activity, but we do not want study participants to change their activity patterns during the course of study, are we obligated to disclose the purpose of the study? Some ethical concerns in public health seem relatively straightforward. For example, few would believe it ethical to randomly assign study participants to an exposure with even moderate evidence of harm, such as radiation, for the sake of research alone. Nonetheless, there are historical examples of studies that proceeded with agency or even government approval and funding that, in retrospect, were clearly unethical.

As a result of past research transgressions, there are guidelines and systems in place to ensure that anyone participating in a research study understands the risks and benefits associated with the study and that the subject consents to be involved in the study, without being bribed or coerced into doing so. The **Nuremberg Code** outlines these and other assurances that must be in place in order to conduct human subjects research. The code arose from the Nuremberg trials of 1946–1947 in which German physicians and their associates were tried, and many convicted, for killing or disabling thousands of people in Nazi concentration camps during World War II[15].

PUBLIC HEALTH CONNECTIONS 1.2
BASIC TENETS OF THE NUREMBERG CODE

The Nuremberg Code comprises ten directives for enrolling people in research studies, summarized below.

1. The study subjects should have legal capacity to give consent, have a choice in participating, and be able to make an informed decision. Study participants should know the purpose of the study and the risks and benefits associated with it.

2. An experiment involving human subjects should be conducted only if there is no other way to arrive at the conclusion and if the study results will benefit society.

3. The experiment should be based on the results of animal studies and knowledge of the natural history of the disease.

4. The experiment should avoid all unnecessary physical and mental suffering and injury.

5. An experiment should not be conducted if there is a reason to believe that death or disabling injury will occur.

6. The degree of risk should never exceed the benefit to society.

7. All precautions should be taken to protect the experimental subject from injury, disability, or death.

8. Only scientifically qualified persons should conduct the experiment.

9. The study participants should be free to withdraw from the study at any time.

10. If at any point during a study the researchers believe continuing the study will cause injury, disability, or death among participants, they should end the study.

The **Belmont Report** was created by the National Commission for the Protection of Human Subjects of Biomedical and Behavioral Research in 1976 with the intent of providing "an analytical framework that will guide the resolution of ethical problems arising from research involving human subjects"[16]. The *Belmont Report* builds upon the Nuremberg Code, distinguishing between research and practice, outlining three basic ethical principles (respect for persons, beneficence, and justice), and listing specific requirements needed to meet the ethical principles (informed consent, assessment of risks and benefits, and fair selection of subjects).

PUBLIC HEALTH CONNECTIONS 1.3

EXCERPTS FROM THE BELMONT REPORT

Part A. Boundaries Between Practice and Research

The purpose of medical or behavioral practice is to provide diagnosis, preventive treatment, or therapy to particular individuals. By contrast, the term "research" designates an activity designed to test a hypothesis, permit conclusions to be drawn, and thereby to develop or contribute to generalizable knowledge (expressed, for example, in theories, principles, and statements of relationships). Research is usually described in a formal protocol that sets forth an objective and a set of procedures designed to reach that research.

Part B. Basic Ethical Principles

1. *Respect for Persons.* Respect for persons incorporates at least two ethical convictions: first, that individuals should be treated as autonomous agents, and second, that persons with diminished autonomy are entitled to protection.... To respect autonomy is to give weight to autonomous persons' considered opinions and choices while refraining from obstructing their actions unless they are clearly detrimental to others.... Respect for the immature and the incapacitated may require protecting them as they mature or while they are incapacitated.... In most cases of research involving human subjects, respect for persons demands that subjects enter into the research voluntarily and with adequate information.

2. *Beneficence.* ...The term "beneficence" is often understood to cover acts of kindness or charity that go beyond strict obligation. In this document, beneficence is understood in a stronger sense, as an obligation. Two general rules have been formulated as complementary expressions of beneficent actions in this sense: (1) do not harm and (2) maximize possible benefits and minimize possible harms....

3. *Justice.* Who ought to receive the benefits of research and bear its burdens? This is a question of justice, in the sense of "fairness in distribution" or "what is deserved." An injustice occurs when some benefit to which a person is entitled is denied without good reason or when some burden is imposed unduly.... Finally, whenever research supported by public funds leads to the development of therapeutic devices and procedures, justice demands both that these not provide advantages only to those who can

(Continued)

PUBLIC HEALTH CONNECTIONS 1.3

EXCERPTS FROM THE BELMONT REPORT (Continued)

afford them and that such research should not unduly involve persons from groups unlikely to be among the beneficiaries of subsequent applications of the research.

Part C. Applications.

1. *Informed Consent.* Respect for persons requires that subjects, to the degree that they are capable, be given the opportunity to choose what shall or shall not happen to them ... the consent process [should contain] three elements: information, comprehension and voluntariness. Information ... include[s] the research procedures, their purposes, risks and anticipated benefits, alternative procedures (where therapy is involved), and a statement offering the subject the opportunity to ask questions and to withdraw at any time from the research.... Because the subject's ability to understand is a function of intelligence, rationality, maturity, and language, it is necessary to adapt the presentation of the information to the subject's capacities.... An agreement to participate in research constitutes a valid consent only if voluntarily given. This element of informed consent requires conditions free of coercion and undue influence.

2. *Assessment of Risks and Benefits.* The assessment of risks and benefits requires a careful arrayal of relevant data, including, in some cases, alternative ways of obtaining the benefits sought in the research. For the investigator, it is a means to examine whether the proposed research is properly designed. For a review committee, it is a method for determining whether the risks that will be presented to subjects are justified. For prospective subjects, the assessment will assist the determination whether or not to participate.

3. *Selection of Subjects.* Justice is relevant to the selection of subjects of research at two levels: the social and the individual. Individual justice in the selection of subjects would require that researchers exhibit fairness: thus, they should not offer potentially beneficial research only to some patients who are in their favor or select only "undesirable" persons for risky research. Social justice requires that distinction be drawn between classes of subjects that ought, and ought not, to participate in any particular kind of research, based on the ability of members of that class to bear burdens and on the appropriateness of placing further burdens on already burdened persons. Thus, it can be considered a matter of social justice that there is an order of

preference in the selection of classes of subjects (e.g., adults before children) and that some classes of potential subjects (e.g., the institutionalized mentally infirm or prisoners) may be involved as research subjects, if at all, only on certain conditions."

Source: Reference 16.

At universities and other research organizations, an **institutional review board (IRB)** or **independent ethics committee (IEC)** is in place to review all research protocols before they begin. The purpose of the IRB/IEC is to protect **human subjects**, the individuals who will be involved in the research study. The IRB/IEC typically is made up of researchers and regulatory experts who understand the federal laws relating to human subject research. The IRB/IEC ensures that potential study participants are given a complete and honest assessment of the activities involved in research and any *potential* positive and negative outcomes. There also must be a method of collecting and documenting that research subjects understand the description of and agree to participate in the study. This can be challenging when studying children or individuals with cognitive disabilities, for example. Often, another person (a legal representative or guardian) provides consent on behalf of the study participant. Careful assessment of the consent process must be ensured any time a vulnerable population is included in research.

In addition to the actual research process, there are ethical standards regarding the personal information and data collected from individuals. Some data may be sensitive and could impact a person's ability to gain employment or insurance (for example, HIV status or health behaviors such as smoking), thus data must be safeguarded against disclosure. The same is true of personal information such as Social Security numbers, which could cause financial loss if inappropriately disclosed. Within the U.S. Department of Health and Human Services (HHS; see Chapter 2 for more details), the Office for Human Research Protections (www.hhs.gov/ohrp) is charged with protecting the rights and welfare of individuals who participate in research funded by HHS, the primary research funding agency of the U.S. government. It provides guidance to researchers and institutions conducting human subject research, registers IRBs and IECs, enforces policies, and educates the public about their rights and responsibilities as research subjects.

Throughout this textbook, we will alert you to cases in which ethical concerns arise in addressing public health problems. As we discuss study designs in

Chapter 5, it is important to think about potential ethical dilemmas that can arise in selecting study participants and providing different treatment options. In our discussion of tuberculosis and other infectious diseases in Chapters 8 and 13, think about the implications of the requirement that specific diseases be reported to public health authorities and the methods used to ensure that individuals take the prescribed medication to prevent the spread of disease.

Summary

Public health is a multidisciplinary field that has evolved over the centuries from basic associations between the environment and health into a field comprising five major disciplines that all work toward preventing poor health outcomes among populations, using the principle of social justice as a core tenet. Public health can be defined in many ways, and public health indeed means something different to different people. Even if it is not identified as such, public health touches people every day through safe food and drug supplies, clean and often fluoridated water, and toxic chemical-free workplaces and homes. A number of individuals have shaped the history of public health, developing the basis for analytic tools and measures we still use to describe and compare health today. In addition, social movements have shaped and continue to direct public health's mission, scope, and activities. Ethical considerations are important in public health, and public health shares its ethical basis with other health and medical fields in landmark works such as the Nuremburg Code and the *Belmont Report*. In the upcoming chapters, we will discuss the structure of public health in the United States, each of the core public health disciplines, and many of the current and future issues public health will face and address.

Key Terms

Belmont Report, 18

biostatistics, 15

endemic, 6

epidemic, 6

epidemiology, 15

environmental health, 15

ethics, public health, 17

etiology, 6

health, 4

health disparities, 6

health management and policy, 16

human subjects, 21

independent ethics committee (IEC), 21

institutional review board (IRB), 21

isolation, 7

mission, public health, 4

morbidity, 11

mortality, 11

Nuremberg Code, 17

pandemic, 6

populations, 14

prevention, 14

public health, 4

quarantine, 7

social and behavioral
   sciences, 16

social justice, 14

social-ecological model, 4

Review Questions

1. Based on what you learned in this chapter, describe how public health and medicine are similar and how they are different.
2. How has sanitation been important throughout the history of public health?
3. How was John Snow able to identify the cause of a cholera outbreak in London in 1848 when the infectious agent that causes the disease was not known at that time?
4. What is the difference between an epidemic, endemic, and pandemic disease? Provide examples of each type of disease, including the area or country in which they occur.
5. Use a reliable source to find information about the Tuskegee Syphilis Trial sponsored by the U.S. Public Health Service from 1932 to 1972. Choose three tenets of either the Nuremberg Code or the *Belmont Report* and describe how the Tuskegee Trial fared in following those tenets.
6. Describe how social justice relates to public health in general and how social justice relates to the ethics of public health research.

References

1. Hearne SA, Locke PA, Mellman M, Loeb P, Dropkin L, Bolger G, et al. Public opinion about public health–United States, 1999. *MMWR*. 2000;49(12):258–260.
2. Preamble to the Constitution of the World Health Organization as adopted by the International Health Conference, New York, June 19–22, 1946; signed on 22 July 1946 by the representatives of 61 States (Official Records of the World Health Organization, no. 2, p. 100) and entered into force on 7 April 1948.
3. Turnock BJ. *Public Health: What It Is and How It Works*. 3rd ed. Sudbury, Mass.: Jones and Bartlett Publishers; 2004.
4. Institute of Medicine. *The Future of Public Health*. Washington, D.C.: National Academies Press; 1988.
5. Hippocrates. Airs, waters, places. In: Buck C, Llopis A, Najera E, Terris M, eds. *The Challenge of Epidemiology: Issues and Selected Readings*. Washington, D.C.: Pan American Health Organization; 1988; 18–19.
6. Rosen GA. *History of Public Health: Expanded Edition*. Baltimore, Md.: The Johns Hopkins University Press; 1993.

7. Parascandola JL. Public Health Service. In: Kurian GT, ed. *A Historical Guide to the U.S. Government*. New York: Oxford University Press, 1998; 487–493.

8. National Center for Health Statistics. 1900–1940 tables ranked in National Office of Vital Statistics, December 1947. Available at: www.cdc.gov/nchs/data/dvs/lead1900_98.pdf. Accessed November 13, 2009.

9. Minino A, Arias E, Kochanek KD, Murphy SL, Smith BL. Deaths: Final data for 2000. *Natl Vital Stat Reports*. 2002;50(15): 8. Available from the National Center for Health Statistics at: www.cdc.gov/nchs/data/nvsr/nvsr50/nvsr50_15.pdf. Accessed November 13, 2009.

10. Centers for Disease Control and Prevention. Ten great public health achievements—United States, 1900–1999. *MMWR*. 1999;48(12):241–243.

11. Institute of Medicine. *Who Will Keep the Public Healthy?* Washington, D.C.: National Academies Press; 2003.

12. Institute of Medicine. *The Future of the Public's Health in the 21st Century*. Washington, D.C.: National Academies Press; 2002.

13. U.S. Department of Health and Human Services. *Healthy People 2010*. 2nd ed. With Understanding and Improving Health and Objectives for Improving Health. 2 vols. Washington, D.C.: U.S. Government Printing Office, 2000.

14. Greenberg Quinlan Rosner Research. Americans overwhelmingly support investment in prevention: Disease prevention plays a lead role in health care reform. Available at: http://healthyamericans.org/assets/files/health-reform-poll-memo.pdf. Accessed June 8, 2009.

15. Nuremberg Code. Reprinted from *Trials of War Criminals Before the Nuremberg Military Tribunals Under Control Council Law*. No. 10, Vol. 2. Washington, D.C.: U.S. Government Printing Office, 1949; 181–182. Available at: http://ohsr.od.nih.gov/guidelines/nuremberg.html. Accessed June 8, 2009.

16. National Commission for the Protection of Human Subjects of Biomedical and Behavioral Research. The Belmont Report: Ethical principles and guidelines for the protection of human subjects of research. April 18, 1979. Available at: http://ohsr.od.nih.gov/guidelines/belmont.html. Accessed June 8, 2009.

CHAPTER 2

MODERN PUBLIC HEALTH SYSTEMS

Lisa R. Chacko, MPH
Sara A. Chacko, MPH

LEARNING OBJECTIVES

- List and define the three core functions of public health and provide a real-life example of each.
- Define the meaning of *population* in the context of public health.
- Describe how the social-ecological model is important when considering public health efforts of prevention.
- Name the three levels of prevention in public health and explain how they differ.
- Identify examples of federal, state, and local public health organizations.
- Briefly describe how the U.S. public health system is organized.

As we discussed in Chapter 1, outbreaks of cholera, dysentery, and typhoid fever were not uncommon in the United States at the beginning of the nineteenth century. The challenging social and economic conditions of the time, including overcrowding, lack of a clean public water supply, lack of waste disposal systems, and a general lack of public hygiene played a large part in the high incidence of these diseases. Over time, however, the development of a public health system, including a public water and sanitation system; the establishment of local, state, and federal public health departments; and the development and distribution of vaccines, led to a dramatic decrease in the incidence of these preventable diseases. Today, these infectious diseases no longer pose significant public health problems in the United States. As this historical account illustrates, public health systems are vital to the prevention of many health issues that directly affect our health and well-being.

This chapter will discuss the fundamentals of public health and the public health system in the United States and will briefly introduce public health systems abroad. The underlying goal of public health is the prevention of disease, and throughout this chapter we will emphasize how the structure and function of public health systems are designed with this goal in mind. The three **core functions** of public health, assessment, policy development, and assurance, form the foundation of all public health activity in the United States, both at the national and local level. It is through these functions that we identify and describe problems within the system, design programs and create new laws to address the issues, and ensure that the programs are implemented as intended. In this chapter, we will consider an example of how these core functions can be applied to the problem of obesity in the United States. We will also discuss the concept of *population* in the context of public health and contrast it with the field of medicine's focus on the individual. In its values, theories, research, and practice, public health is concerned with the health of the group or the population, the factors that shape its health, and the most effective means to positively influence that health. Theories used to conceptualize and understand public health, such as the social-ecological model, will also be addressed. Briefly, the social-ecological model of health attempts to account for multiple and interacting determinants of health by considering individual-, relationship-, community-, and societal-level influences on health, along with their interactions. This model is used to shape public health research and practice, and we will discuss examples of programs based on the social-ecological perspective at the national and grassroots level. The primary goal of public health is prevention. We will discuss how prevention efforts are carried out at three levels, primary, secondary, and tertiary, and we will provide examples of public health activities at each.

In this chapter, we will also briefly introduce the structure of the U.S. public health system and discuss the relationship between jurisdiction at the federal, state, and local levels. In the United States, public health responsibilities are shared between the federal, state, and local governments as well as between private and nonprofit entities. We will introduce the primary agencies that have public health jurisdiction at the federal level, such as the Department of Health and Human Services and its many operating divisions, including the Centers for Disease Control and Prevention (CDC), the National Institutes of Health (NIH), the Food and Drug Administration (FDA), and the Centers for Medicare and Medicaid Services (CMS). We will also discuss the organization and responsibilities of state and local health departments. State health departments work in cooperation with the federal government but are run independently within each state. The state agency in turn operates at the local level through local health departments, which are responsible for the direct provision of public health services. As a final consideration, we will look briefly at examples of public health systems abroad and discuss the challenges and advantages facing other countries, depending on their economic and political systems and availability of resources.

Public Health's Three Core Functions

In Chapter 1, we addressed the question, what is public health?, and we traced the history of public health over time. The field of public health differs from the field of medicine because public health is primarily concerned with the health of the population and the medical field generally focuses on the health of individuals. However, there are similarities in the two fields. In the same way that physicians in the medical field attempt to diagnose and treat diseases in individuals, public health officials make efforts to identify and diagnose health problems in the population, define policies that will treat the problem, and then follow up on the health of the population to make sure the treatment is working effectively. As we saw in Chapter 1, the three *core functions* of public health are assessment, policy development, and assurance. These functions were laid out and defined by the Institute of Medicine over twenty years ago in order to clarify public health's role in society[1]. Here we will explore these core functions in greater depth.

Assessment

Through the process of assessment, the public health community works to identify and understand social and other issues, such as the environment, that affect our health. **Assessment** entails gathering information about a health problem in order to create a clear picture of the situation that needs to be addressed, its potential causes, and which groups of people are most affected. Once a public health issue has been fully assessed, the public health community can use the information to decide whether it is a top priority that should be addressed. If so, officials need to generate a plan to solve the problem, and the process continues into the second core function: policy development. Chapter 3 covers public health surveillance and data issues in more detail.

Policy Development

After a public health issue has been assessed, officials can make decisions about the best way to address the issue and begin the process of problem solving. **Policy development** is the process of formulating the best strategy to approach a public health problem and implementing the new program or law. This process is usually carried out by the local, state, or federal government. During policy development, the importance of the issue being addressed in comparison to other urgent public health issues, the availability of resources, and the feasibility of solving the problem all must be considered. If the problem is deemed a priority with a realistic solution, then a specific plan can be created and resources can be mobilized to carry it out. Policy development is an inherently government-driven process because new laws and public money are often required to carry out the plan or policy. After new programs and policies are created and implemented, it is essential to make sure that they are executed effectively. This leads us to the third core function of public health: assurance.

Assurance

Through the first two core functions, assessment and policy development, a public health issue is first clearly described and a program is designed and implemented to address it. The final step is to assure that public money and resources are being used responsibly to carry out the plan and that the success of public health programs are monitored so they can be changed or discontinued as deemed appropriate. This step is called **assurance**, and it is an ongoing function that loops back into the process of assessment and policy development. For example, during the assessment of a public health issue, public health officials may discover that an existing program is doing little to solve the issue or, even worse, may be exacerbating the problem. In this case, assessment and assurance overlap and in turn inform the development of new policies to replace current programs. Figure 2.1 illustrates the cycle of assessment, policy development, and assurance.

The Three Core Functions in Action

A Real-Life Example: Obesity in the United States

Let's turn to a real-life example to consider how emerging public health issues are addressed at the state and federal level using our understanding of the three core functions of public health. We will review the action of Congress to address the growing obesity epidemic in the United States through a program called the Nutrition, Physical Activity and Obesity Program[3].

First Core Function: Assessment Through data gathered in national surveys in the late 1990s, public health researchers learned that the prevalence of obesity and overweight had increased dramatically over the past few decades among both children and adults. Costs associated with overweight and obesity were

FIGURE 2.1 Public Health Core Functions and Ten Essential Services

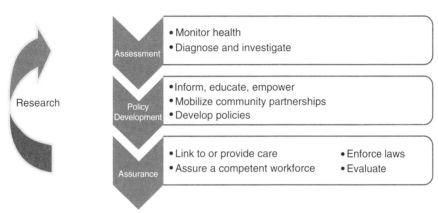

Source: Reference 2.

calculated at almost $80 billion by this time, and the majority of these costs rested mostly upon states.

Second Core Function: Policy Development To address the public health and economic challenges posed by the increased prevalence of overweight and obesity in the United States, Congress established the Nutrition, Physical Activity and Obesity Program (NPAO) in 1999. The program is administered through the Centers for Disease Control and Prevention (CDC), and funding is distributed to participating states. The goal of NPAO is to help states address the problems of poor nutrition and physical inactivity and reduce the burden of obesity and associated chronic diseases by employing evidence-based programs for increasing physical activity, increasing consumption of fruits and vegetables, decreasing TV viewing, and increasing breastfeeding.

Third Core Function: Assurance As part of the program, participating states are required to submit semiannual progress reports summarizing their progress with respect to infrastructure, collaborations, implementation, and evaluation. The CDC uses these reports to manage and improve the program.

Through a process of ongoing assessment, policy development, and assurance, NPAO continues to improve and expand its activities. Today, the program works with twenty-three states to address obesity and other chronic diseases. NPAO seeks to influence the full spectrum of factors that determine these health outcomes, from individual behavior to public policy. This broad approach is called the social-ecological model, a concept we will explore in further detail later in this chapter.

Understanding Population

All of us have been to the doctor's office and met one-on-one with a nurse or physician to discuss our personal health problems and ongoing health promotion and preventive care. We might have discussed weight loss strategies, the need for a vaccine, or how to treat asthma or a sore throat, for example. In this clinical setting, our health is addressed at the individual level. In the public health setting, however, health is addressed collectively, at the population level.

The term *population* has various meanings depending on the context. For example, one might refer to the number of individuals in the country of Mexico by saying that its population is about 110,000,000 people or collectively refer to the U.S. population by saying that the population of the United States is very diverse. However, in the context of public health, a **population** is defined as a group of people who share characteristics such as age, race, gender, geography, income level, and country of origin and who are commonly affected by a public health issue. For an issue to become a public health priority, it must affect a defined group of people, or a population. As an example, a program might identify an urban immigrant community with high rates of obesity living in Washington, D.C., as its target population.

In public health, the population is often discussed in the context of a population focus or **population health**. This usage implies an underlying focus on the group rather than the individual. Public health is uniquely concerned with the group dynamic, and this concern encompasses both small communities and entire countries. The population focus of public health is considered the hallmark of the field. According to the Institute of Medicine[1], "A public health professional is a person educated in public health or a related discipline who is employed to improve health through a population focus." In fact, the key, unifying factor in all public health work is a focus on population-level health.

Promoting population-level health is complicated by the huge number of factors that influence health, well-being, and disease. These factors include complex biological causes and often encompass subtle social dynamics. A broad perspective that can account for this interrelated web of health risks and determinants is required to understand population health, and the need for such an approach gave rise to the social-ecological model of health. This model provides a framework for understanding population health and for carrying out public health's three core functions effectively.

The Social-Ecological Model as a Framework for Prevention

Understanding, influencing, and changing population-level health is a complex and difficult task. For public health professionals, the goal is to identify the important health issues facing populations, understand their underlying causes, design interventions to solve existing problems, and prevent the health issues from arising in the future. To succeed, we need a framework that accounts for multiple, interrelated health determinants and aids our efforts to promote health at the population level.

According to the Institute of Medicine[4], the **social-ecological model** "assumes that health and well being are affected by interaction among multiple determinants of health … and … emphasizes the linkages and relationships among … factors." As mentioned in the previous section, it is important to look beyond biological risk factors to fully understand health. In fact, at least 50 percent of mortality can be attributed to factors other than biology or medical care[5].

What are these other factors? The social-ecological model considers four levels of influence when describing health, identifying public health issues, and designing interventions. These four levels are the individual level, the relationship level, the community level, and the societal level[6]. These four spheres of influence overlap and interact, as depicted in Figure 2.2.

FIGURE 2.2 Levels of Influence

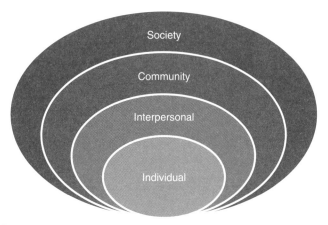

Source: Reference 6.

Four Levels of Influence

Individual Level

Our health is largely determined by personal factors such as our genetic predisposition, behavior, attitude toward health, motivation, beliefs, and family history. Prevention strategies at the **individual level** might include mentoring and education to positively change personal influences on health and illness.

Relationship Level

Our health is also greatly influenced by relationships with peers, partners, and family members. Prevention strategies at the relationship level often include education and peer or family programs to promote relationships that support a positive health outcome. For example, a program designed at the **relationship level** might focus on diet and lifestyle education for both those with diabetes and their families, recognizing that close family members can provide moral and practical support in making the important diet and exercise changes that are critical for the appropriate management of diabetes and the prevention of serious complications.

Community Level

Our health is influenced by our experience in our social environment, such as our neighborhood, school, and place of work. Prevention strategies at the **community level** often seek to change policy and the system as a whole through means such as awareness campaigns or local programs. For example, a program to promote physical activity might aim to make neighborhoods more pedestrian friendly by establishing well-lighted and convenient walking paths and by educating the public about the importance of building exercise into the daily routine.

Societal Level

Finally, our health is shaped by macro-level factors in society as a whole, such as religious and cultural beliefs, economic policies, gender or racial inequalities, and social norms. Prevention strategies at the **societal level** may employ many approaches in combination, such as creating new policies, awareness campaigns, and programs, and they are often carried out by multiple tiers of government and private or nonprofit entities.

The social-ecological model can be used to inform theory, design research studies, create community programs, develop policy, and evaluate existing interventions. Several versions of the model exist, some of which include an additional level of influence called the *institutional* or *organizational* level. This level of influence fits between the relationship and community levels and allows research and

FIGURE 2.3 Multiple Determinants of Health

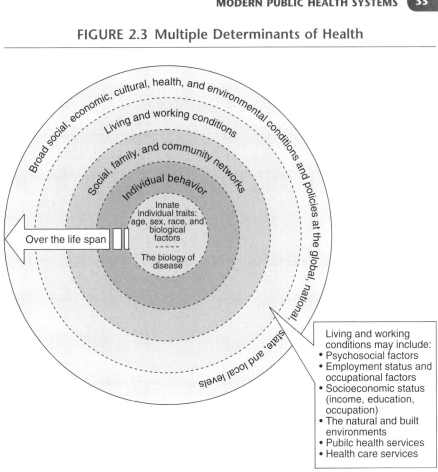

Living and working conditions may include:
- Psychosocial factors
- Employment status and occupational factors
- Socioeconomic status (income, education, occupation)
- The natural and built environments
- Pubilc health services
- Health care services

Source: Reference 4.

interventions to focus more directly on the dynamic within organizations such as schools, churches, or the workplace.

Applying the Social-Ecological Model

Research

A major challenge facing public health researchers is obtaining the data required to define the nature and magnitude of a public health problem. Historically, only simple data such as mortality and morbidity (rates of death and disease) have been collected and used in epidemiological studies. These data are limited in their ability to completely describe health among populations. More recently however, broader recognition of the social-ecological model and the myriad of factors that can contribute to a health problem has supported a shift to more detailed data collection. When smoking was added to the list of reportable diseases and conditions in 1996, it was the first time that a health behavior became part of surveillance. This represented a landmark for public health research[7]. Over time, even more data have become available through the increased reporting and surveillance of demographic and lifestyle risk factors, such as physical activity. This has in turn served to better inform health policy and intervention design. Chapter 3 offers a comprehensive review of public health data collection in the United States.

The merits of the social-ecological model, including its comprehensiveness and ability to account for the complexity of health, create a challenge for research. Public health researchers must make every effort to think in broader terms and address a greater number of research questions in their work. Furthermore, research must often employ interdisciplinary teams of investigators, including social scientists, epidemiologists, biostatisticians, clinicians, and economists in order to bring an appropriate level of expertise to all components of the model.

Programs and Interventions

The complexity of the social-ecological model can make it difficult to apply its principles when designing programs and interventions to address public health issues. Over time, however, the model is being used to design public health programs with increasing success. Two examples of the social-ecological model in practice are discussed below. The first is a large-scale program that addresses violence throughout the United States, and the second is a nonprofit organization that assesses the health needs of an immigrant community.

A Real-Life Example at the National Level: The CDC and Violence Prevention

The **Centers for Disease Control and Prevention (CDC)** is a government agency dedicated to protecting health and promoting quality of life through the prevention and control of disease, injury, and disability. In the late 1970s, the CDC identified violence as a priority area for public health, and throughout the 1980s it established goals and programs for the prevention of violence. By the early 1990s, the CDC established a Division of Violence Prevention (DVP), which monitors violence and related injuries, conducts research on factors affecting violence, creates and evaluates violence prevention programs, and helps state and local governments implement programs. To fully understand violence as a public health issue and to inform these prevention efforts, the CDC relies on the social-ecological model of health. Because violent behavior is extremely complex in its root causes, the CDC has examined the interplay between individual-, relationship-, community-, and societal-level influences on susceptibility to and protection from violent behavior. As a result of this effort, the prevention strategies employed include a continuum of activities, such as community education and awareness efforts, identification of risk and protective factors, and surveillance of violent behavior, to further inform educational prevention programs. These activities address all levels of the social-ecological model in order to create a sustainable approach to violence prevention[6].

A Real-Life Example at the Local Level: Puentes de Salud and Immigrant Health

Puentes de Salud (Bridges to Health) is a nonprofit organization that works as an innovative model for health promotion in the South Philadelphia Latino community. This population has grown dramatically in the past decade, and social support systems targeting this community, including health care, education, and public assistance, have lagged behind. The community has a high prevalence of preventable chronic disease, largely attributable to lifestyle factors. Recognizing multiple and interacting determinants of health, the Puentes de Salud model uses a social-ecological approach to address public health issues facing this community. The model includes providing primary health care, basic dental care and screenings, and referrals to low-cost or free specialist care in the community, as well as health education programs, community outreach, and training of future health care professionals. Through collaborations with private and public organizations, including academic institutions, Puentes offers classes and workshops in immigration legal issues, nutrition, and English as a second language. The Puentes model targets many different angles of the social and health problems of this Latino community and exemplifies the social-ecological model at work at the grassroots level[8].

Three Levels of Prevention

The underlying goal of all public health efforts is **prevention**. Preventing disease before it begins reduces unnecessary suffering and makes the best use of health care resources. Prevention works on multiple levels and in some cases may even apply to certain subsets of the population who already have disease.

There are three levels at which prevention efforts can be focused, known as the primary, secondary, and tertiary levels. At the **primary prevention** level, we seek to prevent disease before it begins. Activities at this level include health promotion and education, as well as provision of primary health care services.

At the **secondary prevention** level, our goal is to detect disease while it is still in its early stages and reduce its progression and effects. This level includes screenings and case finding, followed up by early intervention and control of risk factors. At the **tertiary prevention** level, advanced disease is already present, so we seek to reduce complications and mortality. At this level, efforts are focused on disease management and continuing care. The primary level of prevention is the most effective for many public health issues, and ideally, the majority of resources should be focused at this level. However, people who are already ill can still benefit from prevention efforts at the secondary and tertiary level, as outlined in Table 2.1[9].

Examples of Prevention Levels

Below are two examples of how activities or interventions can target each level of prevention for a public health problem. First, consider the goal of preventing

Table 2.1 The Three Levels of Prevention

Level of Prevention	Primary	Secondary	Tertiary
Who is targeted?	Healthy population	At-risk population	Diseased/affected population
What is the goal?	Prevent the well population from becoming at-risk	Prevent the at-risk population from developing disease and needing hospitalization	Prevent the diseased population from suffering complications, disability, or readmission to hospital
Types of interventions	Promotion of healthy behaviors and environments across the life course Education and public awareness campaigns Vaccinations	Screening Case finding Periodic health examinations Early intervention Risk factor control: lifestyle and medication	Treatment and acute care Disease management (continuing care, maintenance, self-management) Rehabilitation
Who is responsible?	Public health Primary health care Other sectors, i.e., media, community organizations	Primary health care Public health	Hospital care Specialist services Primary health care Community care Public health

Source: Reference 9.

cervical cancer among women. A major cause of cervical cancer is infection with human papillomavirus, or HPV, a sexually transmitted infection (STI). It is estimated that eleven thousand women in the United States are diagnosed with cervical cancer each year, and four thousand women in the United States die of cervical cancer annually[10]. Primary prevention efforts against cervical cancer are intended to prevent the onset of disease and include public awareness and education campaigns, such as public service announcements or commercials about the relationship between HPV and cervical cancer and avoiding STIs, for example by the use of condoms. Also, vaccinating people against HPV is part of primary prevention. (Currently, Gardasil® is the only FDA-approved HPV vaccine, and it is given to young women between the ages of nine and twenty-six.) A screening test, the Papanicolaou or Pap test, can detect changes in cells of the cervix that may indicate cancer. Screening for cervical cancer allows early detection and prevention of disease progression and is an example of secondary prevention of cervical cancer. Finally, tertiary prevention includes chemotherapy, radiation, or surgery to remove cervical cancer, thus reducing complications and mortality due to the disease[11].

Motor vehicle safety is another example of a public health issue for which we can intervene at multiple prevention levels. Primary prevention of motor vehicle crashes includes improving road safety, for example by adding medians or barriers to prevent motorists from crossing into oncoming traffic or running off the road. In addition, installing traffic signs and lights are examples of primary prevention interventions because their purpose is to prevent crashes from occurring. Secondary prevention includes efforts to reduce injury or severity when a crash occurs. To accomplish this, we can install and require the use of seat belts in cars as well as car seats or booster seats for children. We also can establish and enforce speed limits to minimize damage done in a crash. Finally, tertiary prevention in motor vehicle safety involves minimizing disability or injury caused by a crash. This may be accomplished by ensuring that an adequate and responsive Emergency Medical Services (EMS) system exists and that there is access to trauma centers for rapid medical care of crash survivors.

For virtually any public health problem, there are strategies to prevent an outcome from occurring (primary prevention), to limit the negative impact of an event (secondary prevention), and to reduce long-term disability or morbidity associated with the event (tertiary prevention). It is important to recognize and identify action steps at all levels of prevention. Historically, the prevention message and focus of public health has alienated some individuals who felt they were viewed as public health *failures* because some aspect of their life or experience had not been prevented. For example, many primary prevention efforts exist to prevent birth defects and developmental disabilities. Although it is important to educate pregnant women that adequate folic acid intake during pregnancy reduces the risk of giving birth to a child with a neural tube defect (spina bifida), for example, it is also important to have public health measures in place to improve the health of children who are born with such a defect. In a child with spina bifida, secondary and tertiary prevention efforts, including surgery, may be necessary. Primary prevention of other health conditions related to spina bifida, such as urinary tract infections or pressure sores, called *secondary conditions* to convey that they are related to the primary health condition or disability, are also vital and can improve health and quality of life. When designing public health messages about prevention, it is critical to be sensitive to the fact that members of the audience may have the health attribute or condition the message seeks to eliminate.

The U.S. Public Health System

In the United States, public health efforts are organized through a hierarchy of powers shared among the federal, state, and local governments, as well as private and nonprofit entities. Because the responsibility to ensure the public's health is not explicitly delegated to the federal government by our Constitution, public health authority was historically left to state and local government. Over time, the value of federal involvement in public health has been revealed by periods of economic distress, during which the larger infrastructure, budget, and unifying authority of the federal government was necessary to keep public health programs in place. Other advantages to national-level policies and laws have also become apparent through programs such as medication oversight and standards for food safety and additives, automotive crash standards, and water purity. The balance of powers between the federal and state governments with regard to public health and health care continues to evolve and is shaped both by politics and by the needs of society. The past decade has seen a gradual return of power to the states, but with severe budgetary constraints facing states, the United States could return to a more centralized approach to public health planning, as is seen in many other countries.

Public health is tied to government by the very nature of its core functions. As described in previous sections, public health is responsible for assessing public health issues, developing policy, and assuring that policies and programs are carried out. Only our government (at all levels) has the authority to create new laws, regulate programs and industries, and use taxpayer money to fund public health initiatives. Because of this important tie to government, an understanding of the governmental public health infrastructure is essential to your understanding of public health in the United States. In this section, you will learn about the balance of powers between the federal, state, and local governments and be introduced to the many agencies that regulate and ensure our health.

Public Health at the Federal Level

The federal government plays an essential leadership role in the nation's public health efforts. Working in cooperation with state and local governments, federal agencies responsible for public health set the national agenda for research, interventions, and policy. The largest public health agency in the United States is the **U. S. Department of Health and Human Services (HHS)**. This umbrella agency includes a wide range of subagencies whose activities include research, health service provision and financing, industry regulation, health promotion, policy analysis and development, surveillance, and intervention design. In Public Health Connections 2.1, the primary operating divisions of HHS are listed, along with their Web sites and mission statements.

PUBLIC HEALTH CONNECTIONS 2.1

U.S. DEPARTMENT OF HEALTH AND HUMAN SERVICES PRIMARY OPERATING DIVISIONS AND MISSIONS

Administration for Children and Families (ACF), www.acf.dhhs.gov/
To promote the economic and social well-being of families, children, individuals, and communities.
Agency for Healthcare Research and Quality (AHRQ), www.ahrq.gov
To support, conduct, and disseminate research that improves access to care and the outcomes, quality, cost, and use of health care services.
Administration on Aging (AoA), www.aoa.gov
To promote the dignity and independence of older people and to help society prepare for an aging population.
Agency for Toxic Substances and Disease Registry (ATSDR), www.atsdr.cdc.gov
To serve the public by using the best science, taking responsive public health actions, and providing trusted health information to prevent harmful exposures and diseases related to toxic substances.

(Continued)

PUBLIC HEALTH CONNECTIONS 2.1

U.S. DEPARTMENT OF HEALTH AND HUMAN SERVICES PRIMARY OPERATING DIVISIONS AND MISSIONS (Continued)

Centers for Disease Control and Prevention (CDC), www.cdc.gov
To promote health and quality of life by preventing and controlling disease, injury, and disability.

Centers for Medicare & Medicaid Services (CMS), www.cms.hhs.gov
To ensure effective, up-to-date health care coverage and to promote quality care for beneficiaries.

Food and Drug Administration (FDA), www.fda.gov
To rigorously assure the safety, efficacy, and security of human and veterinary drugs, biological products, and medical devices and assure the safety and security of the nation's food supply, cosmetics, and products that emit radiation.

Health Resources and Services Administration (HRSA), www.hrsa.gov
To provide the national leadership, program resources, and services needed to improve access to culturally competent, quality health care.

Indian Health Service (IHS), www.ihs.gov
To raise the physical, mental, social, and spiritual health of American Indians and Alaska Natives to the highest level.

National Institutes of Health (NIH), www.nih.gov
To employ science in pursuit of fundamental knowledge about the nature and behavior of living systems and the application of that knowledge to extend healthy life and reduce the burdens of illness and disability.

Substance Abuse and Mental Health Services Administration (SAMHSA), www.samhsa.gov
To build resilience and facilitate recovery for people with or at risk for substance abuse and mental illness.

Source: Reference 12.

Of the agencies listed in Public Health Connections 2.1, perhaps the most well-known are the CDC, the National Institutes of Health, the Food and Drug Administration, and the Centers for Medicare & Medicaid Services.

In this chapter, we have already discussed the role of the CDC in developing prevention programs such as NPAO and use of the social-ecological model in establishing the Division of Violence Prevention. Established in 1946 and headquartered in Atlanta, Georgia, the CDC's work is often collaborative with states and is essential to disease surveillance in the United States. The CDC monitors infectious disease, including those associated with bioterrorism, and is responsible for our nationwide immunization program and health statistics. The **National Institutes of Health (NIH)** is a world leader in medical research. The NIH provides leadership in setting research priorities for the nation, funds research efforts at private and public institutions, is actively involved in the publication and dissemination of research findings, and supports the training of experts in medical sciences. The NIH employs more than fifteen thousand individuals and is based in Bethesda, Maryland, near the U.S. capital[12]. The **Food and Drug Administration (FDA)** was established in 1906 and is responsible for ensuring a safe food, cosmetic, and medicine supply for the United States. As a regulatory body, the FDA is in charge of an enormous range of industry activities, monitoring an estimated $1 trillion worth of goods each year throughout their manufacture, importation, transportation, storage, and sale[13]. The **Centers for Medicare & Medicaid Services (CMS)** provides health insurance coverage to vulnerable Americans, including children, the elderly, and low-income populations. Medicare, the program that insures Americans age 65 and older, is administered federally, and Medicaid, the program that insures low-income Americans, and the State Children's Health Insurance Plan (SCHIP) are administered in partnership with states. Through CMS, the federal government is the largest purchaser of health-related services in the United States[14].

The **Environmental Protection Agency (EPA)** is the national leader in environmental science, research, education, and assessment efforts. The EPA is responsible for developing and enforcing environmental regulations for such areas as clean air and water; giving grants to fund state environmental programs, nonprofits, and educational institutions; conducting research on environmental issues; teaching the public about the environment; and sponsoring partnerships. The EPA was established in 1970 and employs more than fifteen thousand people nationwide (www.epa.gov). The **Office of the Surgeon General (OSG)** is part of the Office of Public Health and Science and oversees the Commissioned Corps of the U.S. Public Health Service. The Commissioned Corps is a team of more than six thousand public health professionals responsible for the nation's health promotion and disease prevention programs and for advancement of public health science. The surgeon general is the country's chief health educator and provides Americans with the latest scientific information on how to improve their health and reduce the risk of illness and injury (www.surgeongeneral.gov). The **Department of Veteran Affairs (VA)** is responsible for providing military veterans with a wide range of benefits, including health care. The VA health care system is large and well-organized, with health facilities throughout the United States. The VA operates as a single-payer health system, in which the government acts as the financer and provider of health services for the covered population[15].

Public Health at the State Level

Every state and territory in the United States has its own public health agency that operates in cooperation with the federal government and independently from other states. These agencies' structures, responsibilities, and authority vary in accordance with the needs of the state's population and the law by which the agency was first created. In most cases, the **state health department** is an umbrella agency under which local health departments exist and operate, and such departments are funded by a combination of state and federal dollars. Funding received from the federal government is often accompanied by stipulations about its use; for example, it is earmarked to deliver diabetes education programs, operate STI surveillance and treatment, or provide tobacco education and control. State agencies are responsible for supporting the federal government's efforts to carry out public health's three core functions (assessment, policy development, assurance) either directly or through the local public health agencies[4].

Public Health at the Local Level

There are nearly three thousand **local health departments** throughout the United States, with huge variation in size, administrative structure, budgetary constraints, infrastructure, and the populations they serve. Local health departments are often organized at the county level, and most provide a wide range of services, including health screenings, immunizations, community outreach and education, epidemiology and disease surveillance, vital statistics, maternal and child health services, food safety and restaurant regulation, tuberculosis testing, infectious disease control, and some primary health care services. Local health departments often work on extremely limited budgets and are challenged by the needs of the diverse and vulnerable populations they serve. Unlike state and federal agencies, many local-level public health agency staff members have no formal public health training, which represents a constant challenge for the provision of quality services and programs. As mentioned above, local health departments do not typically operate as independent entities but rather work in conjunction with the state health department. Despite chronic underfunding and lack of adequately trained personnel, local health departments form the backbone of the U.S. public health system by acting as the frontline, grassroots level of government action[4].

Public Health Systems Globally

Until now, our discussion has focused on public health within the United States. Let us now consider how health is assured around the world. What unique challenges and advantages do other countries face in their efforts to carry out public health's core functions? Every country establishes its health care delivery and public health systems in accordance with its history, culture, economics, politics, and resources. Often, health systems are built up over time in response to stimuli such as economic changes, outbreaks of infectious disease, or a threat of bioterrorism. Not all systems will or should look alike. In this section, we consider public health systems abroad, and we will consider the public health systems of two of our neighboring countries: Canada, to our north, and Cuba, to our south. We will then turn our attention to the unique challenges facing developing countries as they work to establish new public health systems. See also the example of planning for a new health system in Turkey discussed in Chapter 3.

Public Health in Canada

The **Canada Health Act**, passed in 1980, established a comprehensive single-payer health care system and guaranteed access to *universal* medical care for all Canadians regardless of ability to pay, age, or health status. Even before the new health care system was established, a 1974 report entitled *New Perspectives on the Health of Canadians* recognized that health requires more than a strong health care system and called attention to social influences on health, emphasizing that social inequalities lead to health disparities. This report led to new efforts in health promotion, community outreach and advocacy, and policy development leading toward the goals of public health. The concept of health promotion was further developed in a 1986 report, *Achieving Health for All: A Framework for Health Promotion*. Also known as the Ottawa Charter for Health Promotion, this document called on all countries to emphasize public health through policy and programs. In 2004, the Public Health Agency of Canada was established to centralize the nation's public health activities. This agency is devoted to carrying out disease prevention, health promotion, emergency preparedness, and the strengthening of Canada's public health infrastructure. The agency continues to set the nation's public health agenda and work through collaboration with federal, provincial, and territorial governments[16].

Public Health in Cuba

The current Cuban health system was established in 1959 after the Cuban revolution reshaped the entire nation's infrastructure. The Cuban health system is entirely government run and paid for, and public health and health care are fully integrated[17]. Since its inception, the system has faced many challenges, primarily lack of resources and funding. However, the system has continued to draw the global health community's attention because of its ability to produce excellent public health statistics on a very limited budget. Cuba's approach to public health is the maintenance of an extensive primary care network. Throughout the country, polyclinics (primary care centers that offer a wide range of outpatient services) and neighborhood clinics provide open access to primary care doctors and community health services. Doctors typically live in the same neighborhood they serve, and education and health promotion services are emphasized. Despite severe economic hardship, the Cuban model has been able to reduce morbidity and mortality over the past fifty years by funneling available resources into prevention and primary care[18].

Public Health in Developing Nations

Despite remarkable advances in modern medicine, much of the world's population continues to suffer the consequences of poor nutrition, lack of proper sanitation, and severely limited access to health services. Globally, the leading causes of death in developing nations include preventable diseases such as lower respiratory infections, diarrhea, malaria, and HIV/AIDS. Nations that are beginning to develop health systems face many challenges: lack of money, lack of properly trained health personnel, lack of public health expertise, pressure from international organizations to design systems according to predefined parameters, and inefficient use of resources, to name only a few. Developing nations must make difficult decisions regarding the best way to invest available funds for the development of an appropriate health infrastructure and often look for external advice and support in doing so. Policy makers in developing nations must decide how best to model their own systems on those of other nations. International lending organizations tend to stipulate the way in which loans are spent in favor of free market–style health systems like that in the United States; however, some global health experts argue that it is more realistic to use a Cuban-style model in low-resource contexts such as those encountered in developing nations. While these policy debates continue, countless lives are lost due to poor public health standards and high prevalence of preventable diseases. The establishment of viable health systems throughout the world is an enormous task facing this century's public health community.

Summary

There are three core functions of public health, that of assessment, policy development, and assurance. Public health focuses on population, a group of people who share characteristics such as age, race, gender, geography, income level, or country of origin and who are commonly affected by a public health issue, whereas the medical field focuses on the individual. The social-ecological model of health attempts to account for multiple and interacting determinants of health by considering individual, relationship, community, and societal-level influences on health, along with their interactions. There are three major levels of prevention, primary, secondary, and tertiary, and there are specific programs that target those different levels. In the United States, public health efforts are organized through a hierarchy of powers shared among the federal, state, and local governments as well as private and nonprofit entities. Canada has a comprehensive single-payer health care system and guaranteed access to universal medical care. The Cuban health system is entirely government run and operates on limited resources. Developing nations face many challenges in developing public health systems and must make difficult decisions regarding the best way to invest available funds for the development of an appropriate health infrastructure.

Key Terms

assessment, 27

assurance, 28

Canada Health Act, 43

Centers for Disease Control and Prevention (CDC), 34

Centers for Medicare & Medicaid Services (CMS), 41

community level of influence, 32

core functions, 26

Department of Health and Human Services (HHS), 39

Department of Veteran Affairs (VA), 41

Environmental Protection Agency (EPA), 41

Food and Drug Administration (FDA), 41

individual level of influence, 32

local health department, 42

National Institutes of Health (NIH), 41

Office of the Surgeon General (OSG), 41

policy development, 27

population, 30

population health, 30

prevention, 35

primary prevention, 35

relationship level of influence, 32

secondary prevention, 36

social-ecological model, 31

societal level of influence, 32

state health department, 42

tertiary prevention, 36

Review Questions

1. Describe the three core functions of public health.
2. Provide an example of a current public health policy and trace its creation and implementation using the three core functions of public health.
3. Define the social-ecological model. Identify an example of a local organization that applies this model.
4. What are the four levels of influence of the social-ecological model?
5. What are the three levels of prevention? Define each and give an example.
6. Describe how the U.S. public health system is organized at the federal, state, and local level.
7. What are some of the challenges facing public health systems in developing countries?

References

1. Institute of Medicine. *The Future of Public Health.* Washington, D.C.: National Academy Press; 1988.
2. Public Health in America statement. Available from the Public Health Functions Project Web site. Available at www.health.gov/phfunctions/public.htm. Accessed March 2009.
3. Yee, SL, Williams-Piehota P, Sorensen, A, Roussel, A, Hersey J, Hamre, R. The Nutrition and Physical Activity Program to Prevent Obesity and Other Chronic Disease: Monitoring progress in funded states. *Prev Chronic Dis.* 2006;3(1):A23.
4. Institute of Medicine. *The Future of the Public's Health in the 21st Century.* Washington, D.C.: National Academy Press; 2002.
5. McGinnis JM, Foege WH. Actual causes of death in the United States. US Department of Health and Human Services, Washington, D.C. *JAMA.* 1993;270(18):2207–2212.
6. Centers for Disease Control and Prevention. Violence prevention. Injury prevention & control Web page. Available at: www.cdc.gov/ViolencePrevention/index.html. Accessed March 2009.
7. CDC. Addition of prevalence of cigarette smoking as a nationally notifiable condition. *MMMR.* 1996;45(25):537. Available at: www.cdc.gov/mmWR/preview/mmwrhtml/00042752.htm. Accessed April 27, 2010.
8. Puentes de Salud. An innovative model for health promotion in the South Philadelphia Latino community. Strategic Plan, Aug 2008. Puentes de Salud: Philadelphia, Pa.
9. National Public Health Partnership. *Preventing Chronic Disease: A Strategic Framework.* Background paper. Melbourne, Australia: National Public Health Partnership; 2001.

10. American Cancer Society. *Cancer Facts and Figures 2009.* Available at: www.cancer. org/downloads/STT/500809web.pdf. Accessed April 27, 2010.

11. U.S. Dept. of Health and Human Services. Pap test. National Women's Health Information Center, Office on Women's Health. Available at: www.womenshealth .gov/faq/pap-test.cfm. Accessed April 2009.

12. National Institutes of Health. NIH home page. Available at: www.nih.gov/. Accessed April 2009.

13. Food and Drug Administration. FDA home page. Available at: www.fda.gov/. Accessed April 2009.

14. Centers for Medicare and Medicaid. CMS home page. Available at: www.cms.hhs .gov/. Accessed April 2009.

15. Veterans Affairs. VA home page. Available at: www.va.gov/. Accessed April 2009.

16. Public Health Agency of Canada. *The Chief Public Health Officer's Report on the State of Public Health in Canada 2008.* Ottawa, Ont.: Her Majesty the Queen in Right of Canada, Minister of Health; 2008.

17. MEDICC. The Cuban approach to health care: Origins, results, and current challenges. Available at: www.medicc.org/ns/index.php?s=11&p=0. Accessed April 27, 2010.

18. Swanson KA, Swanson JM, Gill AE, Walter C. Primary care in Cuba: A public health approach. *Health Care Women Int.* 1995;16(4):299–308.

PART
II

ANALYTIC TOOLS
AND METHODS

CHAPTER 3

DATA FOR PUBLIC HEALTH

Elena M. Andresen, PhD
Erin D. Bouldin, MPH

LEARNING OBJECTIVES

- Define surveillance.
- Identify key sources of public health data in the United States, including the United States Census, vital statistics, national surveys, and registries.
- Understand the reasons why topics are chosen for surveillance activities in public health.
- Describe how data apply to the core public health function of assessment.
- Recognize the types of information available through common public health data systems.

This chapter provides an introduction to the vast array of data collected and available for use in public health activities such as planning and research. The majority of this chapter is about surveillance data, that is, information we collect routinely and in an ongoing fashion to inform public health. We touch on some key data sources and describe who is included in each and the population they represent. For example, the United States Census is a data source that is intended to include every person in the country, but most sources of information we use in public health are based on a sample of people or events. Survey-based surveillance systems include the Behavioral Risk Factor Surveillance System and the Youth Risk Behavior Surveillance System, and these two examples demonstrate how surveillance is conducted in practice, what types of data are collected, and how data are used. We will also see how the content and topics are chosen for surveillance, including determining how common a disease is, the potential for intervention, trends in disease, and public opinion.

Public health data are key to performing the core public health function of assessment (see the discussion in Chapter 1 on the Institute of Medicine's report,

The Future of Public Health, and the summary of the core functions of public health[1]. Many of the activities that make up public health assessment and surveillance are conducted by epidemiologists, biostatisticians, and demographers, but other disciplines in public health are involved as well. For example, data may be collected by nurses and physicians as part of their clinical and patient treatment work or by laboratory technicians and medical records specialists in health care settings. We will take a closer look at death certificate data as one key component to public health data. Death certificates form a key part of national vital statistics data (births and deaths).

How Do We Decide What to Include in Surveillance?

Public health **surveillance** is defined as "… the ongoing systematic collection, analysis, and interpretation of outcome-specific data for use in planning, implementation, and evaluation of public health practice."[2, p. 3] Surveillance systems are useful in public health because their ongoing nature provides information over time. Typically, surveillance questions are consistent across populations or geographic areas, and they change infrequently. These attributes allow public health professionals to look at surveillance data and identify trends in the types of people or groups affected by a specific health concern or to identify whether certain health behaviors or health outcomes are changing over time. Surveillance data are therefore useful in making decisions about what health topics to address and how and where to spend public health dollars efficiently.

There are many health problems that we might want to understand. Individuals and even the general public may have strong opinions about what topics are important enough to be included in surveillance systems. Recent public outcry about the problem of medical errors in hospitals raises the question, why don't we have a national list (or data) regarding the problem of medical mistakes? For example, actor Dennis Quaid raised this issue after a massive overdose of a blood-thinning medicine was administered to his newborn twins, a potentially fatal error[3]. He noted that this exact error had occurred before and had even killed newborns. For more information on the problems of medical errors, see the Agency for Healthcare Research and Quality (AHRQ) Web site (www.ahrq.gov/qual/errorsix.htm). The AHRQ estimates that there are as many as ninety-eight thousand deaths each year in the United States due to medical errors, making it the eighth most common cause of death[4]. So why is there no surveillance system for medical errors in the United States? We do collect data on deaths (see below), but this is a slow process to find possible problems and includes only *fatal* events. As we will see below, if a health event is common and serious, it is more likely to be included as an important topic for surveillance activities.

Public health provides some of the input to help set policies, usually at the national level, regarding what to include in surveillance systems. As in other decisions in public health, we live with the real issue of the *public cost* of our decisions. We cannot afford to collect information on all health issues, nor would many people want to have every aspect of our health, our personal medical experiences, and our health behavior monitored. Surveillance systems require substantial time and money to establish and maintain. Therefore, six criteria are generally used to decide what health events should be chosen for surveillance activities: the **frequency of the health event**; the **severity**, **cost**, **preventability**, and **communicability**; and **public interest in the health event**[2].

Let's use the example of medical errors to expand on these criteria. As noted above, the AHRQ has reported that medical errors frequently contribute to death, so the problem is both frequent and severe. In addition, we might assume that even when not fatal, the medical care and treatment necessary to correct the error is likely to be expensive. For example, in the case of the Quaid twins, the mistake required a team of medical care experts and many extra days in the hospital. Are mistakes preventable? This is a complex issue[5], but the answer is yes. We can take steps to prevent errors if we know the common causes at the individual and system levels. For example, clearer and more distinct medication labels might prevent a nurse from delivering the wrong dose to a patient. Improved education for pharmacy technicians and other hospital staff could prevent medication stocking errors in hospitals. Additional monitoring systems in hospitals could help ensure that the correct medications are safely administered more often. Finally, public interest about medical errors is very high. Widespread media coverage of medical errors such as that experienced by the Quaid twins is one measure of interest. Most of us find this personally relevant, and perhaps even know someone who has been affected by a medical error. However, the pragmatic issue of collecting specific information on a routine basis from hospitals demonstrates the formidable problem in routine surveillance. Hospitals are variously funded and are administered privately, publicly, and within federal agencies, such as the Department of Veterans Affairs. Hospitals are not the only place medical errors take place: pharmacies, nursing homes, and clinics would have to be included in surveillance as well. Currently, no consistent data collection or surveillance system for medical errors exists across the many health arenas in which they occur. However, some data are collected, and there is ongoing effort to change policies to reduce medical errors.

One aspect of the criteria for surveillance not included in the category of medical error is communicability of a health event. This criterion is relevant when we talk about infectious disease, and Chapter 8 covers this area of public health in detail. The issue of communicability (the disease passes from one person, object, or animal to another) is important in surveillance because by consistently collecting data about a communicable disease, we may be able to stop its spread. Think about the kinds of public announcements you may have heard on the news. In recent years, new strains of influenza virus have been identified and have spread rapidly around the globe. Influenza surveillance activities have allowed these new strains to be identified quickly and have detected how rapidly and to what areas the virus has spread. This information allows public health officials to alert the public to be vigilant about hand washing and other preventive precautions and also to be alert if traveling to or living in certain areas or participating in specific activities. Likewise, the public may be alerted about more localized communicable disease threats, such as a restaurant employee with hepatitis A or a beach closure because of sewage contamination. Public health surveillance activities are the likely reason that these events are detected. As a result, warnings can be publicized, keeping more people from contracting an illness.

Universal Surveillance Systems and Activities

Typically, it is not feasible to collect surveillance information about every person in a population. However, several examples of universal (all-inclusive) surveillance systems exist, including the United States Census and vital statistics systems.

The Census

We often overlook the decennial (every ten years) United States **Census** as a source of public health information. But in addition to providing a count of how many people reside in the United States, the Census contains information on where and how people live. The Census is used to describe neighborhoods (for example, crowding) and personal conditions (for example, poverty) that can affect health. Some personal conditions, such as disability, are measured also[6]. Figure 3.1 is a county-level map of disability prevalence (the number of people with a disability) in Florida based on questions used on the long form of the 2000 Census. Public Health Connections 3.1 gives the full set of Census questions asked about disability. If we viewed a similar map of the United States, we would see a distribution of *disability inequality* that mirrors distributions of chronic disease such as stroke and heart disease. The reasons for this are not apparent from the Census, but this pattern of poorer health in the southeastern part of our nation has given rise to the description of the area as the **stroke belt**[7,8]. There is, indeed, a higher incidence of this serious vascular disease as well as its associated risk factors, such as smoking and hypertension, in this region. However, geographic patterns are similar for a variety of chronic diseases and conditions, health behaviors, and less access to health care[9] based on data from the Behavioral Risk Factor Surveillance System (see below). The Census also has the advantage of gathering data from very large numbers of people, thus it is one of the few sources of information that can be used for describing small geographic areas, such as counties or even neighborhoods.

FIGURE 3.1 Prevalence of Disability Among Women Age Sixteen to Sixty-four by County in Florida

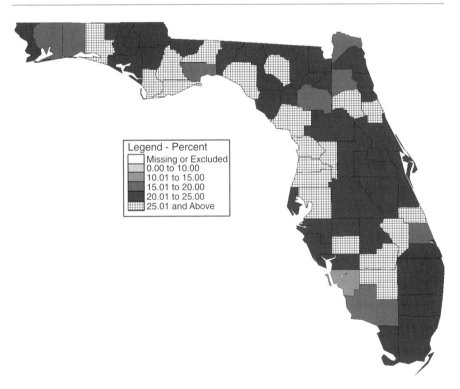

Legend - Percent
- Missing or Excluded
- 0.00 to 10.00
- 10.01 to 15.00
- 15.01 to 20.00
- 20.01 to 25.00
- 25.01 and Above

Source: The United States Census 2000.

PUBLIC HEALTH CONNECTIONS 3.1
CENSUS 2000

During the 2000 United States Census, just six questions were asked about each member of a household who was age five or older. One out of six households were randomly selected to answer an additional fifty-two questions contained in the **long form** of the Census. The head of the household (self-selected) answered questions about himself or herself and then acted as a proxy for other people in the household.

The following questions were used to assess disability status and appeared only on the long form:

Does this person have any of the following long-lasting conditions:

a. Blindness, deafness, or a severe vision or hearing impairment?

b. A condition that substantially limits one or more basic physical activities such as walking, climbing stairs, reaching, lifting, or carrying?

Because of a physical, mental, or emotional condition lasting 6 months or more, does this person have any difficulty in doing any of the following activities:

a. Learning, remembering, or concentrating?

b. Dressing, bathing, or getting around inside the home?

c. (Answer if this person is 16 years old or over.) Going outside the home alone to shop or visit a doctor's office?

d. (Answer if this person is 16 years old or over.) Working at a job or business?

Vital Statistics

In all countries, records about births and deaths, called **vital statistics**, form an important part of public health surveillance. These documents are used primarily as a *legal certification* of births and deaths; that is, they are part of a legal and administrative system of information. For example, you typically need a certified copy of a birth certificate to enroll a child in school, and a widow needs a legal copy of a death certificate to receive pension benefits from her husband's employment. In most countries, the information from these documents is collected and used to examine trends and shifts in population health. From these vital statistics data, we know that the leading causes of death in the United States are heart disease, cancer, stroke, chronic lower respiratory disease, unintentional injuries (accidents), diabetes, and Alzheimer's disease[10]. Let us examine the 1948 Ohio death certificate of our first aviator, Orville Wright (Figure 3.2). It says that Mr. Wright died of a form of heart disease three days after a coronary occlusion from sclerosis (now called atherosclerosis) with possible pulmonary congestion (now called congestive heart failure) at the relatively advanced age of seventy-six.

FIGURE 3.2 Example of a Death Certificate, Orville Wright

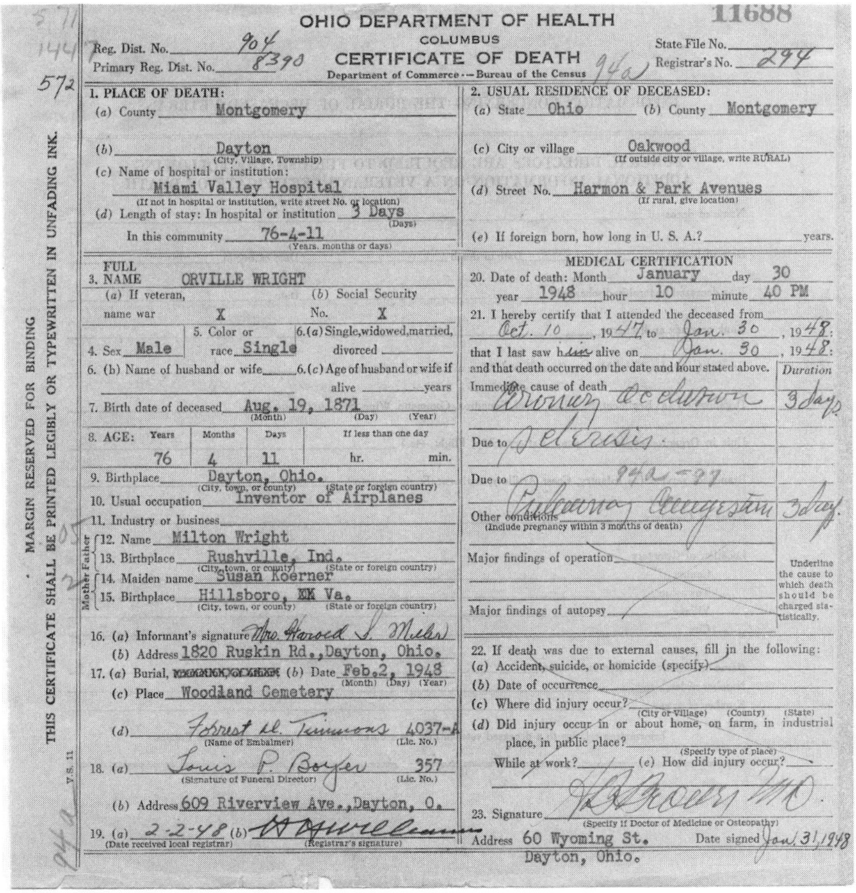

THIS CERTIFICATE SHALL BE PRINTED LEGIBLY OR TYPEWRITTEN IN UNFADING INK. MARGIN RESERVED FOR BINDING

OHIO DEPARTMENT OF HEALTH
COLUMBUS
CERTIFICATE OF DEATH
Department of Commerce—Bureau of the Census

11688

Reg. Dist. No. 904
Primary Reg. Dist. No. 8390
State File No.
Registrar's No. 294

1. PLACE OF DEATH:
(a) County Montgomery
(b) Dayton (City, Village, Township)
(c) Name of hospital or institution: Miami Valley Hospital (If not in hospital or institution, write street No. or location)
(d) Length of stay: In hospital or institution 3 Days (Days)
In this community 76-4-11 (Years, months or days)

2. USUAL RESIDENCE OF DECEASED:
(a) State Ohio (b) County Montgomery
(c) City or village Oakwood (If outside city or village, write RURAL)
(d) Street No. Harmon & Park Avenues (If rural, give location)
(e) If foreign born, how long in U. S. A.? years.

3. FULL NAME ORVILLE WRIGHT
(a) If veteran, name war X (b) Social Security No. X
4. Sex Male
5. Color or race Single
6. (a) Single, widowed, married, divorced
6. (b) Name of husband or wife
6. (c) Age of husband or wife if alive years
7. Birth date of deceased Aug. 19, 1871 (Month) (Day) (Year)
8. AGE: Years 76 Months 4 Days 11 If less than one day hr. min.
9. Birthplace Dayton, Ohio. (City, town, or county) (State or foreign country)
10. Usual occupation Inventor of Airplanes
11. Industry or business
Father 12. Name Milton Wright
13. Birthplace Rushville, Ind. (City, town, or county) (State or foreign country)
Mother 14. Maiden name Susan Koerner
15. Birthplace Hillsboro, Va. (City, town, or county) (State or foreign country)
16. (a) Informant's signature Mrs. Harold S. Miller
(b) Address 1820 Ruskin Rd., Dayton, Ohio.
17. (a) Burial, (b) Date Feb. 2, 1948 (Month) (Day) (Year)
(c) Place Woodland Cemetery
(d) Forrest W. Timmons 4037-A (Name of Embalmer) (Lic. No.)
18. (a) Louis P. Boyer 357 (Signature of Funeral Director) (Lic. No.)
(b) Address 609 Riverview Ave., Dayton, O.
19. (a) 2-2-48 (Date received local registrar) (b) (Registrar's signature)

MEDICAL CERTIFICATION
20. Date of death: Month January day 30 year 1948 hour 10 minute 40 PM
21. I hereby certify that I attended the deceased from Oct. 10, 1947, to Jan. 30, 1948; that I last saw him alive on Jan. 30, 1948; and that death occurred on the date and hour stated above.

	Duration
Immediate cause of death Coronary occlusion	3 days
Due to Sclerosis	
Due to	
Other conditions (Include pregnancy within 3 months of death) Pulmonary congestion	3 days
Major findings of operation	
Major findings of autopsy	

Underline the cause to which death should be charged statistically.

22. If death was due to external causes, fill in the following:
(a) Accident, suicide, or homicide (specify)
(b) Date of occurrence
(c) Where did injury occur? (City or Village) (County) (State)
(d) Did injury occur in or about home, on farm, in industrial place, in public place? (Specify type of place)
While at work? (e) How did injury occur?
23. Signature M.D. (Specify if Doctor of Medicine or Osteopathy)
Address 60 Wyoming St. Dayton, Ohio. Date signed Jan. 31, 1948

V.S. 11

Source: Reproduced with permission from the Ohio Historical Society from the Ohio Divison of Vital Statistics.

In developing nations, documents about births and deaths may not be universally available. For example, in Turkey the government estimates that a formal death certificate is completed for about 60 percent of people who die and notes that death certificates are more common for people who live in major urban centers. By custom, Turkish people are typically buried quickly, often within twenty-four hours. In addition, Turkish religious customs result in medical autopsy (the internal and external examination of a person who has died) being uncommon.

In order to have a more accurate representation of mortality and causes of death, the Turkish government conducted in-person surveys of the health of people from twelve thousand randomly selected households and augmented this with a registry of deaths. When a death was reported in a selected household or in a nearby neighbor's household during the preceding twelve months, a physician visited the house to complete a "verbal autopsy" and determine a cause of death[11–14]. Sixty percent of 1,085 deaths reported during the survey occurred at home. In summarizing the findings, Turkey was able to report accurately that the leading causes of death in rural children aged one month to five years were lower respiratory infections (21.6%), congenital heart disease (16.2%), and meningitis (10.8%). Note that respiratory infections (such as pneumonia) and meningitis are both infectious diseases that are amenable to medical treatment. Among rural adults, the top three causes of death were ischemic heart disease (15.4%), hypertension (12.7%), and myocardial infarction or heart attack (9.1%), all chronic diseases. As Chapter 1 describes, chronic diseases have overtaken infectious diseases in most developed nations as leading causes of morbidity and mortality. For Turkey, data on causes of death in rural areas had been inexact because of the lack of death certificates, and the new data are helping the country with plans for improvements in the national health plan[14]. The data also suggest that Turkey, a country midway in its economic development, experiences health conditions that are midway between developing and developed nations.

In the United States, death certificates have very consistent formats (Figure 3.3). The cause of death section is used to specify the underlying (major) cause of death. These data are collected nationally and add significantly to our ability to understand health trends. For example, the epidemic of lung cancer has finally begun to decrease among men in the United States (Figure 3.4), but continues to increase for U.S. women. We know that this epidemic is largely due to smoking. As smoking rates increased, so did lung cancer, but the lung cancers occurred decades after people began smoking. Because smoking rates decreased, eventually so did the epidemic of lung cancer in men. Widespread smoking occurred later in the United States among women, so the peak of their lung

FIGURE 3.3 A United States Standard Death Certificate

U.S. STANDARD CERTIFICATE OF DEATH

STATE FILE NO.

NAME OF DECEDENT — For use by physician or institution

To Be Completed/ Verified By: FUNERAL DIRECTOR

1. DECEDENT'S LEGAL NAME (Include AKA's if any) (First, Middle, Last)
2. SEX
3. SOCIAL SECURITY NUMBER

4a. AGE-Last Birthday (Years) | 4b. UNDER 1 YEAR — Months | Days | 4c. UNDER 1 DAY — Hours | Minutes | 5. DATE OF BIRTH (Mo/Day/Yr) | 6. BIRTHPLACE (City and State or Foreign Country)

7a. RESIDENCE-STATE | 7b. COUNTY | 7c. CITY OR TOWN

7d. STREET AND NUMBER | 7e. APT. NO. | 7f. ZIP CODE | 7g. INSIDE CITY LIMITS? ☐ Yes ☐ No

8. EVER IN US ARMED FORCES? ☐ Yes ☐ No
9. MARITAL STATUS AT TIME OF DEATH ☐ Married ☐ Married, but separated ☐ Widowed ☐ Divorced ☐ Never Married ☐ Unknown
10. SURVIVING SPOUSE'S NAME (If wife, give name prior to first marriage)

11. FATHER'S NAME (First, Middle, Last)
12. MOTHER'S NAME PRIOR TO FIRST MARRIAGE (First, Middle, Last)

13a. INFORMANT'S NAME | 13b. RELATIONSHIP TO DECEDENT | 13c. MAILING ADDRESS (Street and Number, City, State, Zip Code)

14. PLACE OF DEATH (Check only one: see instructions)

IF DEATH OCCURRED IN A HOSPITAL: ☐ Inpatient ☐ Emergency Room/Outpatient ☐ Dead on Arrival
IF DEATH OCCURRED SOMEWHERE OTHER THAN A HOSPITAL: ☐ Hospice facility ☐ Nursing home/Long term care facility ☐ Decedent's home ☐ Other (Specify):

15. FACILITY NAME (If not institution, give street & number) | 16. CITY OR TOWN , STATE, AND ZIP CODE | 17. COUNTY OF DEATH

18. METHOD OF DISPOSITION: ☐ Burial ☐ Cremation ☐ Donation ☐ Entombment ☐ Removal from State ☐ Other (Specify):
19. PLACE OF DISPOSITION (Name of cemetery, crematory, other place)

20. LOCATION-CITY, TOWN, AND STATE
21. NAME AND COMPLETE ADDRESS OF FUNERAL FACILITY

22. SIGNATURE OF FUNERAL SERVICE LICENSEE OR OTHER AGENT
23. LICENSE NUMBER (Of Licensee)

ITEMS 24-28 MUST BE COMPLETED BY PERSON WHO PRONOUNCES OR CERTIFIES DEATH
24. DATE PRONOUNCED DEAD (Mo/Day/Yr)
25. TIME PRONOUNCED DEAD

26. SIGNATURE OF PERSON PRONOUNCING DEATH (Only when applicable)
27. LICENSE NUMBER
28. DATE SIGNED (Mo/Day/Yr)

29. ACTUAL OR PRESUMED DATE OF DEATH (Mo/Day/Yr) (Spell Month)
30. ACTUAL OR PRESUMED TIME OF DEATH
31. WAS MEDICAL EXAMINER OR CORONER CONTACTED? ☐ Yes ☐ No

CAUSE OF DEATH (See instructions and examples)

Approximate interval: Onset to death

32. PART I. Enter the chain of events--diseases, injuries, or complications--that directly caused the death. DO NOT enter terminal events such as cardiac arrest, respiratory arrest, or ventricular fibrillation without showing the etiology. DO NOT ABBREVIATE. Enter only one cause on a line. Add additional lines if necessary.

IMMEDIATE CAUSE (Final disease or condition --------> resulting in death)   a._____
Due to (or as a consequence of):

Sequentially list conditions, if any, leading to the cause listed on line a. Enter the UNDERLYING CAUSE (disease or injury that initiated the events resulting in death) LAST   b._____
Due to (or as a consequence of):
c._____
Due to (or as a consequence of):
d._____

PART II. Enter other significant conditions contributing to death but not resulting in the underlying cause given in PART I
33. WAS AN AUTOPSY PERFORMED? ☐ Yes ☐ No
34. WERE AUTOPSY FINDINGS AVAILABLE TO COMPLETE THE CAUSE OF DEATH? ☐ Yes ☐ No

To Be Completed By: MEDICAL CERTIFIER

35. DID TOBACCO USE CONTRIBUTE TO DEATH? ☐ Yes ☐ Probably ☐ No ☐ Unknown
36. IF FEMALE: ☐ Not pregnant within past year ☐ Pregnant at time of death ☐ Not pregnant, but pregnant within 42 days of death ☐ Not pregnant, but pregnant 43 days to 1 year before death ☐ Unknown if pregnant within the past year
37. MANNER OF DEATH ☐ Natural ☐ Homicide ☐ Accident ☐ Pending Investigation ☐ Suicide ☐ Could not be determined

38. DATE OF INJURY (Mo/Day/Yr) (Spell Month)
39. TIME OF INJURY
40. PLACE OF INJURY (e.g., Decedent's home; construction site; restaurant; wooded area)
41. INJURY AT WORK? ☐ Yes ☐ No

42. LOCATION OF INJURY: State: | City or Town: | Street & Number: | Apartment No.: | Zip Code:
43. DESCRIBE HOW INJURY OCCURRED:
44. IF TRANSPORTATION INJURY, SPECIFY: ☐ Driver/Operator ☐ Passenger ☐ Pedestrian ☐ Other (Specify)

45. CERTIFIER (Check only one):
☐ Certifying physician-To the best of my knowledge, death occurred due to the cause(s) and manner stated.
☐ Pronouncing & Certifying physician-To the best of my knowledge, death occurred at the time, date, and place, and due to the cause(s) and manner stated.
☐ Medical Examiner/Coroner-On the basis of examination, and/or investigation, in my opinion, death occurred at the time, date, and place, and due to the cause(s) and manner stated.

Signature of certifier:_____

46. NAME, ADDRESS, AND ZIP CODE OF PERSON COMPLETING CAUSE OF DEATH (Item 32)

47. TITLE OF CERTIFIER | 48. LICENSE NUMBER | 49. DATE CERTIFIED (Mo/Day/Yr) | 50. FOR REGISTRAR ONLY- DATE FILED (Mo/Day/Yr)

To Be Completed By: FUNERAL DIRECTOR

51. DECEDENT'S EDUCATION-Check the box that best describes the highest degree or level of school completed at the time of death.
☐ 8th grade or less
☐ 9th - 12th grade; no diploma
☐ High school graduate or GED completed
☐ Some college credit, but no degree
☐ Associate degree (e.g., AA, AS)
☐ Bachelor's degree (e.g., BA, AB, BS)
☐ Master's degree (e.g., MA, MS, MEng, MEd, MSW, MBA)
☐ Doctorate (e.g., PhD, EdD) or Professional degree (e.g., MD, DDS, DVM, LLB, JD)

52. DECEDENT OF HISPANIC ORIGIN? Check the box that best describes whether the decedent is Spanish/Hispanic/Latino. Check the "No" box if decedent is not Spanish/Hispanic/Latino.
☐ No, not Spanish/Hispanic/Latino
☐ Yes, Mexican, Mexican American, Chicano
☐ Yes, Puerto Rican
☐ Yes, Cuban
☐ Yes, other Spanish/Hispanic/Latino (Specify) _____

53. DECEDENT'S RACE (Check one or more races to indicate what the decedent considered himself or herself to be)
☐ White
☐ Black or African American
☐ American Indian or Alaska Native (Name of the enrolled or principal tribe) _____
☐ Asian Indian
☐ Chinese
☐ Filipino
☐ Japanese
☐ Korean
☐ Vietnamese
☐ Other Asian (Specify)_____
☐ Native Hawaiian
☐ Guamanian or Chamorro
☐ Samoan
☐ Other Pacific Islander (Specify)_____
☐ Other (Specify)_____

54. DECEDENT'S USUAL OCCUPATION (Indicate type of work done during most of working life. DO NOT USE RETIRED.)
55. KIND OF BUSINESS/INDUSTRY

REV. 11/2003

Source: Reference 15.

FIGURE 3.4 Lung Cancer Epidemic in the United States 1975–2006

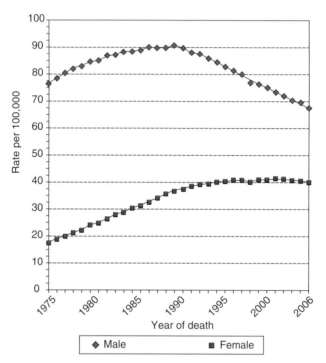

Cancer sites include invasive cases only unless otherwise noted. Mortality source: US Mortality Files, National Center for Health Statistics, CDC. Rates are per 100,000 and are age-adjusted to the 2000 US Std Population (19 age groups -Census P25–1130). Regression lines are calculated using the Joinpoint Regression Program Version 3.3.2, June 2008, National Cancer Institute.

cancer epidemic has not yet been reached. Because smoking rates have declined in women, we expect the lung cancer epidemic among women to decline as well.

Birth certificates are rich sources of health information about childbirth, infant conditions, maternal health, and even social circumstances and medical care. Table 3.1 provides examples of the data collected at the time of birth that are used to describe mothers and their pregnancy experiences, the infant health and condition, and aspects of the delivery and health care. These data have been used to track the prevalence of preterm (delivered at less than thirty-seven weeks) and low birth weight (less than 2,500 grams or 5.5 pounds) infants, for example. Figure 3.5 shows an alarming increase in both preterm and low birth weight in

Table 3.1 Examples of Information Available from U.S. Standard Birth Certificates

Data on mothers	Age, education, height, prepregnancy and weight at birth, smoking before and during pregnancy, diabetes, health insurance status, and prior births
Data on newborns	Weeks of gestation, birth weight, sex, congenital anomalies (e.g., Down syndrome, spina bifida, limb reduction), and breast-fed at hospital discharge
Data about health care	Labor induced, mother's health insurance status, and cesarean section

Source: Reference 15.

FIGURE 3.5 Percentage of infants born preterm or low birth weight, United States 1990–2004

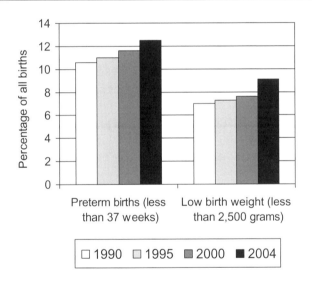

the United States from 1990 to 2004[16]. The reasons for these trends are not entirely clear, but both outcomes are linked to maternal characteristics (very young mothers, mothers who are single, and mothers who live in poverty[17,18]); increases in multiple births (for example twins, triplets[19]); disparities in neighborhood resources (such as available healthy foods in grocery stores[20]); and disparities in access to health care. When infants are born early, or are small, they face much larger risks of mortality and early and late childhood difficulties. As described in Chapter 16, the United States is ranked fairly low in birth outcomes in the global community.

Survey Data

The United States conducts a number of ongoing survey interviews with randomly selected Americans to monitor health with a **representative sample**. These surveys form a vital component of what we know about the nation's health because they are first-hand accounts rather than information from records and observations of others. Three examples are presented here.

Behavioral Risk Factor Surveillance System

The Behavioral Risk Factor Surveillance System, or BRFSS, is the world's largest health survey. Each year, and in each U.S. state, territory, and the District of Columbia, adults age eighteen and older are randomly selected to participate in a telephone survey. The BRFSS is led and funded by the Centers for Disease Control and Prevention (CDC) in Atlanta[21]. In 2007, the BRFSS conducted over 430,000 surveys, and in 2008, that number was over 410,000. The number of surveys conducted in each state varies. In 2007, most states conducted at least 4,000 surveys. The state of Florida conducted over 39,000 surveys in order to provide information to each of its counties for use in local health departments. All states use the same core set of questions each year and then choose supplemental modules representing topics of special interest. Typical core topics include overall health status, tobacco use, alcohol consumption, dietary and physical activity habits, access to health care, and specific health conditions (for example, in 2007 there were questions about diabetes and asthma). These data can be analyzed at the national, state, and sometimes regional or county level. Figure 3.6 shows an example of data collected about the prevalence of adults classified as heavy drinkers (adult men having more than two drinks per day and adult women having more than one drink per day). The states with the lowest prevalence of heavy alcohol use (less than 4 percent) are in the lightest color (Utah, South Dakota), and the darker colors represent increasingly higher levels. The darkest color indicates states with prevalence of heavy drinking at 6.5% or higher (Nevada, Wisconsin, Vermont). Alcohol consumption is a health risk behavior of concern in the United States because it may lead to unintentional injuries (car crashes, falls), violence, or a number of chronic health conditions.

The Youth Risk Behavior Surveillance System

The Youth Risk Behavior Surveillance System (YRBSS) is the complementary CDC survey system for young people[23]. It is a paper and pencil, self-administered survey conducted every other year in school settings for students in grades 9

FIGURE 3.6 Prevalence of Adults Classified as Heavy Drinkers in the United States, by State

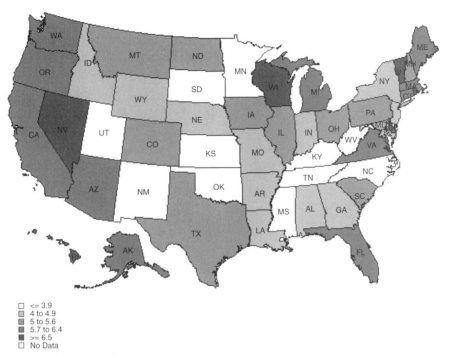

- □ <= 3.9
- ▣ 4 to 4.9
- ▦ 5 to 5.6
- ▩ 5.7 to 6.4
- ■ >= 6.5
- □ No Data

Source: Reference 22.

through 12 throughout the United States. The YRBSS includes questions about health behaviors similar to those in the BRFSS, for example behaviors such as physical activity and smoking, but it also asks about behaviors and experiences that lead to the most common causes of death among young people: intentional and unintentional injuries. Figure 3.7 is a summary of behavioral trends among U.S. students from 1991 to 2007. These survey results suggest that there has been some success in decreasing behaviors that contribute to violence and injury. There was a decrease in weapons in schools during the 1990s, although the decrease has leveled out (and maybe even risen again) since 2000. Fully 35 percent of students said they had been involved in a physical a fight in the last twelve months in 2007, and close to 5 percent said they had been treated for an injury because of a physical fight. At the beginning of this chapter, we said that criteria for choosing to conduct surveillance include severity and preventability. Carrying weapons and physical fights are serious, and can even cause deaths. Are they preventable? As described in Chapter 11, public health educators work

FIGURE 3.7 The Youth Risk Behavior Survey, 1991–2007

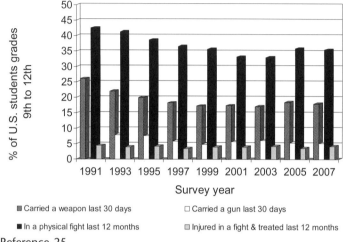

Source: Reference 25.

on educational campaigns to help change our behaviors to improve the health of the public. School-based violence prevention programs are recommended as a method to reduce violence[24]. More examples of these kinds of YRBSS survey questions are listed in Public Health Connections 3.2. To view these and other data for your state, see the Review Questions at the end of the chapter.

PUBLIC HEALTH CONNECTIONS 3.2

YOUTH RISK BEHAVIOR SURVEY QUESTIONS ABOUT BEHAVIORS THAT MAY LEAD TO VIOLENCE

- During the past 30 days, on how many days did you carry a weapon such as a gun, knife, or club?

- During the past 30 days, on how many days did you carry a gun?

- During the past 30 days, on how many days did you carry a weapon such as a gun, knife, or club on school property?

- During the past 30 days, on how many days did you not go to school because you felt you would be unsafe at school or on your way to or from school?

- During the past 12 months, how many times has someone threatened or injured you with a weapon such as a gun, knife, or club on school property?

- During the past 12 months, how many times has someone stolen or deliberately damaged your property such as your car, clothing, or books on school property?

- During the past 12 months, how many times were you in a physical fight?

- During the past 12 months, how many times were you in a physical fight in which you were injured and had to be treated by a doctor or nurse?

- During the past 12 months, how many times were you in a physical fight on school property?

- During the past 12 months, did your boyfriend or girlfriend ever hit, slap, or physically hurt you on purpose?

- Have you ever been physically forced to have sexual intercourse when you did not want to?

Source: Reference 25.

Registries

A registry is a different type of data source from that which we have discussed up to now. Rather than collecting information from everyone in a population (U.S. Census, vital statistics) or selecting a representative sample of the population (surveys), **registries** seek to identify all individuals in a population with a specific exposure or health condition. Perhaps the most well-known example of a registry in the United States is the Surveillance Epidemiology and End Results (SEER) Program, maintained by the National Cancer Institute (NCI)[26]. SEER actually is a group of registries that collects population-based information about cancer diagnoses, treatment courses, and outcomes. The SEER Program covers about a quarter of the U.S. population, with eighteen registries covering metropolitan areas (for example, Seattle-Puget Sound and San Francisco-Oakland), states (for example, Connecticut and New Mexico), and specific ethnic groups (Alaska Native Tumor Registry and Arizona Indians).

Establishing and maintaining a registry is time intensive and costly. A registry must begin with a clear **case definition**, a thorough description of quantifiable and objective clinical symptoms or diagnostic criteria or exposure classification, depending on the type of registry. This ensures the registry contains the individuals with the exposure or disease of interest, limiting misclassification. Ideally, registries include a mechanism of **active surveillance** for new cases, that is, seeking out people newly exposed or diagnosed by contacting health care providers or by searching medical records. **Passive surveillance**, in contrast, occurs when health care providers or patients are encouraged to report the exposure or disease to the registry, but no case-finding effort is made by the registry personnel. Once a case definition is established, other data elements must be decided. For example, will the registry include demographic information, diagnostic information, treatment data, and long-term follow-up? The purpose of the registry must be considered when establishing the information to be collected from registry participants. For example, we would collect different information if our goal is to understand the etiology of a disease than if our goal is to compare the effectiveness of different treatment strategies. These decisions also incorporate the pragmatic aspects we discussed at the beginning of this chapter regarding the choice of surveillance activities. For example, long-term follow-up for mortality of persons in a cancer registry can use vital statistics data with special permission and fairly low cost, but following up with cancer patients by telephone for their self-reports of symptoms and quality of life would be an expensive undertaking.

Two exposure-based registries in the United States are the National Exposure Registry and the World Trade Center Health Registry[27–29]. Both registries are managed by the Agency for Toxic Substances and Disease Registry (ATSDR) within the Department of Health and Human Services (HHS) in cooperation with other federal or local agencies.

The National Exposure Registry (NER) seeks to identify health risks associated with exposures, especially long-term exposures, to various hazardous substances, such as metals (lead, cadmium) and other naturally occurring contaminants, and man-made chemicals used in industrial processes or produced as by-products of these processes (trichloroethylene, dioxin, benzene)[27]. The NER identifies sites known to be contaminated with a particular hazardous substance and then includes in the registry individuals who have been exposed to the substance in the environment. Substances included in the NER are chosen based on the number of sites in which they are known to be a contaminant, how toxic they are, and the likelihood that humans would be exposed to them. In addition to collecting data for research, the NER is also used as a mechanism to contact individuals who have been exposed with updated research findings to educate them about potential health risks[27]. Chapter 10 describes aspects of human exposures and risk in detail.

The World Trade Center (WTC) Health Registry, the largest such registry in the United States, was established in 2002 to follow individuals who were exposed to the World Trade Center disaster on September 11, 2001[28]. Individuals who were in the buildings or the surrounding areas and those who responded to the disaster (firefighters, police, construction workers, journalists) were exposed to a number of potentially hazardous compounds, including building debris (concrete dust, asbestos, glass shards, fiberglass), jet fuel, and combustion products[29]. In addition, these individuals experienced events that could negatively impact mental health. The WTC Health Registry was established to understand and identify poor physical and mental health outcomes associated with exposure to the disaster and at this time is expected to continue for twenty years. Data on 71,437 individuals are available through the WTC Registry. Like the NER and other registries, the WTC Health Registry provides information and research findings back to participants. In addition, the registry can help enrollees link to medical and other benefit programs for which they are eligible, and it has begun a smoking cessation program for registry members. To date, a number of studies have been published using WTC Registry data. Among the findings are higher rates of newly diagnosed asthma and post-traumatic stress disorder (PTSD) for exposed individuals compared to the unexposed population, a high prevalence of psychological distress, and high rates of acute and chronic respiratory problems[29–31]. Rates of these outcomes varied based on the type of exposure experienced. For example, individuals who were in the dust cloud, the heavy plume of debris created when the buildings fell, were more likely to develop asthma than were other individuals exposed to the disaster but who were not enveloped by the cloud[30].

Reporting Systems

In addition to the many data systems and sources outlined above, there are additional reporting systems maintained at the federal, state, and local levels. These systems typically rely on passive surveillance and thus do not seek out participants, but they allow reporting to a centralized system on a specific health topic. Three examples of these are the county-level reportable disease system, the Vaccine Adverse Events Reporting System, and the Adverse Event Reporting System.

The local reportable disease system is an important component of tracking and assessing infectious disease in the United States. The CDC maintains a list of Nationally Notifiable Infectious Diseases (see www.cdc.gov/ncphi/od/AI/phs/infdis.htm) for which all health care professionals and laboratories are required to notify their local (usually county or city) health department if an individual tests positive or is presumed to have one of the diseases listed. States may choose to add conditions to the list, and most have a note that any disease believed to be part of an outbreak or any disease considered a public health threat also must be reported. We will discuss reportable diseases further in Chapter 8.

The Vaccine Adverse Events Reporting System (VAERS) is a Web-based, voluntary reporting system managed jointly by the CDC and the Food and Drug Administration (FDA). The system includes all licensed vaccines in the United States and allows anyone, individuals or health care providers, to report any **adverse events** (negative side effects) they believe to be linked with receipt of a vaccine. As with reportable infectious diseases, the law requires that health care providers report adverse vaccine-related events through VAERS. Data are publicly available through the VAERS Web site (http://vaers.hhs.gov/info.htm) and can be searched by type of vaccine, reaction, age of the vaccine recipient, vaccine manufacturer, and a variety of other factors. Reports on the VAERS site should not be considered *causative*; in other words, VAERS reports include incidents that may not have been related to the vaccine, and a cause and effect relationship between vaccine and outcome is not implied. However, these data can be useful in identifying potential negative effects of vaccines and might be a warning system for new or emerging reactions.

The Adverse Event Reporting System (AERS) is nearly identical to VAERS, except that it is used for the reporting of negative effects associated with exposure to approved medications. The FDA maintains the AERS, and reporting is possible through its Web site[32]. Individuals or health care providers may report adverse events voluntarily, and drug manufacturers who are alerted to adverse events are legally obligated to report them. As with the VAERS system, events reported in AERS may not actually be caused by the drug, but the data can provide important clues to potential problems and may encourage further research.

Summary

In this chapter, we have seen how we decide what information to collect and how to collect it for the core public health function of assessment. Although in theory many types of adverse exposures, health problems, and experiences are important, in practice the public funds for public health data are applied to problems that are common, serious, costly, preventable, and communicable and for which there is broad public support. Surveillance and other public health data sources provide information about trends over time and can be analyzed for different groups or populations, including countries, states, local areas, or people with specific demographic characteristics or exposures. These data come from a number of systems, including those that collect information about everyone, or nearly everyone, in a population, such as the United States Census or vital statistics; those that survey a random sample of citizens, such as the Behavioral Risk Factor Surveillance System or Youth Risk Behavior Survey; and those that rely on reports from health professionals and the public or medical records review, including the National Exposure Registry and the Adverse Event Reporting System. Taken together, these sources provide the backbone of our understanding of health issues and the data to set policy and evaluate public health programs.

Key Terms

active surveillance, 66

adverse events, 68

case definition, 65

Census, 54

communicability of a
    health event, 53

cost of a health event, 53

frequency of a health
    event, 53

long form, 56

passive surveillance, 66

preventability of a health
    event, 53

public interest of a health
    event, 53

registries, 65

representative sample, 62

severity of a health event,
    53

stroke belt, 55

surveillance, 52

vital statistics, 56

Review Questions

1. The Youth Risk Behavior Surveillance System (YRBSS) includes information on health habits. Select either smoking or alcohol use, and answer a question about your state or district compared to national data on this behavior. For example, do students in grades 9–12 in your area report they are current smokers more or less often than do students nationally?
    Web sites:
    CDC Youth Risk Behavior Surveillance System (YRBSS) main page www.cdc.gov/healthyyouth/yrbs/index.htm.
    YRBSS Comparisons Between State or District and National Results (Fact Sheets) www.cdc.gov/healthyyouth/yrbs/state_district_comparisons.htm.

2. The Behavioral Risk Factor Surveillance System (BRFSS) includes information on health behaviors, health, and personal characteristics. Select one condition or characteristic from the list below and describe the trend over the past five years.

Diabetes

Health care coverage (for adults aged eighteen to sixty-four)

Annual influenza (flu) shots for adults aged sixty-five and older

Web sites:

CDC Behavioral Risk Factor Surveillance System (BRFSS) main page www.cdc.gov/brfss/.

BRFSS Prevalence and Trend Data (compare over time or by area) http://apps.nccd.cdc.gov/brfss/.

3. Using the six criteria for identifying health events on which to conduct surveillance, explain why cancer is one of the health conditions for which we do surveillance in public health.

4. Describe any limitations in generalizing the findings of the data from each of the following data systems to the entire U.S. population.

Census

BRFSS

YRBSS

Other Web sites to explore for more information on health statistics:

The National Center for Health Statistics National Health Interview Survey, www.cdc.gov/nchs/nhis.htm.

The Agency for Healthcare Research and Quality Medical Expenditure Panel Survey, www.meps.ahrq.gov/mepsweb/.

The World Health Organization Global Health Atlas, www.who.int/globalatlas/.

References

1. Institute of Medicine (IOM). *The Future of Public Health*. Committee for the Study of the Future of Public Health. Washington, D.C.: National Academy Press; 1988.

2. Teutsch SM, Churchill RE. *Principles and Practice of Public Health Surveillance*. New York: Oxford University Press; 1994.

3. Dennis Quaid recounts twins' drug ordeal. Interview with Steve Kroft. *60 Minutes*. Updated August 22, 2008. Available at: www.cbsnews.com/stories/2008/03/13/60minutes/main3936412.shtml. Accessed September 30, 2009.

4. Medical Errors: The Scope of the Problem. Fact sheet, Publication No. AHRQ 00-P037. Agency for Healthcare Research and Quality, Rockville, Md. Available at: www.ahrq.gov/qual/errback.htm. Accessed August 26, 2008.

5. Institute of Medicine (IOM). *To Err is Human. Building a Safer Health System*. Kohn LT, Corrigan JT, Donaldson MS, eds. Committee on Quality of Health Care in America. Washington, D.C.: National Academies Press; 2000.

6. Andresen EM, Fitch CA, McLendon P, Meyers A. Reliability and validity of disability questions for U.S. Census 2000. *Am J Public Health*. 2000;90(8):1297–1299.

7. Glasser SP, Cushman M, Prineas R, et al. Does differential prophylactic aspirin use contribute to racial and geographic disparities in stroke and coronary heart disease (CHD)? *Prev. Med.* 2008;47(2):161–166.

8. Voeks JH, McClure LA, Go RC, et al. Regional differences in diabetes as a possible contributor to the geographic disparity in stroke mortality: The Reasons for Geographic and Racial Differences in Stroke Study. *Stroke.* 2008;39(6):1675–1680.

9. Kilmer G, Roberts H, Hughes E, et al. Surveillance of certain health behaviors and conditions among states and selected local areas—Behavioral Risk Factor Surveillance System (BRFSS), United States, 2006. *MMWR Recomm Rep.* 2008;57(7):1–188.

10. Centers for Disease Control and Prevention (CDC). Leading causes of death. National Center for Health Statistics, FastStats home page. 2006. Available at: www.cdc.gov/nchs/fastats/lcod.htm. Accessed October 30, 2009.

11. Bang AT, Bang RA. Diagnosis of causes of childhood deaths in developing countries by verbal autopsy: Suggested criteria. The SEARCH Team. *Bull World Health Organ.* 1992;70(4):499–507.

12. Chandramohan D, Maude GH, Rodrigues LC, Hayes RJ. Verbal autopsies for adult deaths: Their development and validation in a multicentre study. *Trop Med Intl Health.* 1998;3(6):436–446.

13. Mirza NM, Macharia WM, Wafula EM, Agwanda RO, Onyango FE. Verbal autopsy: A tool for determining cause of death in a community. *East Afr Med J.* 1990;67(10):693–698.

14. Ministry of Health (Turkey), Başkent University. *National Burden of Disease and Cost-Effectiveness Project.* Inception Report. Refik Saydam School of Public Health Directorate, Ankara, Turkey; November 2002.

15. Centers for Disease Control and Prevention (CDC). 2003 Revisions of the U.S. Standard Certificates of Live Birth and Death and the Fetal Death Report. National Vital Statistics System page. Available at: www.cdc.gov/nchs/nvss/vital_certificate_revisions.htm. Accessed April 29, 2010.

16. Martin JA, Hamilton BE, Sutton PD, Ventura SJ, Menacker F, Kirmeyer S. Preterm births for 2004: Infant and maternal health. Health E-stats. Hyattsville, Md.: National Center for Health Statistics. November 15, 2005. Available at: www.cdc.gov/nchs/products/pubs/pubd/hestats/prelimbirths04/prelimbirths04health.htm. Accessed March 6, 2009.

17. Alexander GR, Wingate MS, Bader D, Kogan MD. The increasing racial disparity in infant mortality rates: Composition and contributors to recent US trends. *Am J Obstet Gynecol.* 2008;198(1):51.e1–51.e9.

18. Colen CG, Geronimus, AT, Bound J, James SA. Maternal upward socioeconomic mobility and black-white disparities in infant birthweight. *Am J Pub Health.* 2006;96(11):2032–2039.

19. Kochanek, KD, Martin JA. Supplemental Analyses of Recent Trends in Infant Mortality. Health E-Stats. Hyattsville, MD: National Center for Health Statistics. Available at: www.cdc.gov/nchs/products/pubs/pubd/hestats/infantmort/infantmort.htm. Accessed September 29, 2009.

20. Lane SD, Keefe RH, Rubinstein R, et al. Structural violence, urban retail food markets, and low birth weight. *Health Place.* 2008;14(3):415–423.

21. Centers for Disease Control and Prevention (CDC). Behavioral Risk Factor Surveillance System page. Available at: www.cdc.gov/brfss/. Accessed September 29, 2009.

22. Centers for Disease Control and Prevention (CDC). Behavioral risk factor surveillance system prevalence and trends data. Available at: http://apps.nccd.cdc/brfss/. Accessed May 21, 2010.

23. Centers for Disease Control and Prevention (CDC). Methodology of the Youth Risk Behavior Surveillance System. *MMWR Recomm Rep.* 2004;53(RR-12):1–13.

24. Guide to Community Preventive Services. Violence prevention focused on children and youth: School-based programs Web page. Available at: www.thecommunityguide.org/violence/school.html. Accessed March 6, 2009.

25. Centers for Disease Control and Prevention (CDC). National Center for Chronic Disease Prevention and Health Promotion, Division of Adolescent and School Health. 2003 National school-based Youth Risk Behavior Survey. Available at: http://ftp.cdc.gov/pub/data/yrbs/2003/yrbs2003codebook.txt. Accessed May 21, 2010.

26. National Cancer Institute (NCI). Surveillance epidemiology and end results (SEER) Web page. Available at: http://seer.cancer.gov/. Accessed May 21, 2010.

27. *U.S. Department of Health and Human Services. Agency for Toxic Substances and Disease Registry. NTIS Database Web page. What is the National Exposure Registry?* Available at: www.ntis.gov/products/ntisdb.aspx. Accessed May 21, 2010.

28. Schwartz J. *World Trade Center Health Registry Annual Report 2008.* New York: World Trade Center Registry; 2008. Available at: www.nyc.gov/html/doh/wtc/downloads/pdf/registry/WTC_AnnualReport.pdf. Accessed June 8, 2009.

29. Herbert, R, Moline J, Skloot G, et al. The World Trade Center disaster and the health of workers: Five-year assessment of a unique medical screening program. *Environ Health Perspect.* 2006;114(12):1853–1858.

30. Farfel M, DiGrande L, Brackbill R, et al. An overview of 9/11 experiences and respiratory and mental health conditions among World Trade Center Health Registry enrollees. *J Urban Health.* 2008;85(6):880–909.

31. DiGrande L, Perrin MA, Thorpe LE, et al. Posttraumatic stress symptoms, PTSD, and risk factors among lower Manhattan residents 2–3 years after the September 11, 2001 terrorist attacks. *J Trauma Stress.* 2008;21(3):264–273.

32. U.S. Food and Drug Administration. Adverse Event Reporting System (AERS). FDA Web site. Available at: www.fda.gov/Drugs/GuidanceComplianceRegulatory Information/Surveillance/AdverseDrugEffects/default.htm. Accessed September 29, 2009.

CHAPTER 4

EPIDEMIOLOGY
INTRODUCTION AND BASIC CONCEPTS

Erin D. Bouldin, MPH
Elena M. Andresen, PhD

LEARNING OBJECTIVES

- Define epidemiology and describe what epidemiologists do within the area of public health.
- Outline historical developments important to the field of epidemiology.
- Identify the exposure and outcome in a public health research question.
- Describe the difference between descriptive and analytic epidemiology.
- Identify counts, proportions, and rates in reported data.
- Calculate the incidence rate or the prevalence of a health event in a population.
- Identify potential confounders in a research study and understand their influence on results.

Epidemiology deals with the study of the causes, distribution, and control of disease in populations[1]. Rather than focusing on the health of an individual person or a patient, however, epidemiologists focus on the health of groups of people. The field of epidemiology is a relatively young one, although the methods of statistics and other branches of mathematics, along with general scientific inquiry, form its basis. Epidemiology can be used in two broad ways: to describe where, when, and to whom a health event occurs or to quantify the amount of risk associated with a particular exposure or behavior. Epidemiologists use a variety of measures to describe the health of populations and to identify risk factors for health outcomes and disease, including counts, proportions, and rates. These measures are described in more detail in this chapter, and the methods for identifying risk factors appear in Chapter 5.

What Is Epidemiology?

Epidemiology, derived from the Greek, translates to "the study of that which is upon the people" (*epi*, "on, upon"; *demos*, "people"; *logos*, "word, statement"). Thus epidemiologists are concerned with understanding health outcomes not in individuals, but in populations, or groups of people. Typically, an epidemiologist investigates the relationship between two things: the *exposure* and the *outcome* of interest. In statistics, the **exposure** would be called the independent variable; it is the health behavior, toxic substance, or other event or material a person encounters or experiences. The outcome, on the other hand, is the dependent variable. In epidemiology, we are interested in understanding how the exposure changes the chance someone will experience the outcome. An **outcome** can be a disease or other health outcome, or it could be a health behavior. For example, if an epidemiologist is interested in whether smoking causes lung cancer, smoking is the exposure and lung cancer is the outcome. Likewise, an epidemiologist may investigate whether eating a specific type of food (exposure) causes infection with *Salmonella* (outcome). The research question determines whether a given behavior or health outcome is the exposure or outcome. In some cases, smoking could be an outcome. Perhaps an epidemiologist is interested in looking at whether teens in rural areas are more likely to start smoking compared to teens in urban areas. In that case, rural residence is the exposure and smoking is the outcome. An outcome does not have to be a disease state; it can be any health event or health outcome of interest to the investigator. Likewise, outcomes do not have to be negative. An outcome may be a positive health behavior, such as eating the recommended five servings of fruits or vegetables per day, or it may be a positive health outcome, such as giving birth to a baby who is considered normal weight.

Epidemiologists may work to identify the causes of disease, also known as disease **etiology**[2]. An underlying assumption is that diseases and health outcomes are **multifactorial**, or caused by many different variables or factors. These factors may be physical, such as a virus or bacteria; they may be inherent or individual, such as genetic components or demographic characteristics; or they may be environmental, including neighborhood characteristics or governmental policies. Epidemiologists, like other public health professionals, conceptualize health outcomes using the social ecological model described in Chapter 2. In addition to elucidating disease etiology, epidemiologists commonly work to identify factors that increase or decrease a person's likelihood of having a particular health outcome[2]. This leads to a second underlying assumption in epidemiology: health outcomes are not randomly distributed in a population.

In other words, the multiple factors that cause a disease are measurable and identifiable. If health events occurred at random, the prevention work of public health would be futile. We know, however, that there are a multitude of variables that can be linked to health outcomes. Epidemiologists seek to find these variables so that they and other public health professionals can work to intervene and prevent poor health in populations. Epidemiologists also may study how a disease progresses over time, or its natural history, from onset, through treatment, and possibly to death[2]. Furthermore, some epidemiologists work to compare different ways of preventing a health outcome or treating a disease to determine which methods are most effective[2]. Finally, epidemiologists work to determine and describe how much of a health event or health outcome occurs in a population and also among whom it is more common[2]. Ultimately, epidemiology is concerned with improving the health of populations. Therefore, a final area in which epidemiologists may work is promoting or developing public health policies that are based on the data epidemiologists collect and analyze[2].

History of Epidemiology

Epidemiology often is referred to as one of the sciences of public health. Although individuals have been applying epidemiological principles for many centuries, the formal field called *epidemiology* is a relatively young one. As you may recall, we discussed some early epidemiologists in our history of public health in Chapter 1. William Petty (1623–1687), Gottfried Achenwall (1719–1772), and Adolphe Quetelet (1796–1874) were all important in beginning the field of statistics and creating standards for analysis. John Graunt (1620–1674) published the first statistical analyses of a population's health, noting associations between demographic variables and disease, and created the first calculations of life expectancy[3].

The amount of data available for developing epidemiology methods grew tremendously during the nineteenth century. It has been argued that much of the basis of modern epidemiology was borne out of France during the nineteenth century after the French Revolution[4, pp. 28–38]. Perhaps the most notable figure in the French movement was Pierre Charles-Alexandre Louis (1787–1872). Louis, drawing on the work of earlier scientists and statisticians, worked to understand the etiology (cause) and natural history of various diseases and to compare the effectiveness of different treatments. His concepts of epidemiology and epidemiological methods are much the same as those today, recognizing the importance of random sampling, confounding, and error, topics we will discuss later in this chapter and in Chapters 5 and 6. Louis counted among his students some of the most important figures in the development of epidemiology in England, where the field was greatly expanded, and in the United States[4, pp. 28–38]. One of Louis' students, William Farr (1807–1883), served as the chief statistician in England's General Register Office. In this position, Farr had access to great quantities of vital statistics data and used these data to develop models that predicted the number of cases of disease over time during an outbreak or epidemic. Farr also worked to measure and predict morbidity (illness) in the same way others had predicted mortality (death). Like Louis, he also worked to develop methods to compare the effectiveness of different treatments. Although he would not have identified it as such, Farr thought about health and disease in terms of the social-ecological model, recognizing the importance of environmental influences, namely living conditions, on health[4, pp. 1–21].

In addition to the improvement of statistical methods by Louis, Farr, and others, epidemiology was advanced by the broad acceptance of the germ theory of disease, that a specific, living, contagious agent was responsible for each infectious disease, in the middle to late nineteenth century. As long as alternate theories such as miasma (bad air) were widely accepted, identifying the causes of disease was challenging. As you may remember from Chapter 1, John Snow was able to identify the likely cause (water contamination) of several cholera outbreaks in London before the causative agent of the disease was known. This illustrates that epidemiology allows for the interruption of disease transmission even when the underlying cause is unknown. Nonetheless, targeted measures that more successfully control the spread of disease can be more easily developed when the causative agent is known.

During the twentieth century, epidemiological studies became commonplace as sophisticated methodologies for studying the relationships between exposures and outcomes developed. A number of large, epidemiological studies such as the Framingham Heart Study (discussed in more detail in Chapter 5) have allowed us to identify risk factors for such chronic diseases as heart disease, stroke, and others. Increasingly sophisticated technology and scientific study have allowed us to identify the causative agents for many infectious diseases.

Types of Epidemiology

The first step in understanding a health outcome often includes **descriptive epidemiology**, which depicts the health event by *person*, *place*, and *time* variables. Person, or "who" variables, include the demographic characteristics age, sex, and race or ethnicity. For example, a health outcome may occur only among women, or it may affect children under the age of five more often than any other age group. It may impact people of a certain race, ethnicity, or country of origin more frequently than other groups. Place variables tell the "where" of the health outcome. Are rural populations more likely to experience the outcome compared to urban dwellers? Perhaps an illness strikes in settings where many people come into close contact, such as schools, prisons, or nursing homes. A physical factor such as a river or a salt marsh may be the center of a cluster of outcomes. All of these examples illustrate the use of place variables in describing a health outcome. Finally, time, or "when" variables, provide information about trends in a health outcome across years or seasons, and in the case of infectious diseases, time variables may be used to help identify the source of an infection based on the timing of reported symptoms. Diseases such as influenza are cyclical in nature and commonly occur during specific seasons. Tracking the timing of influenza cases may alert public health officials to an early start to a flu season or to a possible epidemic or pandemic strain of the virus. Lyme disease cases spike substantially during the summer months, when people are more likely to be outdoors and in contact with the deer ticks that transmit the disease. In other cases, there may be a point in time after which the outcome of interest became increasingly common. For example, a contaminated potato salad at a company picnic may lead to an outbreak of *Salmonella*. In this example, we might describe the outbreak epidemiology in reference to the day of the picnic and track and identify those who began exhibiting symptoms thereafter. In epidemiology, it is useful to monitor trends over time to understand the nature of health outcomes and to evaluate whether interventions or control strategies are having an impact because the time of their implementation is known. The descriptive person, place, and time information about a health outcome is helpful in designing studies or interventions to address it.

Figure 4.1 shows the prevalence of obesity, defined as a body mass index (BMI) greater than or equal to 30, by state for the years 1990, 2000, and 2008. All data are from the Behavioral Risk Factor Surveillance System (BRFSS). From this figure, we have descriptive epidemiology information about obesity in the United States, namely place and time. From 1990 to 2008, obesity prevalence increased dramatically across the United States. Certain areas of the country, particularly the Southeast, appear to have higher obesity prevalence than do others. From these figures, we see that over time obesity has increased in the United States and that people living in certain places (states or regions) have a higher prevalence of obesity than people living in other places.

Figure 4.2 adds the dimension of *person* to the descriptive epidemiology of obesity in the United States. Based on data from 2006–2008, we see that obesity prevalence is higher among people of certain racial or ethnic groups. The maps show that in all states reporting data, the prevalence of obesity is highest among

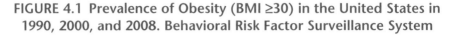

FIGURE 4.1 Prevalence of Obesity (BMI ≥30) in the United States in 1990, 2000, and 2008. Behavioral Risk Factor Surveillance System

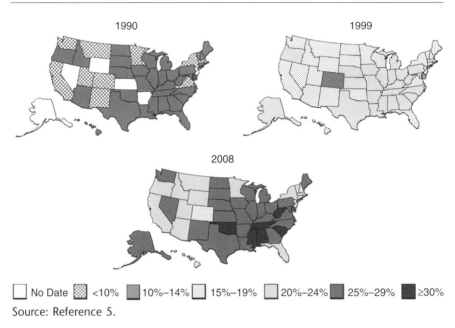

☐ No Date ▨ <10% ▧ 10%–14% ▨ 15%–19% ☐ 20%–24% ▨ 25%–29% ■ ≥30%

Source: Reference 5.

people who reported their race and ethnicity as Black, non-Hispanic. Taken together, these two figures provide some descriptive epidemiology of obesity in the United States; specifically, obesity has been increasing over the past two decades and people in the southeastern United States and who report Black, non-Hispanic race and ethnicity have higher obesity prevalence than do people in the West or who report White, non-Hispanic race. This information may be useful to researchers designing a study of obesity prevention or to public health professionals working to implement a health promotion program.

Analytic epidemiology goes a step beyond a description of a health problem or health outcome and seeks to identify *risk factors* or *protective factors* for the outcome. A **risk factor** is any personal attribute, environmental exposure, or other feature of a person or his or her environment that increases the likelihood that he or she will experience a given health outcome. **Protective factors** are any of the same types of variables that reduce the chance a given outcome will occur. Often, we use the term *risk factor* to include characteristics that impact the likelihood of a given outcome, whether positively or negatively. In order to identify and quantify risk factors, we design epidemiological studies. There are

FIGURE 4.2 Prevalence of Obesity (BMI ≥30) in the United States by Race and Ethnicity, 2006–2008. Behavioral Risk Factor Surveillance System

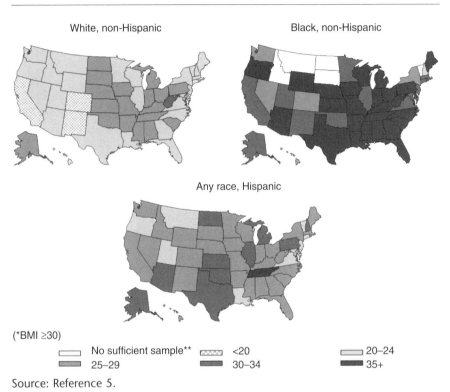

White, non-Hispanic

Black, non-Hispanic

Any race, Hispanic

(*BMI ≥30)

No sufficient sample**	<20	20–24
25–29	30–34	35+

Source: Reference 5.

many types of studies, some of which will be detailed in the next chapter, but all studies share some basic characteristics.

Research studies begin with a question, such as one of the following: Are caregivers less likely than noncaregivers to have recommended cancer screenings? Are children whose parents wear bicycle helmets more likely to regularly wear a bicycle helmet compared to children whose parents do not use bicycle helmets? These research questions each include an exposure, the independent variable of interest, and an outcome, the dependent variable of interest. In the first question, caregiving is the exposure and cancer screenings are the outcome. In the second question, parents' helmet use is the exposure and children's helmet use is the outcome. The researcher next examines similar work that has been completed on the topic and forms a **hypothesis**, a statement of the investigator's expectation of the relationship between exposure and outcome. In the case of bicycle helmets, the researcher may hypothesize that children are more likely to wear a bicycle helmet regularly if a parent wears a helmet. The next step in analytic epidemiology, designing and conducting a study to test the hypothesis, will be covered in Chapter 5.

Basic Epidemiological Measures

Epidemiology deals largely with numbers, or **quantitative data**. There are many ways to express numbers of health events, and epidemiologists have a set of measures they typically use to report health numerically. You probably are familiar with many of these already, although the terminology for some measures may be new to you.

Expressing Data: Counts and Rates

One simple way to report health data is to provide a **count**. For example, in 2007 there were 13,293 cases of tuberculosis reported in the United States[6]. Although this simple count does provide some information about tuberculosis in the United States, it would be much more helpful if we had additional information, a denominator, to go along with this count. As you recall from Chapter 3, the United States Census can give us the number of people in the United States in 2007. By dividing the number of cases of tuberculosis in 2007[6] by the number of U.S. residents in 2007[7], we get the **proportion** of U.S. residents who had tuberculosis in 2007:

Proportion of U.S. population with tuberculosis in 2007:

$$\frac{13,293}{301,290,332} = 0.000044$$

If we multiply this number by 100, it gives us the percentage of the population with tuberculosis in 2007: 0.0044%.

When the term **rate** is used, the denominator includes a measure of time during which the events in the numerator occurred. For example, a mortality rate is the number of deaths for a given change in time, typically one year. Mortality rates are perhaps the most common rates used in public health. The **infant mortality rate** is the number of infants who die within the first year of life per 1,000 live births. Thus the infant mortality rate does not include infants who die in utero or infants who are not alive at birth, or stillborn. The infant mortality rate is widely considered to be a useful measure of the overall health and development of a nation. Death in the first year of life reflects prenatal and postnatal health care practices, the nutritional status of mothers and infants, the prevalence of serious birth defects or health conditions at birth, and other factors. Figure 4.3 shows the infant mortality rate in the United States by race and ethnicity from 1995 to 2005.

When a rate is expressed as its actual value, it is called a **crude rate**. For example, the infant mortality rates expressed in Figure 4.4 represent the crude

FIGURE 4.3 Infant Mortality Rate (death in the first year of life) per 1,000 Live Births for the United States, 1995–2005, by Race and Ethnicity

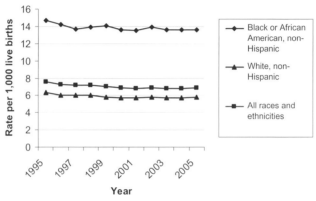

Source: Reference 8.

FIGURE 4.4 Infant Mortality Rate (death in the first year of life) per 1,000 Live Births for the United States, 2000–2006

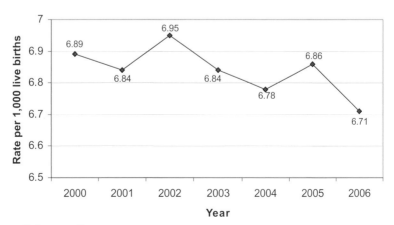

Source: Reference 9.

Table 4.1 Number of Deaths and Crude and Age-adjusted Mortality Rates in the United States in 1980 and 2005

Year	Number of Deaths	Crude Mortality Rate (per 100,000)	Age-adjusted Mortality Rate (per 100,000)
1980	1,989,841	878.3	1,039.1
2005	2,448,017	825.9	798.8

Source: Reference 10.

infant mortality rates for the years 2000–2006 in the United States. These crude rates are taken directly from **vital statistics** records, or birth and death certificates, from those years.

Crude rates provide an accurate picture of rates of an event, disease, or death in a population, but in some cases it is useful and preferable to calculate an **adjusted rate**, especially when comparing across populations or over time. Table 4.1 illustrates the difference between crude and adjusted mortality rates.

Table 4.1 first shows the importance of expressing numbers as rates as well as counts and also the difference between a crude rate and an adjusted rate. Based on the data in the table, there were over 450,000 more deaths in 2005 than there were in 1980. You may know that the population of the United States increased substantially from 1980 to 2005, so this increase in the number of deaths may not be surprising. In fact, once we express the counts as rates (column three), we see that the difference in the number of deaths is in large part a function of the different population sizes in the two years. When expressed as a mortality rate per 100,000 residents, the United States mortality rate in 1980 looks similar to the mortality rate in 2005. The 2005 rate even is slightly lower, a positive sign indicating that perhaps public health and other measures are reducing the number of deaths in the United States over time.

You may have heard recently that the aging baby boom generation is leading to an overall increase in the average age of the U.S. population. You also may expect that as one ages, the chance of dying increases. So, if the U.S. population was getting older during the period 1980 to 2005, you might expect that the mortality rate would increase rather than decrease over the same time. Because people are more likely to die when they are older than when they are younger, this difference in age distribution during the two years should be accounted for when comparing morality rates. The final column in Table 4.1 provides the age-adjusted mortality rates for the United States in 1980 and 2005. The methods used to adjust data are beyond the scope of this textbook, but the

FIGURE 4.5 Crude and Age-adjusted Death Rates: United States, 1960–2005

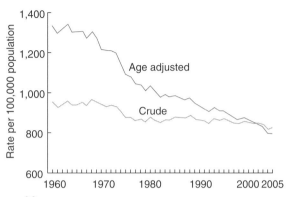

Source: Reference 10.

purpose of adjustment is to convert the crude rate to the rate that would be observed if both populations were identical in their age structures. In this example, and in many cases in practice, the standard U.S. population from the 2000 Census is used as the basis for age adjustment. A **standard population** is one for which the age and sex distribution is known, in this case from the 2000 Census[1, p. 236]. Once age differences between the years are adjusted for, the 2005 mortality rate looks much lower than the 1980 mortality rate. In 1980, the age-adjusted death rate in the United States was 1,039.1 per 100,000 population, whereas in 2005 it was 798.8 per 100,000 population. Figure 4.5 illustrates the difference between the crude and age-adjusted mortality rates in the United States over a longer period, from 1960 through 2005. The decline in age-adjusted mortality over this period is quite striking, a trend that is obscured when looking at only the crude mortality rate.

An alternative to calculating adjusted rates is to **stratify** data based on a variable of interest. For example, in the case of comparing mortality rates in 1980 and 2005, we could present mortality rates for residents age 0–25, 26–50, 51–64, and 65 and older in these two years. This allows us to compare across years within specific age strata and helps us identify any groups that differ over time. Figure 4.3, which shows the infant mortality rates in the United States by race and ethnicity, is an example of a stratified presentation of data. The figure illustrates that there is a large racial disparity in infant mortality rates between non-Hispanic African Americans and non-Hispanic Whites in the United States.

There are various ways to express epidemiological data, and each method conveys a different piece of information. It is important to consider the circumstances in which data are used to determine whether a count or a rate is the best expression of the information and whether crude or adjusted data should be reported.

Quantifying Disease Frequency: Prevalence, Incidence, and Risk

The term **prevalence** is used to describe the amount or frequency of a health outcome that exists in a population at a certain point or over a certain period of time[1, p. 191]. For example, we might say that 49.7 million people in the United States age five and older are living with a disability according to Census 2000[11]. Prevalence is defined as the number of existing cases divided by the total population at risk of the health outcome a given point in time.

$$\text{Prevalence} = \frac{\text{Number of existing cases at a specified point in time}}{\text{Size of population at risk}}$$

$$\text{Prevalence of disability in the United States} = \frac{49.7 \text{ million}}{257.2 \text{ million}} \text{ or } 19.3\%$$

You may recognize from our discussion of proportions above that prevalence is a proportion. Prevalence has no units, and it is not a rate. The denominator used in a measure of prevalence may be the size of the population at risk at the point of interest. Alternatively, the denominator may be the size of the population at risk at the midpoint of the period of interest, often a year. As is typical of proportions, people in the numerator also are in the denominator in a measure of prevalence.

It is important when calculating measures such as prevalence and incidence (below) to include in the denominator only the **population at risk**. A person is at risk for the disease if it is biologically plausible for him or her to develop it in the immediate future. If you calculate the incidence of ovarian cancer in a community, the denominator should include only individuals who have ovaries. Thus we would exclude men and any women who have had their ovaries removed. Whether a person is at risk for a given outcome may change over time. *At risk* does not necessarily imply *at high risk* relative to others. Rather, it means that there is a nonzero chance of developing the outcome. *Not at risk* means an individual is considered to have a zero chance of developing the outcome. Some diseases or diagnoses last throughout an individual's life, such as AIDS or Alzheimer's disease. Once a person develops such an outcome, the person is no longer considered to be at risk. Other outcomes or infections are not lifelong but rather leave the individual no longer susceptible to a recurrence, for example, mumps or other infectious diseases that confer lifelong immunity. These people would be treated the same as those who do not recover from an outcome; they are no longer at risk and are not counted in the denominator of a prevalence or incidence measure. Other outcomes can affect an individual multiple times, including urinary tract infection, the common cold, depression, or angina pectoris (chest pain). Therefore, it is important to consider the attributes of the health outcome when deciding who is included in the population at risk.

Incidence is the number or frequency of new health outcomes or health events over time. Incident cases of disease are those of persons who are free of the health outcome at the beginning of a defined time period and who subsequently develop the disease or experience the health event during a specified observation time. Although we know that 49.7 million people age five and older in the United States were living with a disability in the year 2000, we may be interested to know how many people in the United States have developed a disability since 2000. This number would represent the incidence of disability in the United States since 2000. Usually, each person is counted only once when calculating incidence, even if she or he experienced two or more disease events during the observation period. Using the disability example, a woman may have been living with a vision disability in 2000 and thus would be included in the prevalence measure of disability in that year. However, she may also have developed a mobility disability resulting from a fall in 2004 and therefore could be considered to have incident disability since 2000 as well. Because we are interested in the broad category of disability, this person would be counted only once, in the prevalence measure of disability, and not as an incident case of disability. The reason we count only the first event when calculating incidence is because subsequent events may not be independent of the first. In other words, it often is true that having one health event, such as a myocardial infarction (heart attack), is a risk factor for having another heart attack. In the example above, the woman may have fallen and developed a mobility disability because of her vision disability. Clearly, this is not always the case, so the researcher must determine for each question whether individuals should contribute more than one event to a measure of incidence.

In contrast to prevalence, incidence is expressed as a rate; it includes a measure of time. Specifically, the **incidence rate** includes the number of new cases of disease (numerator) divided by the amount of time during which these cases arose (denominator):

$$\text{Incidence rate} = \frac{\text{Number of new cases or events}}{\text{Person-time at risk}}$$

This formula includes **person-time**, a measure of the amount of time during which a person is at risk of developing the outcome of interest. Person-time can be collected directly for each person followed over the time period of interest. For example, if we want to calculate the incidence rate of cervical cancer in New York City, we would include only women (men do not have a cervix) and only women who are free of cervical cancer. Each woman is followed for a given period of time, and whatever length of time she remains free of cervical cancer goes into the denominator. Often, person-years are used as the denominator, and fractions of a year can be used. Therefore, if a woman develops cervical cancer after six months, she would have contributed 0.5 person-years to the denominator and would be counted as one case in the numerator. If we are calculating the incidence of cervical cancer in New York City over a period of twenty years and some women never develop cervical cancer during follow-up, their person-years (twenty) are included in the denominator, but they do not contribute to the numerator. Incidence rates can also be calculated using population estimates from sources such as the Census as the denominator. In this case, person-time is calculated as the average size of the population at risk multiplied by the length of time of interest. Mortality rates are an example of this: the numerator is the number of deaths, and the denominator is the average size of the (living) population multiplied by the time period of interest (often just one year).

Prevalence and incidence, although different, are related. Once a person has an incident case of the outcome of interest, he or she will be counted as a prevalent case at future time points. Thus incidence contributes to prevalence. However, the relationship between these two measures in a population varies based on the specifics for a health outcome. For example, if the health outcome of interest is spinal cord injury, we would expect that new or incident cases of injury would be counted as prevalent cases for the rest of their lives. Spinal cord injury is not something one recovers from in most cases, so an increase in spinal cord injury incidence leads to an increase in spinal cord injury prevalence. The same may not be true for an infectious disease such as influenza. If the incidence of influenza is high in the winter, the time typically considered flu season, then the prevalence of influenza the following summer may still be low. Influenza infection is not chronic or long lasting, so although incidence may spike, prevalence measured just months later would not reflect the high incidence. You can imagine other cases in which the prevalence of a health outcome would increase, such as the availability of therapies or treatments that prolong the life expectancy of people with the outcome or improved reporting systems for the health outcome.

Assessing and Interpreting Data

We already have seen some examples of **trends** in data, or the movement of a measure in one direction over time. Trends are useful in epidemiology because they can help predict future needs and can alert public health officials to areas that need further investigation or intervention. Often, measures such as mortality rates, incidence rates, and prevalence are plotted over time on a graph (as in Figure 4.4), allowing us to assess trends in these measures.

In infectious disease, the terms *epidemic* and *pandemic* are used to describe the occurrence of disease in greater frequency than expected. As you may recall from Chapter 1, **endemic** diseases are those that occur with expected frequency in a population; there is some standard background rate of disease present. A disease becomes **epidemic** when the amount of disease exceeds the standard or expected levels. A **pandemic** is a disease that has reached epidemic levels and spreads around the world. There are methods specific to infectious disease epidemiology used to assess the level of disease and to track and understand disease outbreaks. These methods will be discussed in more detail in Chapter 8.

Confounding

One definition of *confound* is to mix up or confuse[12]. This is the sense meant by the term **confounding** as it is used in epidemiology. A **confounder** is any variable that confuses the relationship between the exposure and outcome of interest. In the comparison of mortality rates in the United States in 1980 and 2005 above, is there a confounder? Begin by identifying the exposure and outcome of interest. Recall that we were interested in comparing the mortality rates among two time periods. In other words, we wanted to quantify the risk of death based on which year (1980 or 2005) people lived. Therefore, year is the exposure; specifically, one could identify living in the United States in 1980 as being exposed and living in the United States in 2005 as being unexposed, and death is the outcome. Upon first inspection of the crude mortality rates, it appeared that exposed people (U.S. residents in 1980) were about equally as likely to die as unexposed people (U.S. residents in 2005). However, once we adjusted for age differences in the United States in the two years, we saw that, in fact, the chance of dying in 2005 was much lower than it was in 1980. In this example, age is a confounder. Age, a factor other than the exposure or outcome, was misleading us, making us think that the mortality rate was not much different in 2005 than it was in 1980. However, once we controlled or adjusted for

Table 4.2 Alcohol Consumption and Lung Cancer Diagnosis
Among 1,000 Men Age 65 and Older

Alcohol Consumption	Lung Cancer (outcome)	No Lung Cancer (no outcome)
Heavy (exposed)	10	110
Not heavy (unexposed)	50	830

Table 4.3 Alcohol Consumption and Cigarette Smoking Status
Among 1,000 Men Age 65 and Older

Alcohol Consumption	Current or Former Smoker (potential confounder)	Non-Smoker (potential confounder)
Heavy (exposed)	90	30
Not heavy (unexposed)	270	610

age, we saw that the mortality rate in the United States decreased substantially from 1980 to 2005.

Another example of confounding is the relationship between alcohol consumption and lung cancer. Look at the data in Table 4.2. Assume we asked 1,000 men over age 65 about their alcohol consumption and whether or not they have been diagnosed with lung cancer. As you can see, lung cancer is not common (60/1,000 or 6% of the sample has lung cancer). Likewise, most men are not heavy drinkers (120/1,000 or 12% of the sample drinks heavily). You may also notice that among heavy drinkers, 10 out of 120, or 8.3%, have lung cancer. Among non-heavy drinkers, 50 out of 880, or 5.7%, have lung cancer. From these data, it appears that older men who drink heavily have a higher chance of having lung cancer.

Your first instinct may be to say that heavy alcohol consumption causes lung cancer. Based on your knowledge, is there any biological reason that drinking alcohol might cause lung cancer? Are there any other risk factors for lung cancer of which you are aware? You may know that years of research show smoking cigarettes greatly increases the risk of lung cancer. Is it possible that smoking status could be confounding the relationship between alcohol consumption and lung cancer we see in Table 4.2? To answer this question we need more data. We need to ask those same 1,000 men whether or not they smoke now or have ever smoked cigarettes regularly. Table 4.3 shows these results.

Table 4.3 shows us that men who drink alcohol heavily also smoke more commonly than men who do not drink heavily. Specifically, 75% of heavy drinkers are smokers whereas 31% of non-heavy drinkers are smokers. This suggests that, indeed, smoking may be causing the relationship between alcohol consumption and lung cancer we saw in Table 4.2.

We will discuss some of the analytic methods available to adjust for confounding in the following chapters. For now, you should simply have an understanding of what confounders are and be aware of possible confounders when reading studies. Confounders can be difficult to identify and to measure. When designing a study, it is important to read other research studies to identify potential confounders based on others' work. Confounders create a number of problems in epidemiological studies, and we will continue to discuss them in the next two chapters.

Epidemiology in Public Health

Epidemiology provides much of the empirical evidence of relationships between exposures and outcomes and allows us to track health over time. This epidemiological information allows us to make better decisions about resource allocation, prevention efforts, and policies in public health. Much of the activity of epidemiology falls within the **assessment** core function (Chapter 2) of public health. Specifically, the following essential services of public health describe epidemiology's activities:

- Monitor health status to identify and solve community health problems

- Diagnose and investigate health problems and health hazards in the community

- Research to gain new insights and innovative solutions to health problems

Epidemiologists, often working with other public health professionals, use research and data to design and implement programs or policies that prevent the spread of disease or prevent poor health outcomes. You can find epidemiologists in local public health agencies such as county and state health departments where they may trace infectious disease outbreaks and work to prevent the spread of disease. They also track chronic diseases over time and assess preventive health behaviors in communities to identify areas in which interventions may be most beneficial. Epidemiologists also work in academic settings such as colleges and universities where they conduct research to identify risk factors for disease or poor health among populations and train the next generation of public health professionals. Hospitals and other health care facilities employ epidemiologists to assess safety and quality within their practices. There, epidemiologists use medical records and laboratory reports to track nosocomial (hospital-acquired) infections, such as resistant bacteria, or to track secondary infections that could be prevented, such as infections at the site of a surgical intervention. Epidemiologists work in many settings within public health and focus on a variety of health issues.

Summary

This chapter has introduced you to the field of epidemiology and some of the measures commonly used by epidemiologists when reporting public health data. Epidemiology can be divided into two broad divisions: descriptive and analytic. In this chapter, we focused on descriptive epidemiology, or providing information about a health outcome based on *person, place,* and *time* variables. Person variables include attributes of a population such as age, gender, race, or ethnicity; place variables describe where an outcome occurs geographically or by some other social boundary; and time variables include those that describe trends in an outcome across days or years or whether an outcome occurs with a seasonal variation. In describing the epidemiology of a health event, a variety of measures can be used to convey information. You may provide a simple count of the events in a population, you could add the number of people from which those cases arose and report a proportion, or you could report an incidence or prevalence number using only the population at risk of the outcome in the denominator. Prevalence is the proportion of people who have the health outcome at a given point in time (existing cases), and incidence is the rate of disease that develops over a given time period (new cases). Incidence contributes to prevalence, but the magnitude of this contribution depends on the attributes of the health outcome of interest. The incidence of an infectious disease that resolves quickly may be very high over a given time period, but prevalence at any one point may be lower because cases are not cases for very long. On the other hand, diseases that last throughout one's life and have a low mortality rate may be relatively rare (low incidence), but because people may live with them for many years, the prevalence of the disease may be high.

When calculating measures of disease, it is important to consider the influence of confounders, variables other than the exposure and outcome of interest that may influence the exposure and outcome. Confounders, by definition, confuse the relationship between the exposure and outcome in which you are interested. We saw in Figures 4.1 and 4.2 that obesity prevalence is highest in the southeastern United States and among people who report Black, non-Hispanic ethnicity. Therefore, if we are doing a study of obesity prevention across the United States, we may need to account for the race and ethnicity of each state's population. This accounting or controlling for confounding variables creates an adjusted rate. Adjusted rates often are preferable to the crude rate of an outcome because they allow for more direct comparisons across populations that have different age, gender, race, or other distributions.

Epidemiology is an important component of public health. Most of the activities of epidemiology fall into the assessment core function, allowing public health professionals to monitor health and investigate the relationships between exposures and outcomes.

Key Terms

adjusted rate, 82

analytic epidemiology, 78

assessment, 89

confounder, 87

confounding, 87

count, 80

crude rate, 81

descriptive epidemiology, 76

endemic, 87

epidemic, 87

epidemiology, 73

etiology, 74

exposure, 74

hypothesis, 79

incidence, 85

incidence rate, 85

infant mortality rate, 80

multifactorial, 74

outcome, 74

pandemic, 87

person-time, 86

population at risk, 84

prevalence, 84

proportion, 80

protective factor, 78

quantitative data, 80

rate, 80

risk factor, 78

standard population, 83

stratify, 83

trends, 87

vital statistics, 82

Review Questions

1. How was the development of vital statistics data important in the development of the field of epidemiology?
2. Figure 4.6 is John Snow's map of London during the 1848 cholera outbreak. How does this map illustrate descriptive epidemiology?
3. Using the data in the following table, fill in the following measures:
   a. Count of diabetes cases among adults in Anytown in 2010: _____
   b. Prevalence of diabetes among adults in Anytown in 2010: _____
   c. Sex-specific prevalence of diabetes among adults in Anytown in 2010:
      Male: _____ Female: _____

FIGURE 4.6 John Snow's Cholera Mortality Map from an 1848 Outbreak in London

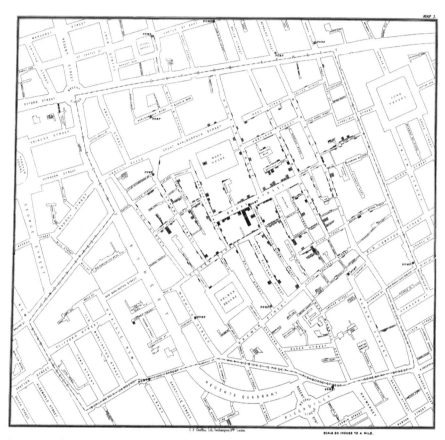

Source: Reference 13.

d. Incidence of diabetes in Anytown during 2010 (assume that all 2009 cases also have diabetes in 2010): _____

Population Size and Number of Diabetes Cases by Sex Among Adults in the Hypothetical Anytown in 2009 and 2010

Year	Male Population	Female Population	Total Population	Male Diabetes Cases	Female Diabetes Cases	Total Diabetes Cases
2009	100,000	110,000	210,000	8,000	9,900	17,900
2010	105,000	112,000	217,000	8,925	10,080	19,005

4. If calculating an incidence or prevalence measure for testicular cancer, who would be included in the population at risk used in the denominator?

5. Assume the data in the following table came from a twenty-year study of skin cancer among women who work outdoors. (This represents a partial list.) Complete the empty column (Person-years contributed) and calculate the incidence of skin cancer among women, using the information below. A maximum of one skin cancer diagnosis was allowed for each woman.

Follow-up Information for Ten Women from a 20-Year Study of Skin Cancer Among Women Who Work Outdoors

Participant ID	Enrollment Date	Skin Cancer Diagnosis Date	End of Follow-up Date	Person-years Contributed
M164	June, 1990	—	April, 2004	
M288	August, 1990	January, 2001	January, 2001	
M298	August, 1990	—	June, 2010	
M314	September, 1990	—	October, 2008	
M398	September, 1990	—	June, 2010	
M433	September, 1990	—	June, 2010	
M568	October, 1990	April, 1996	April, 1996	
M570	October, 1990	—	February, 1995	
M659	November, 1990	—	June, 2010	
M682	December, 1990	—	March, 1998	
Total:				

References

1. Porta M, ed. *A Dictionary of Epidemiology*. 5th ed. New York: Oxford University Press; 2008.
2. Gordis L. *Epidemiology*. 2nd ed. Philadelphia, Pa.: W.B. Saunders; 1996.
3. Rosen G. *A History of Public Health*. Expanded ed. Baltimore, Md.: The Johns Hopkins University Press; 1993.
4. Lilienfeld AM. *Times, Places, and Persons: Aspects of the History of Epidemiology*. Baltimore, Md.: The Johns Hopkins University Press; 1980.
5. Centers for Disease Control and Prevention. Overweight and obesity: U.S. obesity trends. Available at: www.cdc.gov/obesity/data/trends.html. Accessed November 16, 2009.

6. Pratt R, Robison V, Navin T, Menzies H. Trends in tuberculosis—United States, 2007. *MMWR*. 2008;57(11);281–285.

7. United States Census Bureau. National and State Population Estimates. Table 1: Annual estimates of the resident population for the United States, regions, states, and Puerto Rico: April 1, 2000 to July 1, 2008. (NST-EST2008–01). Available at: www.census.gov/popest/states/NST-ann-est.html. Accessed June 9, 2009.

8. United States Department of Health and Human Services (US HHS), Centers of Disease Control and Prevention (CDC), National Center for Health Statistics (NCHS), Office of Analysis and Epidemiology (OAE), Division of Vital Statistics (DVS). Linked Birth/Infant Death Records 1995–1998, 1999–2002, and 2003–2005 on CDC WONDER online database. Available at: http://wonder.cdc.gov/lbd-icd9.html. Accessed on June 4, 2009.

9. MacDorman MF, Mathews TJ. Recent trends in infant mortality in the United States. NCHS Data Brief, no 9. Publication and Information Products. Hyattsville, Md.: National Center for Health Statistics; 2008. Available at: www.cdc.gov/nchs/data/databriefs/db09.htm#infantmortality. Accessed May 10, 2010.

10. Kung HC, Hoyert, DL, Xu J, Murphy SL. Deaths: Final data for 2005. *Nat Vital Stat Rep*. 2008;56(10)L1–120.

11. Waldrop J, Stern SM. Disability status: 2000. *Census 2000 Brief*. Washington, D.C.: US Department of Commerce, US Census Bureau; 2003.

12. Confound. Merriam-Webster Online Dictionary. Available at: www.merriam-webster.com/dictionary/confound. Accessed March 26, 2009.

13. Frerichs, R. University of California Los Angeles, Department of Epidemiology, School of Pubic Health, John Snow Web site. Available at: www.ph.ucla.edu/epi/snow.html. Accessed February 24, 2010.

CHAPTER 5

STUDY DESIGN

Elena M. Andresen, PhD
Erin D. Bouldin, MPH

LEARNING OBJECTIVES

- Identify and define the primary research designs used in public health epidemiology.
- Describe how experimental and observational research studies differ and the strengths of each.
- Calculate and interpret a relative risk for cohort studies and an odds ratio for case–control studies.
- Define the elements of causal inference in evaluating the relationship between an exposure and a health outcome.
- Evaluate observational research for causal inference of risks and health outcomes.

In Chapter 4, we introduced you to some of the measures used to quantify the health of a population. You now know how to assess changes in health over time and how to compare measures across populations. You can determine whether infant mortality is higher in Georgia than it is in Nevada and whether this trend is changing over time. You may recall this is known as *descriptive epidemiology*. But why is there a difference in infant mortality, and what factors increase or decrease the risk of death in the first year after birth? In this chapter, we will cover the basics of quantifying the relationship between *exposure (independent variable)* and *outcome (dependent variable)* within a population, or what is known as *analytic epidemiology*.

In epidemiology there are several common categories of **quantitative study** designs. These types of studies rely on measures that can be described by discrete numbers. For example, age and months of employment are two pieces of information that have specific numbers associated with them. For other topics with less obvious links to numbers, we can create categories of answer choices and assign them a number, making them into **categorical variables**. For example, we might ask people to rate their general health using a 5-point scale in which 1 represents poor health and 5 represents excellent health. In this way, we are able to quantify measures that seem subjective or are not intuitively numerical. Quantitative data are analyzed using statistical methods introduced in Chapter 6.

In contrast, **qualitative study designs** collect rich, descriptive information that does not fit into clearly defined categories. Qualitative studies and qualitative data are discussed in Chapter 12.

Within quantitative studies, there are two broad categories: observational and experimental studies. In *observational studies*, the researcher does not intervene in any way regarding the subjects' exposures or actions; he or she simply observes them. These studies are then analyzed based on the experiences of the subjects and assessment of their outcomes. In *experimental studies*, the researcher does intervene, controlling subjects' exposures. Study participants are divided into groups, and each participant receives the exposure randomly prescribed to that group. Perhaps the most commonly reported type of experimental study is the randomized trial, of which drug trials may be most familiar (see Chapter 7). In these trials, study participants may be given a *placebo* (an inactive pill), an established drug, or a new drug to compare their effectiveness. Below we will introduce you to some of the most common observational studies: ecological, cross-sectional, cohort, and case–control. We also will discuss two types of experimental studies: the aforementioned randomized trial and the community trial (Figure 5.1).

Finally, in this chapter we will discuss *causal inference*. As mentioned above, the purpose of **analytic epidemiology** is to identify and quantify risk factors

FIGURE 5.1 Major Types of Study Designs within Epidemiology

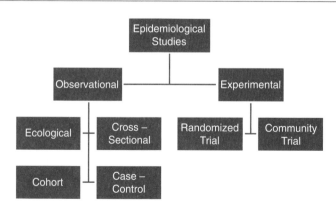

for health outcomes. However, a single study is rarely enough to make us confident in this relationship, and different studies may have different results. Therefore, criteria exist to assess whether there is a cause and effect relationship between two variables. It is important to understand the criteria for causal inference no matter what your career goals are because, as a consumer, you must make decisions based on evidence presented by sources such as the media, industry, and health care providers.

In Chapter 3, we discussed some of the many ongoing data collection systems in the United States. Below you will see reference to some of these systems again; please refer back to Chapter 3 for detailed descriptions of each.

Observational Studies

An **observational study** is one in which the researcher simply observes people and collects information about their behaviors and health choices to determine whether these factors influence their chances of having a particular health outcome. The researcher does not assign research participants to any particular exposure group but instead follows people and allows them to make their own choices about whether or not they are exposed to various activities or substances. Observational studies are useful in public health because it would not be ethical to assign to people many exposures in which we are interested. For example, low birth weight is a public health problem because infants born small are at an increased risk of a number of poor health outcomes, including mortality. We do not fully understand all the causes of low birth weight, so research is ongoing to identify risk factors for low birth weight in the United States. Some of the exposures that may cause low birth weight include cigarette smoking, drug use (legal or illegal) during pregnancy, and certain pesticides. We know that cigarette smoking causes other poor health outcomes; we know that people should not use medications that are not prescribed for a health reason; we know that some drugs are illegal to use; and we know that some pesticides increase the risk of cancer. Clearly, it would not be ethical to expose pregnant women, or anyone else, to these substances intentionally. For this reason, we must use an observational study design, one in which we look at the birth weight of infants born to women who have been exposed to these various substances of their own accord, and compare their infants' health to the health of infants born to women who were not exposed to these substances. You may be thinking that women who smoke during pregnancy may be different from women who do not smoke during pregnancy in ways that influence their chances of giving birth to a low birth weight infant. This concern, the possibility of **confounding**, is a common one in observational studies and must be carefully accounted for when analyzing data from this type of study[1–7]. Confounding occurs when some factor other than the exposure of interest obscures or confuses the relationship between the exposure and outcome of interest. In all observational studies, it is vital to measure possible confounders such as health conditions and health behaviors, which are other exposures that may be related to the outcome of interest. Because the investigator is not controlling exposures in observational studies, participants may engage in activities or behaviors that contribute to the development of the outcome, and this must be distinguished from the exposure of interest in the study. We will address confounding later in this chapter and again in Chapter 6.

The first two types of observational study designs we will discuss, ecological and cross-sectional studies, often make use of readily available data. We will see below that both types of studies can have design flaws that may make them more useful as descriptive studies than as analytic studies. The next set of observational studies we will discuss, cohort studies and case–control studies, are the most common classes of analytic epidemiological studies conducted in public health, and they have design features that make them superior to most ecological and cross-sectional studies.

Ecological Studies

Ecological studies vary from all the other observational studies we will discuss in one important way: they make use of **group-level data** rather than individual-level data[1–2,4,7]. This means that instead of collecting information from individuals about an exposure and an outcome of interest, in an **ecological study** we have summary exposure and outcome information for the entire population[8]. In ecological studies, we are comparing entire groups: the average level of exposure for the group is correlated to the group's average outcome. In these studies, the **independent variable** (x, or **exposure**) is the percentage of people exposed in the group, and the **dependent variable** (y, or **outcome**) is the rate or risk of disease in the group. The **unit of analysis** in ecological studies is the group rather than the individual.

By nature, these studies must be interpreted at the group rather than the individual level. In fact, there is a term that refers to making individual-level inferences based on group-level (ecological) data: **ecological fallacy**[7,9]. The ecological fallacy occurs for a number of reasons. First, it may be that although a population looks as though it has high exposure, it may be only a group of individuals within the population who have the exposure, and they may or may not be the same individuals with the outcome of interest. Second, there may be confounders (other factors) that are not measured in the data that coincide with the exposure of interest. We will come back to the concept of confounding again later.

For example, imagine we are interested in the relationship between high levels of particulate matter in the air and severe asthma attacks. Particulate matter (PM) is a combination of very small solid particles and liquid droplets that have the potential to negatively affect human health (see Chapters 9 and 10 for more details about environmental health). PM may be made up of dust or debris emitted from vehicles, power plants, forest fires, or construction sites, and they can contain compounds such as metals and sulfates. PM is a concern because these small particles can be inhaled into the lungs and may cause or exacerbate breathing and other health problems. Data on PM concentration are available for certain areas through the U.S. Environmental Protection Agency's Ambient Air Monitoring Program, created to comply with the Clean Air Act (see www.epa.gov/oar/oaqps/qa/monprog.html#NAMS for more details). Let us say that we decide to use air quality data for the city of Los Angeles to measure the relationship between exposure to high levels of PM and severe asthma attacks. In order to quantify the outcome, in this case severe asthma attacks, we access the intake data from emergency rooms at several Los Angeles hospitals in conjunction with air quality data. This is an ecological study because we are using data for groups of individuals from the same population to measure exposure and outcome. In other words, we are not measuring an individual's exposure to PM and also assessing whether that individual has a severe asthma attack. Rather, we are measuring PM concentrations in an area (Los Angeles) and also measuring the number of emergency department visits due to severe asthma attacks in that area. Assume these data show that on days in which PM levels were high, emergency room visits due to asthma attacks also increased. If we conclude that exposure to high levels of PM causes severe asthma attacks in individuals in Los Angeles, we may be making a statement based on the ecological fallacy. We did not measure the PM exposure of those individuals who visited the emergency room for asthma attacks, and thus we cannot be sure those visits were related to air quality at all. It is possible that the PM concentration near the collection station was high on the day the individual visited the emergency room, but perhaps PM concentration was quite different at the individual's home or school where he or she was actually exposed. There also could be a number of confounders in this scenario for which we have no measurements. Perhaps the asthma attack is related to air quality, but not PM; rather, the asthma attack is related to something else in the air that is not measured. It could also be that other factors, such as an individual's activity patterns, medication use, or exposure to smoke in the home, occurs in tandem with changes in PM concentration and is the actual cause of the asthma exacerbations. Based on this study, there appears to be a relationship or a **correlation** between high levels of PM in the air and increased emergency room visits for severe asthma attacks at the group level. At the individual level, however, we cannot confidently say that high PM concentrations in the air increase the risk of having a severe asthma attack.

Ecological studies typically are better for *generating hypotheses* than testing them, as illustrated by the example above. There is a correlation between PM concentration in the air and asthma attacks in Los Angeles, and we can now generate a hypothesis and test it using individual-level studies. Ecological studies often are a good first stage in an analytic strategy because easily accessible data may be available from a public source such as a state or federal agency. Although public health focuses on populations, group-level data are often not the best source of data for uncovering cause and effect relationships between exposures and outcomes. There are some exceptions to this statement, and it may be argued that for some exposures (such as neighborhood) or perhaps some environmental exposures (such as air pollution), group-level data are indeed appropriate, perhaps in combination with individual-level data[10–15]. The advantages of thinking about influences from the standpoint of multiple levels are described by the social-ecological public health model (see Chapters 2, 11, 12).

Ecological data are useful for assessing **time trends** and may provide hints of exposure–outcome relationships[7]. If there is a spike in mortality for example, you may also plot relevant events such as the introduction of a new drug or exposure to new food additives along the curve and take note of the correlation. The graph in Figure 5.2 shows an example of plotting group data over time. It shows the prevalence of **spina bifida** and anencephaly at birth (also called incidence) from 1995 to 2005 in the United States. Spina bifida and anencephaly are both **neural tube defects** caused by the incomplete closure of the spinal column during early pregnancy. The graph also shows the change in folic acid fortification of the grain supply in the United States. The data in Figure 5.2 represent an ecological study. We do not have information about the folic acid intake of mothers and their birth outcomes; rather, we have the overall population trend in two neural tube defects along with changes in the food supply. Presumably, adding folic acid to grain products will increase the folic acid consumption of the general population, including pregnant women. Based on this figure, it appears that higher levels of folic acid reduce the incidence of neural tube defects, particularly spina bifida.

Cross-Sectional Studies

As the name implies, **cross-sectional studies** collect information at a single time point, providing a snapshot of a population at a given time[1–2,4,7]. These

FIGURE 5.2 Prevalence of Spina Bifida and Anencephaly at Birth in the United States from 1995 to 2005 and Phases of Folic Acid Fortification of the Grain Supply

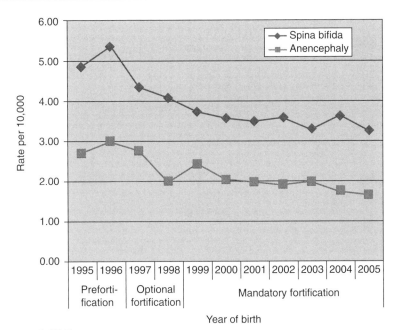

Courtesy of CDC.

studies collect information about both exposure and outcome at a single point in time. Often, cross-sectional studies include data obtained from surveys or interviews that occur only once or data obtained from a publicly available source such as a government agency. The Behavioral Risk Factor Surveillance System (BRFSS), discussed in Chapter 3, is an example of a data source for a cross-sectional study. Although the BRFSS occurs every year, it does not sample and interview the same individuals annually to gain information about their health over time; rather, a new set of randomly dialed households are contacted, and an individual in each household completes the survey once. When interviewed, they report both health conditions and behaviors at the same time, or in a cross-sectional manner.

Cross-sectional studies are useful as basic prevalence studies, providing information about the amount of a health problem in a population. These types of cross-sectional studies would be considered descriptive, designed to provide information about the person, place, and time variables of a health outcome, but not designed to identify risk factors for that outcome. For example, the Youth

Risk Behavior Surveillance System (YRBSS), a CDC survey administered to students in high schools, asks questions on a variety of topics, including sexual activity, alcohol and drug use, and violence, as described in Chapter 3. Based on 2007 data, 9.0% of males and 1.2% of females reported they carried a gun to school on at least one day in the past thirty days. These data are helpful in public health planning (in this case, injury and interpersonal violence prevention) and also provide evidence that there is a difference by sex in the numbers of those who carry a gun.

A study based on the BRFSS demonstrates the potential analytic use as well as some caveats regarding cross-sectional studies: investigating the effect of early onset disability (mobility impairment) on participation later in life. Participation includes being employed, going to school, engaging in social activities, and so on. Some developmental theories suggest that if a child has a significant disability and his or her parents treat the child as if he or she is very dependent upon them, that child's participation in life activities as an adult will be lower. The theory considers the time before age two as the vulnerable time period. Rebecca Selove and colleagues of Saint Louis University conducted a study looking at the BRFSS data from ten states and Washington, D.C., combined over two years to test the hypothesis that having a disability before the age of two increases the risk of being unemployed later in life. How could she construct anything like a historical exposure variable using the BRFSS? The BRFSS disability module used in these ten states included a question about duration of the impairment. If a person reported mobility impairment on the BRFSS and reported its duration, Selove subtracted the duration from current age and **dichotomized** (divided into two groups) people with mobility impairment before age two and after age two. Selove found that individuals with current significant mobility limitation with onset prior to age two were about twice as likely to be unemployed than similar individuals with onset after age two[16]. The positive aspects of this study include the random sample of individuals representing the population. In fact, a population-based perspective of the relationship between early-onset disability and adult employment status was not available before Selove's study.

There are some problems with this study. The depth of information collected was limited. Questions about family characteristics and the severity of the impairment were not included and would have been useful for testing the hypothesis more directly. In addition, the questions used to define mobility impairment were broad and may have caused people to be misclassified.

As we see in this example, researchers must weigh benefits against drawbacks when designing a study. For example, if Selove had designed a study specifically to investigate the relationship between age at disability onset and adult employment status, she would have been able to ask more detailed and targeted questions, but likely would not have been able to sample enough people to make the study represent the entire population of ten states.

Perhaps the biggest flaw associated with cross-sectional data is a temporal sequence issue, or the order of exposure and outcome in time. Because data on exposure and outcome are collected simultaneously, there can be a problem distinguishing which came first in a cross-sectional study. For example, if we use a cross-sectional design to investigate whether clinical depression increases the risk of being overweight, we would not be assured that depression preceded overweight; the relationship could, in fact, be the reverse. In some cases, it is possible to phrase a question in such a way that this temporal sequence problem is minimized. From the example above, we could ask about weight before and after the depression diagnosis and determine whether weight or body mass index (BMI, a measure combining weight and height) had changed. Selove's study also relied on reports of historical events to reconstruct the temporal sequence. This type of questioning, however, relies on the person's memory and may introduce other issues associated with poor recall. In other cases, temporal sequence is not a concern because there is no way the relationship could plausibly be reversed. This is true when the exposure is something innate or is a variable that the outcome could not possibly change, such as age, or as in the example of carrying a gun discussed above, sex. In other words, carrying a gun to school could not possibly precede or alter a high school student's sex; the exposure, the student's sex, came before the behavior.

Finally, cross-sectional studies do not provide the full experience of individuals across time; they do not capture future disease and sometimes may exclude past disease. This is the nature of prevalence studies. It is not a problem per se, but it should be noted when using cross-sectional studies in analytic work. Figure 5.3 illustrates this point. In the figure, the lines may represent a survey assessing exposure or outcome. In either case, it is clear that if we collect data at only one time point, as occurs in cross-sectional studies, we may not sample people during the period of exposure or outcome. Let us assume that the figure shows data for obesity, defined as a BMI of 30 or higher. Solid lines indicate time periods during which a person is not obese, and dotted lines indicate time periods during which a person is obese. If we collect our cross-sectional data at the point indicated by the vertical line, we will calculate an obesity prevalence of 2 in 6, or 33.3%. However, we see that one person was obese at an earlier point in his life, and another person will become obese later in life. Also, one of the two people included in our prevalence estimate fluctuates over time between being classified as obese and not obese. Depending on the research question of interest, it may be important to know whether someone has ever been obese rather than knowing

FIGURE 5.3 Generic Cross-sectional Study Design Showing the Various Points in Exposure or Disease Process at which Individuals May Be Surveyed

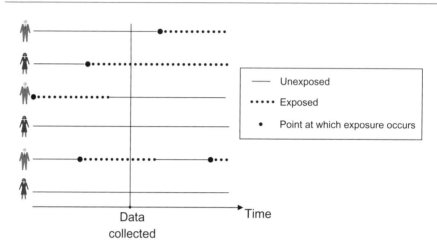

only if he or she was obese at the time of data collection. In some studies, this may not be a limitation, but it is a factor that researchers designing a study should consider.

Cohort Studies

Cohort studies may be the most intuitive of the observational studies. If told to observe a group of people to determine the relationship between an exposure and an outcome, one would naturally choose two groups, a group exposed and a group not exposed to the substance or event of interest, and then would follow those groups over time to look at the occurrence of the outcome. This describes a cohort study. In a **cohort study**, we compare the occurrence of a health outcome in persons who are exposed and persons who are not exposed[1–4,6–7,17]. The follow-up may be **prospective** (into the future)[1] or **retrospective** (in the past)[1], sometimes called historical cohorts[7]. Observational studies are always called *cohorts* if the study participants are divided into groups based on their exposure status (Figure 5.4).

Cohort studies begin with individuals who all are free of the outcome of interest. Thus in a cohort study, we have an exposed group and an unexposed group, and we follow them over time to compare the development of the outcome of interest, or **incidence** of the outcome. In a cohort study, the inves-

FIGURE 5.4 Generic Scheme of Cohort Study Design in which All Participants Are Free of the Outcome at the Beginning of the Study

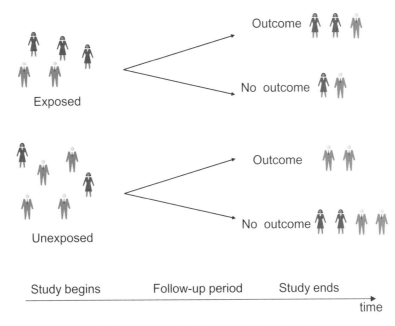

Participants are divided into groups based on the exposure of interest, and followed over time to assess which participants develop the outcome in each group and which do not.

tigator often begins by identifying the exposed group, for example, people who are engaged in a behavior such as smoking or people who are exposed to a chemical compound such as arsenic. The unexposed group should be drawn from the same **population** as those exposed. (Recall that *population* in this sense will be defined by the researcher and may include attributes such as place of residence, demographic characteristics, or other factors.) For example, the study population may consist of workers in a specific industry, so the exposed and unexposed members may be drawn from the same plant or shipyard but have different job duties and thus different exposures.

Ideally, the unexposed comparison group should resemble the exposed members of the cohort in every way except exposure, but in practice this rarely occurs. Perhaps the clearest potential problem in the evidence of exposure–disease relationships from cohort studies is that the differences between the exposed and unexposed people might be related to the outcome you are studying and may confound your answer. If there are important differences between the exposed and unexposed members of the cohort *and* these differences are causal factors for the outcome of interest, the association of interest will be confounded. Measurement of all potential confounding factors in a cohort study is a must. Methods exist to control the effects of confounding, which we will discuss later, but an unmeasured confounder is an uncontrollable confounder[1–4,6,7].

Sometimes it is possible to compare the risk or rate of disease among those exposed to some known risk or rate rather than construct an unexposed group for the cohort. For example, we might compare the risk of asbestosis (an asbestos-related lung disease) among a special group of occupationally exposed workers to the risk of asbestosis among the general population.

Especially in occupational cohorts, you may have a problem with the **healthy worker effect**[2,7,18]. Individuals who are working tend to be healthier than individuals who do not work, and they also are advantaged in other ways, socially and economically, because of employment. Meanwhile, statistics from the general population reflect both employed and unemployed persons. The healthy worker effect can make an exposed working group appear to be at less risk for some adverse outcome than they actually are if the comparison group includes both working and nonworking individuals. Recently, the healthy worker effect has been suggested to occur in other groups, for example among individuals who become caregivers for a family member or friend with a health condition or disability[19]. These caregivers often report high levels of stress associated with their caregiving duties, but their health does not appear to be poorer in comparison to population-based samples of noncaregivers. The explanation for this may be that those people who become caregivers are healthier at baseline than are other family members, so they are selected into the caregiver role based on a higher level of health. This could be called a "healthy caregiver effect."

Cohort studies can be very complex, expensive, and time consuming to conduct. Usually, National Institutes of Health (NIH) grants are funded for five years only, which can be a challenge in establishing a cohort and collecting adequate follow-up data. For this reason, many large cohorts are established by a federal agency. For example, the Health ABC Study is a large prospective cohort study looking at aging[20,21]. It is one of the most expensive studies ever mounted, including aspects such as imaging (MRIs) of subjects. The Women's Health Initiative is another very large study of over 160,000 women, with an observational (cohort) arm and many exposures and outcomes of interest, including cancer and cardiovascular disease[22]. The Women's Health Initiative was initiated by the NIH and involved a number of recruitment centers across the United States. Finally, the Framingham Heart Study, which we will discuss in more detail below, is a long-term cohort study that seeks to identify the causes of cardiovascular disease. These long-standing cohort studies that occur over time are sometimes known as **longitudinal** studies.

Cohort Study Examples

Below we discuss two cohort studies, the Framingham Heart Study and the Rochester Radiation Cohorts, in more detail to provide concrete examples of some of the methods and challenges associated with these types of studies.

The Framingham Heart Study The **Framingham Heart Study**, or simply the Framingham Study, is perhaps the most well-known cohort study in the United States. It began in 1948 around the time when infectious diseases were subsiding in the United States and chronic diseases, specifically cardiovascular diseases, were becoming the most common causes of death and disability. The study continues today and has followed three generations of adults in Framingham, Massachusetts, to identify the causes of and risk factors for cardiovascular disease, including heart disease and stroke. This kind of long-term longitudinal study is very costly, and in this case it is a joint project between the National Heart, Lung and Blood Institute (one of the National Institutes of Health) and Boston University[23–25].

At the study's start in 1948, investigators recruited 5,209 Framingham residents who had not had a heart attack or stroke and who did not have any evidence of cardiovascular disease. At the beginning of the study, these participants were between 30 and 62 years of age. The Framingham Study includes personal interviews, physical examinations, and laboratory tests at baseline (the point when a person is enrolled in the study) and every two years thereafter. The second Framingham generation was sampled in 1971 ($n = 5,124$), and the third generation was enrolled in 2002 ($n = 4,095$). These second- and third-generation study participants were the children and grandchildren (and their spouses) of the original Framingham Study cohort.

The Framingham Study has been vital to our understanding of the natural history of cardiovascular disease and in identifying important causes and risk factors that public health interventions can target. To date, the Framingham Study has been instrumental in linking smoking, cholesterol, blood pressure, physical activity, and obesity to cardiovascular disease risk. In addition, the study has been used to provide incidence measures and to create predictive risk models for heart disease. More details about the study's history, design, findings, and cohort members are available on its Web site, www.framinghamheartstudy.org.

The Rochester Radiation Cohorts The Rochester Radiation Cohorts in New York exemplify the strengths, complexity, and cost of cohort studies[26–30]. Begun in the mid-1950s, the **Rochester Radiation Cohorts** were an ambitious series of studies used to determine whether adverse effects, specifically cancer, are related to medical irradiation. A number of irradiation therapies were in vogue at the time of the study's commencement. The study enumerated all persons treated with irradiation for postpartum mastitis (breast infection) and enlarged thymus in Monroe County, New York. New mothers with breast infections (mastitis) were treated with X-rays. Infants judged to have a large thymus gland, usually at birth, were believed to have an increased risk for crib death (now called sudden infant death syndrome), and X-rays were used to shrink the gland.

To identify exposed subjects, investigators searched the records of all ten facilities in Monroe County that used medical irradiation for these conditions. Researchers abstracted information on all treated patients. If the subjects were children, the information about their parents was also recorded. Data were recorded on note cards in the handwriting of the abstractor, often in pencil; these cards served as the primary research record. Initially, exposure was classified as a dichotomous (yes/no) outcome. The dose of exposure for X-rays was calculated based on the number of treatments and the radiation level of the machines. Questionnaires were used to measure self-reported exposures to other medical radiation and a number of other relevant exposures: for example, smoking history, the use of oral contraceptives, and family history of breast cancer.

For the thymus groups, other children in the same family were enumerated during the first mailed survey, and these untreated siblings became the unexposed comparison group. For the mastitis group, sisters not treated for mastitis were used as the primary unexposed group. A second unexposed group was later created composed of women with mastitis who had delivered at New York City hospitals, where X-rays were not used to treat mastitis, and their sisters.

The primary method of ascertaining cancer outcomes was by mailed surveys. In addition, the names of cohort members were compared to the New York State Tumor Registry. New York's tumor registry is rated as excellent, with good case ascertainment, and checking cohort members' names against it ensured that the exposed persons were not reporting cancer outcomes differently compared to those who were not given X-ray treatments (see Chapter 3 for more discussion of registries). Most subjects granted permission for their medical records to be released, and these records and pathology reports were used to code specific histological types of cancers and to verify reported diagnoses.

Maintaining a cohort is in itself a science. As of the last survey of the mastitis and thymus cohorts (1985–1987), six surveys had been conducted, approximately every five to six years. Locating subjects was accomplished by some of the techniques listed below. In addition, some new methods are described that were not available at the time[31,32].

1. Postal inquiry of the last-known address. Although useful in earlier decades of the cohort, this has become very expensive and yields low success, except in rural or small-town areas.

2. Merging subject files with New York State driver's license data files. During the life of the studies, participants' location of residence was fairly stable. As of the late 1980s, over 50 percent resided in Monroe County and about 70 percent in New York State. Note that in areas with frequent population transition (e.g., big cities or areas with rapid economic growth), this would be a challenge.

3. The responses of siblings on surveys. At each survey, respondents were instructed to list their siblings and their current whereabouts.

4. Previously reported friends, employers, and relatives. On later surveys, respondents were instructed to list a friend or relative who would always know the respondent's whereabouts. Also, employment information was collected. This remains a favorite way of tracking research participants but is subject to close scrutiny by ethics reviews (**institutional review boards**, or **IRBs**) of research proposals because of concerns about subjects' confidentiality.

5. Reverse directories (city directories). Formerly done with published paper directories, this tracking and tracing is now easier using the Internet features of reverse directories. By examining the address of a participant, one can call current residents or neighbors for more information.

6. Subject-finder services (for example, Equifax). These companies use methods similar to (and are usually connected with) credit report companies. Like other services, once the social security number (SSN) of a subject is obtained, it will be easier to find the subject later. However, it is hard to convince IRBs to allow the use of SSNs because of increasing ethical and identity theft concerns. There are some Web-based services that will run names against some subscriber data resources, but they are expensive (about $20–$40 per request, with a few hours to twenty-four-hour turnaround).

7. Web-based services. More recently, Web-based services and personnel with expertise (e.g., Battelle Corp., PhoneDisc, Reference USA, Trans Union's RE-TRACE and TRACE[31]) are available at a cost. None of these services were available for the last Rochester Radiation Cohort survey.

8. National Death Index (NDI). This technique was not used in the Rochester Radiation Cohort studies but can be used in long-standing cohorts where mortality data can help ascertain health outcomes. The NDI is a national data source of death certificates from all states[33–35]. As with other methods of tracing and tracking, its use requires careful review and approval by an IRB.

The survey of 1985–1987 consisted of a five-page booklet. After multiple mailings and follow-up phone calls, success (sometimes called **response rate**) was over 90 percent. Contrast this with the reported response of the BRFSS in Chapter 3, which hovers around 50 percent.

The results of the Rochester Radiation Cohorts showed an increased risk of thyroid cancers immediately and persistently in the thymus cohort[29–30]. Excess breast cancers in the mastitis and thymus cohorts also have been detected[27,28]. An important component of maintaining these cohorts is that irradiated subjects were alerted to increased risks of cancer, a practice that is clearly ethical given the opportunity for early detection and treatment, but which may be criticized for producing some bias in ascertaining cancers[26].

Analyzing Cohort Studies

In both cohort studies and case–control studies, which we will discuss in the next section, the basic analysis begins with the construction of a **two-by-two (2 × 2) table**. These tables have two rows, one for the exposed and one for the unexposed subjects, and two columns, one for those with the outcome and one for those without the outcome. The number of people who fall into each row by column category are represented by the letters a, b, c, and d as shown in Table 5.1.

In cohort studies, the **relative risk (RR)** is calculated as the **measure of effect** or the **measure of excess risk**, the amount by which exposure increases (or decreases) the risk of the outcome. The relative risk is sometimes called the risk ratio or rate ratio, but relative risk will be used in this text. The RR is the incidence in the exposed group divided by the incidence in the unexposed group; thus we are comparing the rate of new disease among the exposed and the unexposed groups.

$$RR = \frac{a/(a+b)}{c/(c+d)}$$

If the RR equals 1.0, there is no difference in risk of the outcome based on exposure. In other words, someone with the exposure of interest is equally as likely to develop the outcome as someone without the exposure of interest. If the

Table 5.1 Generic 2 × 2 Table for Analyzing Epidemiological Study Data

	Outcome	No Outcome
Exposed	a	b
Unexposed	c	d

Table 5.2 Two-by-two Tables with Data and Relative Risk (RR) Calculations for a Hypothetical Cohort Study Investigating whether Wearing a Seat Belt During a Crash (exposure) Is Associated With Traumatic Brain Injury (TBI; outcome)

(a)

	TBI	No TBI
Seat belt	50	300
No seat belt	95	305

$$RR = \frac{50/(50+300)}{95/(95+305)} = 0.60 \text{ (less likely or protected)}$$

(b)

	TBI	No TBI
No seat belt	95	305
Seat belt	50	300

$$RR = \frac{95/(95+305)}{50/(50+300)} = 1.66 \text{ (more likely or increased risk)}$$

RR is greater than 1.0, we say the exposure increases the risk of outcome. For example, if smoking was the exposure and lung cancer the outcome, and we calculate an RR of 4.3, we would say smokers are 4.3 times as likely as nonsmokers to be diagnosed with lung cancer. Likewise, if the RR is less than 1.0, the exposure is protective against the outcome. In another scenario (Table 5.2a), we may be looking at seat belt use during a crash as the exposure and traumatic brain injury (TBI) as the outcome. If we calculate an RR of 0.6 in this study, we would say that individuals wearing a seat belt at the time of a crash were 0.6 times as likely (less likely) to have a TBI compared to individuals who were not wearing a seat belt during a crash. We can also invert the rows of a 2×2 table and reverse the interpretation of the relative risk. Table 5.2b illustrates this feature.

In part (a) of Table 5.2, the 2×2 table is set up in the standard fashion as described in Table 5.1, with the exposed group (wearing a seat belt during a crash) on the top row and the unexposed group below. The RR in this hypothetical cohort study is 0.6, meaning that individuals wearing a seat belt at the time of a crash were 0.6 times as likely to have a TBI compared to individuals not wearing a seat belt. In some cases, it is easier to explain a relationship or more useful to report a result with an RR greater than 1.0. In part (b) we see this alternate approach, listing the unexposed group in the first row and the exposed group in the second row. Note that the RR in part (b) is simply *the inverse* of the

RR obtained in part (a). The appropriate interpretation of the RR in (b) is that individuals who were *not* wearing a seat belt at the time of a crash were 1.7 (1/0.6) times more likely to have a TBI compared to individuals who were wearing a seat belt at the time of a crash. The data provide the same information, but one explanation may be easier for the audience or the public to understand.

Also note that identical numbers of individuals in the exposed and unexposed groups in a cohort study are not required. Often, the frequency of exposure will influence the number of subjects who can be identified, and this may result in an imbalance in numbers. There are statistical measures that can show whether a study has a sufficient number of subjects to detect significant differences in risk; these are beyond the scope of this textbook, however.

Cohort Analysis Example

To illustrate the use, analysis, and interpretation of RRs from 2×2 tables, we revisit the Rochester Radiation Cohorts. As described above, the Rochester Radiation Cohorts showed an excess number of cancers among study participants who had been irradiated for enlarged thymus as infants. Tables 5.3 and 5.4 show the data for extrathyroid malignant tumors, or cancerous tumors in sites other than the thyroid, from the cohort after an average of twenty-nine years of follow-up. Table 5.3 shows the data in a standard 2×2 format. In Table 5.4, the data are presented in a different way and provide an alternate method of calculating relative risk. Instead of using individual people as the denominator for the study, Table 5.4 presents **person-years** at risk for the outcome. (Recall the discussion of **person-time** that appeared in Chapter 4 and the calculation of incidence based on person-time.) Because the RR is the ratio of incidence in

Table 5.3 Number of Malignant Extrathyroid Tumors Among Individuals Irradiated for Enlarged Thymus During Infancy and Their Nonirradiated Siblings, Rochester Radiation Cohorts

	Malignant Extrathyroid Tumors	No Malignant Extrathyroid Tumors
Subjects irradiated in infancy	52	2,804
Nonirradiated siblings	46	5,007

Source: Reference 36

$$RR = \frac{52/(52+2,804)}{46/(46+5,007)} = 2.00$$

Table 5.4 Number of Malignant Extrathyroid Tumors and Person-years at Risk for Individuals Irradiated for Enlarged Thymus During Infancy and Their Nonirradiated Siblings, Rochester Radiation Cohorts

	Number of Malignant Extrathyroid Tumors	Person-Years at Risk
Subjects irradiated in infancy	52	66,877
Nonirradiated siblings	46	117,899

Source: Reference 36

$$RR = \frac{52/66,877}{46/117,899} = 1.99$$

the exposed to incidence in the unexposed, we can still calculate this measure using person-years.

The study included 2,856 subjects who had been irradiated and 5,053 who had not. This explains why there were more person-years at risk represented by the nonirradiated siblings group. As you can see from Tables 5.3 and 5.4, the RR for malignant extrathyroid tumors is around 2.0 regardless of the denominator used (individual people or person-time at risk). In other words, subjects who were treated with X-rays for an enlarged thymus as infants were *twice as likely* as their nonirradiated siblings to develop cancerous tumors in a site other than the thymus later in life. Although there is no random assignment to exposure, cohort studies otherwise resemble experiments (randomized trials) in their scientific design, methods, and analyses.

Case–Control Studies

In case–control studies, participants are selected based upon their outcome status, and exposure frequencies (or levels) are compared between groups (Figure 5.5). People with the outcome are called *cases*, and people without the outcome are called *controls*. In other words, **case–control studies** compare the exposure histories of ill persons to those of persons who are at risk of developing the illness[1–7,37].

In order to successfully conduct a case–control study, it must be possible to identify members of the population who are at risk for the outcome; in other words, controls from the population from which the cases arose must be found. Alternatively, one could use a group of controls whose exposure histories represent that of the population at risk. It must also be possible to measure the history

FIGURE 5.5 Generic Scheme of a Case–control Study Design in which Participants with and without the Outcome are Identified (cases and controls, respectively)

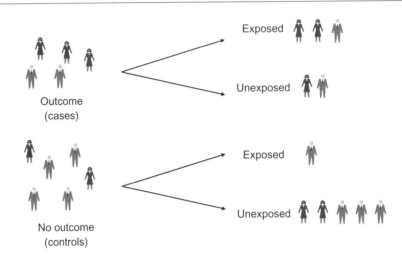

The exposure status for each individual is then assessed, either through an interview or through historical records, if available.

of exposure in a valid way in both cases and controls. If these two conditions are met, and if the condition under study, the cases, are not too common (an assumption we examine below), a case–control study will provide the same result as a properly done cohort study.

Establishing Case and Control Definitions

Cases The criteria for selecting individual cases in a case–control study must be objective. Specific diagnostic criteria or other parameters should be defined prior to case selection to limit bias in the results of the study. **Bias** is a systematic difference in the results of a study from what in fact is occurring[1,2,6,38,39]. Bias occurs for a variety of reasons that will be examined in more detail in Chapter 6, but these reasons include problems in the way subjects were selected for a study, the measurements used in the study, or the analysis of the data. The criteria for case selection must have high sensitivity and specificity (accuracy) in order to minimize misclassification. **Sensitivity** in this case refers to the ability to correctly identify people who have the outcome (labeling cases as cases), and **specificity** means that people without the outcome are correctly identified as not having the outcome (labeling controls as controls). **Misclassification**, categorizing someone as a case when he or she is not or improperly classifying a control as a case, can **attenuate**, or dampen, the results of the study. In epidemiological studies, attenuation results in the RR or odds ratio (OR) estimate moving closer to 1.0 (the level of no effect or association).

By extension, the case–control study design may be a poor choice for some conditions with broad case definitions or for syndromes that include several heterogeneous kinds of cases. However, if the exposure–outcome relationship is strong enough, case–control studies may still offer the advantage of (1) smaller sample sizes than cohort studies, (2) larger numbers of suspect exposures from the same outcome examined, and (3) a shorter study period, allowing completed follow-up of the subjects. These advantages are demonstrated in examples below.

Controls Controls ideally are selected from the same population as that from which the cases arose. It is best if controls are selected randomly from the population, as in random digit dialing, the method used for the BRFSS and other studies. Controls may be persons identified through the same means as the cases; for example, controls may have been admitted to the same hospital as cases but for different reasons. There are potential problems with this method of selecting controls, which will be discussed below. Controls may be persons without the outcome who are related in some way to the case, such as a friend, a relative, or a neighbor of the case. As with our discussion of using siblings in the Rochester Radiation Cohorts, this would presume the exposure of interest was not strongly linked in some manner to these controls, such as through genes or environment.

Case–Control Study Example: Control Selection

The first case–control study example illustrates why we are careful in selecting controls, in this case using hospital-based controls. This study evaluated the association between artificial sweeteners and lower urinary tract cancers in men[40]. Investigators suspected that taking control subjects from a hospital-based study might overestimate the population's use of artificial sweeteners because of obesity and diabetes-related diseases. If that were true, then a real association between sweeteners and cancer would be reduced compared to results achieved when the controls were selected randomly to represent the population exposure to sweeteners.

As Table 5.5 illustrates, there is a difference in exposure (use of artificial sweeteners) among the different control groups. Specifically, artificial sweetener use is higher among hospital controls with an obesity-related disease. We can understand why this would be true because these men might have a tendency

Table 5.5 Exposure Data for Male Controls in a Case–control Study of Artificial Sweetener Use and Urinary Tract Cancer, Detroit, Michigan, 1978

Ever Used	Population Controls (*n* = 296)	Hospital Controls (*n* = 234)	Hospital Controls Without Obesity-Related Disease (*n* = 152)	Difference Between Hospital Controls With and Without Obesity-Related Disease
Any artificial sweetener	38%	44%	38%	−6%
Tabletop sweetener	24%	29%	26%	−3%
Diet drinks	24%	30%	26%	−4%
Diet foods	13%	16%	11%	−5%

to avoid sugar. The exposure levels of population controls are similar to hospital controls who do not have an obesity-related disease; for example, 38% of controls in each group had used any artificial sweetener, and 13% of population controls and 11% of hospital controls without obesity-related disease used diet foods. Artificial sweetener use was 3% to 6% *higher* among hospital controls with obesity-related disease compared to hospital controls without obesity-related disease. The message here is that when using hospital controls in a case–control study, there may be important differences between these controls and population controls due to the health conditions that caused the controls to be in the hospital. Hospitals can be a good source of controls for a case–control study, but the researcher must carefully assess the relationship between hospitalization and exposure to ensure these controls represent the population accurately. This example also reminds us of what our expectations are in case–control studies: the controls represent the population experience of those at risk, but they have not experienced the disease.

PUBLIC HEALTH CONNECTIONS 5.1

DISTINGUISHING COHORT STUDIES AND CASE–CONTROL STUDIES

Many students find cohort studies and case–control studies difficult to distinguish. Indeed, there are similarities: both collect individual-level information and use information over time rather than at a single time point (as in cross-sectional studies). The defining difference between these two types of studies is the manner in which subjects are selected. In cohort studies, participants are selected based on exposure, whereas in case–control studies, participants are selected based on outcome. Perhaps the most confusing distinction is between case–control studies and retrospective cohort studies because they can seem nearly the same. In both cases, we already know the outcome status of study participants and must go back in time to construct exposure. Again, the difference comes in the analysis of these data: were the participants broken into groups based on whether or not they were exposed or whether or not they have the outcome of interest? This requires that you correctly identify the exposure of interest and the outcome of interest in the study in question. If the researchers set up a group of exposed and a group of unexposed subjects, it is a cohort study (in this case, a retrospective cohort). For example, imagine we search hospital records for individuals who have a specific type of brain tumor, and we are interested in whether or not people who worked in air traffic control towers are at increased risk for these tumors. The exposure is working in an air traffic control tower, and the outcome is having a brain tumor. If we use the hospital records to identify a group of people with the brain tumor and a group without the brain tumor of interest, then interview them (or use other data sources) to classify whether or not they worked in an air traffic control tower, we would be conducting a case–control study. Conversely, if we contact people and find out whether or not they worked in an air traffic control tower (interview or other data sources), then use medical records to determine whether or not they had a brain tumor, we would be conducting a retrospective cohort study. In these retrospective cohort studies, the researcher behaves as if he or she does not know the outcome status of the individuals when dividing participants into groups. There is still an exposed and an unexposed group, but there also is information about outcomes at the start of the study so that follow-up time is not required.

Another point of confusion can occur when reading scientific journal articles. As we have described in this chapter, the relative risk (RR) is the appropriate measure of excess risk in cohort studies, whereas the odds ratio (OR) should be used for case–control studies. However, there are many published cohort studies that report results as ORs. What is going on here? The OR in a cohort study is an artifact of using the analytic methods of **logistic regression** modeling. This method will be described in more detail in Chapter 6, but essentially it allows the researcher to go beyond the basic 2×2 table and model exposure and outcome while controlling for confounding. As described in this chapter, confounding can be a substantial problem in cohort studies (and observational studies in general), so logistic regression is a common tool in observational epidemiology. However, ORs are not a universally acceptable replacement for the RR: the OR only approximates the RR if the outcome (disease) is rare, somewhere around 5 percent. In this text, you are expected to use RR calculations when working with data from cohort studies.

Table 5.6 Generic Example of a 2 × 2 Table and Formula for Odds Ratio (OR)

	Outcome	No Outcome
Exposed	a	b
Unexposed	c	d

$$OR = \frac{a \times d}{b \times c}$$

Analyzing Case–Control Studies

In case–control studies, we begin analysis by setting up a 2 × 2 table, just as we did with cohort studies. However, in case–control studies, we must use the **odds ratio (OR)** approximation to the relative risk, as shown in Table 5.6.

The interpretation of the OR is similar to the RR, except we are talking about the *odds* of an outcome rather than the *risk* of an outcome. For example, if we calculate an OR of 2.9 for competitive running (exposure) and knee replacement (outcome), we would say the odds of having a knee replacement for competitive runners was 2.9 times the odds of knee replacement in noncompetitive runners.

The reason we cannot calculate a relative risk in case–control studies is that we do not have a measure of incidence. Recall that in a case–control study we select people based on the presence (case) or absence (control) of the outcome, so the researcher is artificially establishing the number of cases and controls: rarely does the distribution match the actual incidence of the outcome in the underlying population. Because we cannot measure incidence in a case–control study, we must instead calculate the odds of an event occurring in each exposure group. If the outcome is rare, often defined as occurring in 5 percent of the population or less, the OR will closely approximate the RR (called the *rare disease assumption*)[5,41].

As in all observational studies, analysis of case–control studies must include rigorous assessment and control of confounding variables. There are some additional issues of which to be keenly aware in case–control studies as well, and recall bias is one of the most notable. **Recall bias** occurs if cases and controls remember past exposures differently, with cases potentially having more recently considered their exposures because of the diagnosis or event that makes them a case[2, 5–7,39]. Recall bias does not necessarily imply that cases overreport exposure because they attribute their outcome to a particular exposure; rather, cases may in fact recall their exposures more accurately than do controls.

Recall bias can lead to **differential misclassification**, that is, inaccurately classifying study participants and making a different assignment based on

Table 5.7 Hypothetical Case–control Study of Maternal Illicit Drug Use and Birth Defects Showing the Effect of Differential Misclassification Caused by Recall Bias on the Odds Ratio (OR) Estimate

	True Classification	
	Birth Defect	No Birth Defect
Maternal drug use	10	10
No maternal drug use	90	90
	OR = 1.0	

	Observed Classification	
	Birth Defect	No Birth Defect
Maternal drug use	19	5
No maternal drug use	81	95
	OR = 4.5	

either exposure or outcome status[1,2,6]. The following example illustrates differential misclassification by outcome (case or control) status[39]. In a hypothetical study of maternal use of illegal drugs during pregnancy and infant birth defects, case mothers who did take drugs are 100 percent accurate in their reporting, but control mothers are more likely to *not* mention their drug use. Case mothers who did not take drugs during their pregnancy also tend to report drug use from before their pregnancy as occurring during their pregnancy, a phenomenon called **telescoping**, reporting more distant events as being closer to the present and during the exposure window of interest (Table 5.7).

As we noted earlier, one of our major concerns in an observational design, including case–control studies, is confounding. To deal with confounding we sometimes use a **matched case–control study** design[1,2,5,7]. In this practice, one control subject is identified who matches a case on a factor or factors, such as age, gender, race, or hospital admission date. When a factor is matched, it can no longer be investigated as an exposure because the researcher has manipulated its distribution to be equal across cases and controls. Thus if we are conducting the study about illicit drug use during pregnancy and birth defects, and we decide to match on the age of the mother at conception, we can no longer investigate the impact of a mother's age at conception on her risk of having a child with a birth defect. However, this matching assures us that age is not confounding the relationship between maternal drug use and birth defects because age is the same across both groups of women. One benefit of matching is that more than one control may be matched to each case to decrease the number of

Table 5.8 Necessary Sample Sizes for a Given Effect Size Measuring the Relationship between Hypothetical Contaminant X and Spina Bifida Using Various Study Designs*

Exposure Effect Size (RR or OR)	Cohort Sample Size	1:1 Case-Control Sample Size (number of cases)	3:1 Case-Control Sample Size (number of cases)
1.1	572,000	21,266 (10,633)	28,508 (7,127)
1.2	151,000	5,734 (2,867)	7,720 (1,930)
1.3	71,000	2,736 (1,368)	3,700 (925)
1.4	42,000	1,648 (824)	2,232 (558)
1.5	28,200	1,124 (562)	1,528 (382)
2.0	8,700	374 (187)	512 (128)
3.0	3,000	146 (73)	200 (50)
5.0	1,200	68 (34)	92 (23)
10.0	430	36 (18)	48 (12)

*Assumptions: $p = 0.05$, power $= 0.80$; for cohort, equal number of exposed and unexposed; base frequency of spina bifida in the unexposed is 0.58 per 1,000 births; for case–control, base frequency of exposure to contaminant X in controls is 20%.

cases needed to achieve adequate statistical **power** (also known as minimizing type 2 errors, which will be discussed in Chapter 6). In this instance, the matching design increases the sample size in a specific way, adding more controls to the study sample, which increases the chance of finding a real statistical association when one exists (study power). This is illustrated, in part, in Table 5.8. If one control is matched to each case, it is notated as a 1:1 case–control study, whereas a 3:1 study would indicate three controls were chosen for each case.

Case–control studies are particularly good for rare outcomes because study subjects are chosen based on the outcome. This is in contrast to a cohort study, in which rare outcomes are more inefficient because follow-up of many people is needed to identify an adequate number of individuals who develop the outcome of interest. For example, spina bifida, which occurs in about 0.58 per 1,000 births in the United States, is a rare outcome and would require that we follow a very large number of pregnant women in order to identify just a few children born with this condition. Table 5.8 illustrates this, showing the required study size for identifying whether contaminant X causes spina bifida. The table shows the sample sizes required for a cohort study, a 1:1 case–control study, and a 3:1 case–control study with the same effect size (RR for cohort study, OR approximation to RR for case–control study).

As Table 5.8 shows, smaller effect sizes (small RR or OR) require a larger sample size to detect the difference between two groups. As noted above, case–

control studies require a fraction of the sample size required by a cohort study for the same exposure effect size. Finally, although a 3:1 case–control study requires *more total subjects* be enrolled than a 1:1 case–control study, the 3:1 study requires that *fewer cases* be identified to achieve the same statistical power. In general, case–control studies are faster and cheaper to conduct than cohort studies because there is no follow-up time needed and sample sizes may be smaller.

PUBLIC HEALTH CONNECTIONS 5.2

CHOOSING AN OBSERVATIONAL STUDY DESIGN

Cohorts are a good choice when exposures are rare, the outcome occurs quickly (i.e., pregnancy), and the outcome is common (large incidence). Retrospective cohorts can overcome some of the problems of rare outcomes and long duration but depend on good follow-up information and prior records of exposure.

Case–control studies are a good choice when the outcome is rare, there is good exposure history, and appropriate controls can be identified from the population under study.

Choice of an Observational Study Design

Characteristic	Favors
Frequency of exposure is:	
High	*All (especially case–control)*
Low	*Cohort*
Frequency of outcome is:	
High	*Cohort*
Low	*Case–control*
Expensive to ascertain in specific individuals	*Case–control*
Unable to accurately assess prior exposure given presence of outcome (e.g., recall bias is serious, altered biological state)	*Cohort*
Availability of	
Follow-up mechanism	*Cohort*
Exposure records	*All (especially cohort)*
Duration between exposure and outcome	
Long	*Case–control*
Short	*Cohort*

Experimental Studies

Thus far we have discussed observational studies, those in which the investigator simply collects data on groups or individuals without influencing the factors under observation. As we discussed, observational studies are appropriate for many questions, especially when we cannot ethically assign exposures, for example, randomly assigning car seat use to test whether they protect infants in vehicle crashes. In contrast, in **experimental studies** the researcher assigns study participants to a particular exposure group (exposed or unexposed). Experimental studies have a number of strengths, namely that they limit confounding[4,6]. There are a number of types of experimental studies. Here we will discuss only randomized controlled trials and community trials.

Randomized Controlled Trials

Often termed the *gold standard* of epidemiological studies, **randomized controlled trials** (**RCTs**) provide strong evidence of cause and effect when designed and conducted well[2,42]. The term *gold standard* comes from the practice of guaranteeing paper money with gold and applies to a standard that is judged to be the truth. In practice, very few science standards are really golden. (We even use the term *alloyed gold standard* to suggest that we have a standard that probably needs improving.) These studies are called *randomized* because study subjects are assigned at random, without respect to demographic or other factors, to a specific exposure group. Each subject has the same probability of being assigned to a given exposure group. The random nature of this assignment serves to distribute potential confounding factors across each exposure group equally. If confounding factors are similar across exposures, then any difference in the outcomes can be attributed to the exposure itself. In practice, it is often necessary to control for confounding even after randomization because the randomization process is not perfect and some confounding factors may not have been equally distributed between exposure groups. As in observational studies, this control of confounding can be achieved using methods described in Chapter 6.

The word *controlled* refers to the characteristic that RCTs have a standard or control group to which the new or hypothesized better treatment is compared. The control group may be individuals who receive no treatment at all when that is ethically appropriate. Often in pharmaceutical trials, the control group is given an inactive substance that looks like the treatment, which is called a **placebo**. In some RCTs, the study does not compare nothing and something but rather compares the current standard of care and a new method of care. In this case, the control group receives standard care and the treatment group receives the new method.

In addition to these features, many RCTs have some level of **blinding**, or concealing the subject's exposure status. A **single-blind study** is one in which the study participant does not know whether he or she is in a treatment or control group. In a **double-blind study**, neither the participant nor the investigator knows whether the subject is in a treatment or control group. By blinding those involved in the study, it is more likely that all participants will be assessed in the same way, decreasing the opportunity for misclassification or bias[8].

RCTs may target any of the three levels of prevention. Those studies that aim at **primary prevention** (preventing a disease from occurring) often are called **preventive trials**[8]. Preventive trials may include testing the efficacy (ability to produce an effect) of a vaccine in healthy individuals, for example. **Intervention trials** are those that test the impact of drugs or other efforts to reduce the severity of a disease in individuals who are at high risk of the outcome (**secondary prevention**)[8]. Finally, **therapeutic trials** are designed to improve outcomes once an individual has a disease (**tertiary prevention**)[8]. In therapeutic trials, it is unlikely that subjects would receive no treatment; rather, standard care may be compared to additional levels of treatment or intervention. An example of a therapeutic trial might be one that tests ways to help smokers stop smoking (the outcome of interest). If we were working in a clinic setting, the standard of care might be to recommend a smoking cessation class offered by health educators and to provide a free or low-cost nicotine substitute, such as a nicotine patch or chewing gum. The new treatment might add a prescription medication that is believed to help with cravings, and the standard group might receive either no new drug or a placebo that looks like the new drug.

As in observational studies, before beginning an RCT the investigator must define the population of interest and select a representative sample from this population to participate in the experiment[8]. Often, RCTs have very specific inclusion and exclusion criteria that may limit the population to which the results can be generalized. For example, in a study investigating the effectiveness of a cholesterol-lowering drug, researchers may exclude individuals with existing conditions such as heart disease or hypertension. Even though this exclusion may allow a more precise biological estimation of the effect of the drug, the results may be applied only to the population of people with high cholesterol and no existing heart disease or hypertension. Once this drug is licensed for general use, many of the individuals who take it may in fact have comorbid conditions (heart disease or hypertension). There is the potential that this group of individuals who were not included in the clinical trial population will not respond as well to the drug or will have adverse reactions. This occurs somewhat rarely, but caution should be exercised when generalizing the results of any study beyond the study population. In recent years, it has become common, and even required in some countries, that **postmarketing surveillance**, or drug monitoring after agency approval, occurs for drugs newly introduced to the market. As with other surveillance activities, postmarketing surveillance can provide useful time-trend data and may alert researchers, clinicians, and pharmaceutical producers to unexpected side effects associated with a drug. Pharmacoepidemiology, the specialized field of epidemiology that deals with pharmaceutical drugs and postmarketing surveillance, is detailed in Chapter 7.

RCTs can have limitations, the most important of which is the ability to use these studies in public health research. In many cases, it is unethical to randomize individuals to the exposure of interest. For example, one cannot randomize women to illegal drugs during pregnancy to understand the impact of drug use on the risk of birth defects. We know that drug use is harmful to the woman and that it may cause other poor birth outcomes, so the only way to assess this relationship is through an observational study design. Another ethical consideration in RCTs is the local standard of care. Some RCTs are conducted in developing countries, in part because the outcome of interest may occur more frequently there. This is not necessarily unethical, unless the results of the trial will not be of use to the population on which the trial was conducted. Recall from Chapter 1 that the *Belmont Report* includes justice as one of its tenets, which includes equal distribution of risks in research. In other words, if one population assumes all of the risk associated with testing a new drug, that population should also have access to the benefits of that drug after the trial ends.

RCTs often are time and cost intensive. As with prospective cohort studies, RCTs require follow-up to assess the outcome, sometimes for many years. In addition, RCTs may require intense medical care or procedures, such as frequent visits and laboratory tests. The issues of noncompliance and loss to follow-up are important in RCTs: discarding participants because they do not take their drugs as instructed or do not comply with the intervention may compromise the very benefits of the randomization of exposures and make them more like observational studies. For example, patients who do not take a trial medication as instructed (**noncompliant**) or who leave a study early (**lost to follow-up**) may do so because of negative side effects. If these individuals are then excluded from analyses, their negative experience may be lost, and the results of the study would be less accurate[43].

Community Trials

The major difference between RCTs and **community trials** is the unit of analysis[8]. In community trials, as in ecological studies, the unit of analysis is a group rather than an individual. The community under study represents a larger population, such as a school district, a city, or a county. These trials may test an etiological hypothesis or the impact of a program or intervention[8]. In a community trial, one or more communities serve as the intervention group and another community or communities serves as the control. As in all epidemiological studies, the intervention and control groups should be as similar as possible, except for the exposure status, and they should represent the same underlying population. Ideally, the populations of the study communities will be relatively stable to ensure changes seen in the outcome are due to the exposure under study rather than to changes in the community's population[8]. Community trials are different from ecological studies in that the exposure is manipulated by the investigator rather than occurring naturally.

The process of a community trial is similar to that of an RCT except groups are assigned to an exposure rather than individuals. Whenever possible, allocation to intervention or control should be done at random in community trials. Once the treatment group is assigned, the intervention begins, and the groups are followed over time to evaluate changes in the outcome of interest. The outcome may be the incidence of disease, the use of specific medical care, or the prevalence of a preventive health behavior, for example. In a community trial of smoking and low birth weight, we might randomize prenatal care clinics by adding a health educator who conducts smoking cessation programs. We would compare smoking rates or quit rates among women attending the intervention clinics that have a health educator and women attending control clinics with **usual care** (no health educator).

Community trials are an especially good choice when social constructs are expected to influence the effectiveness of an intervention[8]. For example, drinking laws, law enforcement, social norms, and retailer practices (such as verifying age upon purchase) may all influence whether a teenager has access to alcohol. In a study of the effectiveness of an educational campaign to prevent underage drinking, a community trial may provide a better understanding of the actual impact of the campaign on teen alcohol use in a real-world setting than would an individual-level RCT or observational study. In addition, community trials may have a larger public health impact than RCTs because many more people can be reached during an intervention trial than during an individual-level RCT[8].

Community trials have some weaknesses, including the potential for confounding. Changes in a community related to frequent in- and out-migration may cause a change in the outcome that is not related to exposure. Likewise, baseline differences in the communities chosen may influence the effectiveness of the intervention. Because the unit of analysis is the group in community trials, the ecological fallacy is possible. This might lead us to see an association at the group level and apply that association to the individual level when, in fact, that relationship does not hold. Finally, community trials can be time intensive and costly because a large number of people (the entire sample community) must receive the intervention and be followed over an adequate time period[8].

Causal Inference

We noted that experimental study designs are considered the gold standard in epidemiological research. These studies provide strong evidence of cause and effect because the exposures are not self-selected by study participants. For this reason, confounding is likely to be less of an issue, and any relationship we observe between exposure and outcome is likely to be a causal one. By design, experimental studies also are prospective in nature so that in a well-designed trial we begin with people who are free of the outcome and follow them over time to assess whether the experimental and control groups have different rates of incident outcome.

When we move to observational studies, we need to consider more carefully if we feel confident about making a **causal inference**, a statement about the exposure causing the outcome, based on the evidence[1,2,6,7,44,45]. In assessing causation, it is important to not only consider studies individually but also to look for patterns of evidence. In simple terms, causal inference requires that we examine the research and ask the following: how good is the scientific evidence? Authors list the elements of causation somewhat differently and with greater details and examples. However, there are five basic criteria to consider when assessing causal inference in the absence of definitive experiments, as summarized in Table 5.9.

In all observational studies, we need to think carefully about the possible problems in the time or **temporal sequence**. As mentioned above, the concern about which came first, exposure or outcome, occurs in cross-sectional studies when both are assessed simultaneously. The concern is also raised in case–control studies when we know the outcome and seek to assess a past exposure. These studies must be designed carefully to assure exposure information relates to prior experiences rather than current habits that might have been influenced by the outcome. For example, in a cross-sectional study, if people are asked to report their weight and whether they have been diagnosed with diabetes, we might identify obesity as a cause of diabetes because people with diabetes are, on average, heavier than the general population. But what if the reverse were true: what if having diabetes led to obesity? Not all exposure–outcome relationships assessed in cross-sectional studies create a temporal problem, however. When

Table 5.9 Criteria for Assessing Causal Inference in Observational Epidemiological Studies

Criterion	Definition
Temporal sequence	Time sequence: the exposure occurs before the outcome.
Strength of association	The association between exposure and outcome is strong based on magnitude or size of the OR or RR.
Dose-response	A gradient in exposure results in a gradient in outcome; for example, increasing levels of exposure result in increasing levels or risk of the outcome.
Plausibility	Biologically (or socially, behaviorally), there is an explanation, a pathway, for the exposure causing the outcome.
Consistency	The association between exposure and outcome is present in a variety of settings and study designs.

using cross-sectional data to examine the relationship between family heritage and risk of skin cancer, the outcome cannot possibly alter or precede the exposure. In summary, some observational study designs are prone to generating concerns about temporal sequence, but the time relationship must be assessed in each case. When there is a concern about the temporal sequence of exposure and outcome in a study, be cautious about making a causal inference.

We have seen examples of studies with RRs or ORs and know that as the difference between the groups gets larger, the RR and OR get larger. **Strength of association** in general terms means that the larger the difference between exposure groups, the easier it is for us to infer that something else (a confounder) is not responsible for the association. That is, the association is stronger as the estimate of effect size (RR or OR) gets farther away from 1.0. There is no cutoff value for what is a large effect, but when a dichotomous (two-level categorical) exposure generates an RR of 1.05, that would not be considered to be a strong association because it is only a 5 percent relative increase in risk. However, an RR of 10.5 is very, very large: it indicates that the risk of the outcome among the exposed is ten times the risk of the outcome among the unexposed. What constitutes a strong association is different in studies that look at continuous rather than dichotomous variables. In a study using age as the exposure, the risk of heart disease increased by a factor of 1.07 per year between ages forty and fifty. Even though an RR of 1.07 is small, a cumulative increase each year would begin to look like a large increase in risk of heart disease. Finally, although the statistical significance of the measure of effect is not technically part of our list or criteria, we might look at the size of the relative risk and consider if the result might be due to chance (P value > 0.05; see Chapter 6, Biostatistics, for more details).

It is easy to confuse strength of the association with the size of the study, the number of people taking part in the study. A remarkable case–control study helps us view the issue more clearly. In a very small case–control study published in 1971, investigators reported on eight cases of a rare vaginal cancer in young women and compared their exposures to thirty-two control women[46,47]. Remarkably, seven of the eight cases were the daughters of mothers who had taken a specific drug called diethylstilbestrol (DES), and none of the control women had been exposed. The association would never have been detected in a cohort study because it would have taken decades of follow-up for such a rare event to occur. And although the case–control study was very small, it indeed identified a strong link between DES exposure and vaginal cancer.

In some exposure–outcome relationships, we expect there to be a biological or social reason that more of an exposure will cause more of an outcome or a larger risk of the outcome. In these cases, it is helpful to measure exposures as a gradient or dose and look at the pattern that emerges, namely whether there is a **dose response**. A clear example of this is smoking. If we are investigating lung cancer risk, the risk may be higher for smokers than for nonsmokers, but if we quantify the amount of smoking, we might expect to see increasingly larger RRs for lung cancer as we move from nonsmokers to light smokers to heavy smokers. Some exposures are simply categorical, such as sex or state of residence or the clinic one goes to for health care. In these cases, we would not rank one category above another and therefore would not be able to assess a dose response. There may be differences by category (men are more at risk for heart disease, for example), but these would not be classified as a dose response if there are only two categories or if the categories do not have an intuitive rank.

Observational studies sometimes provide evidence of an exposure–outcome relationship well before we understand the mechanism for it. For example, there was a very strong association between cigarette smoking and lung cancer before we had a clear picture of the biological carcinogens responsible. Thus even in the absence of the specific mechanism, common sense indicated that when a foreign substance, smoke, was inhaled into the lungs, the lung cells were more likely to become cancerous. The association makes biological sense, or the evidence is **biologically plausible**. Sometimes the biological evidence comes from animal studies, for example studies in which rodents are randomly exposed to tobacco smoke. Sometimes we consider information other than pure biology in making the case for inference. For example, it is plausible that traumatic events, such as interpersonal violence, can lead to an increased chance of symptoms of stress and mental health problems[48,49] or that living in a neighborhood with limited access to fresh produce can increase the amount of saturated fats in one's diet[50,51]. Although these relationships may seem to have less biological or mechanistic explanations underlying them, there is nonetheless plausibility to the relationships.

With all studies, we find the cause and effect argument improves as we see more evidence, and more studies, that have similar results. There may be some studies that do not hold to the pattern, but generally, as we look at studies on the same exposure–disease relationship, the **consistency** of the story is built. In any one study, the evidence of other studies should be part of the introduction and the discussion section of the report or article (see Public Health Connections 5.3). For example, two 1970s British studies on the use of oral contraceptives (birth control pills) and heart disease both showed an increased risk[52,53], helping to build the causal inference for the relationship. Keep in mind that this consistency criterion refers to *between* studies rather than *within* a study.

It is not necessary that all five criteria (Table 5.9) be in place and be strong in order to make a causal inference. These are general guidelines for assessing whether an exposure causes an outcome in an observational study. Experimental data also tend to need repetition (consistency) before causal inference can be accepted, and as discussed earlier, experiments can also have problems in confounding and generalizability.

PUBLIC HEALTH CONNECTIONS 5.3

READING SCIENTIFIC JOURNAL ARTICLES

Often, reports you hear in the news linking a food to decreased cancer risk or describing the negative health impacts of engaging in specific behaviors are based on research published in peer-reviewed journal articles. These journals require that other individuals in the field (peers) read and comment on the design of the study and the interpretation of data before the results are published. This helps to ensure accuracy and scientific merit in published work.

Most journals have a similar format regardless of the field in which it publishes. Journal articles begin with a **background** or **introduction** that describes work that has occurred in the past that relates to and has informed the current study. The author usually includes the hypothesis of the study. Following the background or introduction section, the article moves into **methods**, which details the steps taken in the current study. In an epidemiology article, this would

(Continued)

PUBLIC HEALTH CONNECTIONS 5.3

READING SCIENTIFIC JOURNAL ARTICLES (Continued)

include the data source(s), a description of how study participants were selected (**inclusion** and **exclusion criteria**), and details about the measures and analyses used in the study. After describing the study's construction in methods, the author discusses the **results**, sharing the findings of the study. The results section often includes tables and figures that provide data from the analyses. The text of the results section puts these data into words, but does not explain their meaning. Instead, the interpretation of the data is included in the next and often final section, the **discussion**. The discussion may cite other studies that have found similar or different results and suggest reasons for these differences. It often includes a synopsis of the study's strengths and weaknesses. Finally, it describes the meaning of the work in the larger context of the field and may suggest future areas of study. Some journal articles also include one last section, the **conclusion** for these summative remarks. An **abstract** is a brief summary of the entire article, typically comprising a sentence or two from each section of the work to provide readers a brief overview of the design and findings of the study.

Today, many journals are available online in addition to print. University libraries hold licenses for various journals, and individuals may purchase annual subscriptions or individual issues. Many scientific societies produce leading journals in their fields, and membership to the society may include a subscription to the journal. When searching for articles on a specific topic, it is helpful to use one of the many search engines, such as PubMed (National Library of Medicine, www.ncbi.nlm.nih.gov/PubMed) or Web of Science (Thomas Reuters, http://thomsonreuters.com/products_services/science/science_products/scholarly_research_analysis/research_discovery/web_of_science) to search across journals for a specific topic or author of interest.

Example: Applying Causal Inference Criteria

We now return to the cohort study example from Rochester, New York, in which infants who were treated with X-rays were followed-up for tumors and compared to their brothers and sisters who had no treatment. This is an observational study, so the causal inference criteria should be applied.

First, let us consider the *temporal sequence*. We described this study as a prospective cohort, meaning we began with infants or young children, none of whom had any cancers or tumors, and followed them for many years. This is an excellent example of the exposure coming before the disease and unambiguously

Table 5.10 Risk of Benign Thyroid Adenomas (Tumors) After X-ray Irradiation for Enlarged Thymus Gland at Birth

Group	Number of Tumors	Tumor Incidence per 100,000 per Year	Relative Risk (RR)*
All exposed infants	86	102.2	14.1
Dose groups			
0.01–0.049 Gy	19	43.6	6.0
0.50–3.99 Gy	27	124.5	17.2
4.0 and up	30	310.0	42.7
Unexposed siblings	11	7.3	1.0
			(reference group)

*Overall, the average dose was 1.36 Gy for the thymus-irradiated group. The RRs are calculated by the ratio of each exposure group compared to the unexposed, for example, overall, 102.2/7.3, and for the middle dose group, 124.5/7.3. (Source: Reference 29.)

giving us a sound temporal association. Next, let's consider *strength of association*. We calculated an RR of 2.0 for malignant extrathyroid tumors, which is considerably large, a doubling of risk for infants exposed to irradiation compared to their nonirradiated siblings. In other reports using these data, there are even larger estimates of risk, including an RR of 14.1 for thyroid tumors when comparing all the subjects that had the X-rays and their siblings (Table 5.10). This is evidence of a strong association between exposure to X-rays in infancy and a risk of various benign and malignant tumors at multiple body sites later in life. Even more striking is the evidence that when the RR is calculated for exposed infants based on how much radiation they received, we see increasingly larger relative risks in Table 5.10. Although the overall RR is large, this *dose response* gives us even more evidence to consider when making an inference. For *plausibility*, we consider the biological effects of radiation. Even without consulting specific scientific and animal studies, we know that radiation can cause cancer. In this study, we also know that the X-rays were directed at the same area of the body as the thyroid, so this really makes biological (and common) sense: the highest RR for tumors was in the site that received radiation. Finally, we consider if the evidence is *consistent*, that is, whether we see the same kind of association in other studies. A literature search would tell you that there is evidence that large amounts of X-rays seem to cause cancers. This was an unusual cohort study, so there is no direct evidence from similar observational studies, but there have been cohort studies that assess tumor and cancer incidence among people exposed to atomic bombs, for example. Can we make a causal inference about X-ray radiation for enlarged thymus in infancy and thyroid and other tumors later in life? Yes. The overall summary of the causal criteria is very compelling.

Summary

In this chapter, we have discussed the basic epidemiological study designs, the components of analytic epidemiology, and criteria for assessing the exposure–outcome relationship investigated in these studies. We distinguished observational studies, those in which the researcher simply collects information about exposure and outcome from people who self-select their exposures, from experimental studies, those in which the researcher assigns participants to a particular exposure group. Observational studies include ecological, cross-sectional, cohort, and case–control studies. Experimental studies include randomized controlled trials and community trials. We also have covered the basic analytic tools for these studies and have described how to interpret measures of effect. For most study designs, we calculate a relative risk, a ratio of the incidence among the exposed to incidence among the unexposed. However, in a case–control study, the researcher selects people based on outcome, and therefore incidence cannot be calculated. As a result, we must use a different measure, the odds ratio, as the measure of effect in case–control studies. There are many variations on the types of studies presented in this chapter and advanced methods of analyzing study data that are beyond the scope of this textbook, but with this introduction you likely will be able to understand many scientific journal articles and media reports based on these articles. The epidemiological methods and caveats presented in this chapter will make you a more informed consumer and a more prepared professional, if you plan to go into a health-related career. If you are watchful, you will see epidemiology everywhere.

Key Terms

abstract (data), 130

analytic epidemiology, 96

attenuate, 115

background, 129

bias, 114

biologically plausible, 128

blinding, 123

case-control study, 113

causal inference, 126

cohort study, 104

community trial, 124

conclusion, 130

confounder/confounding, 97

consistency, 129

control (subject), 115

correlation, 100

cross-sectional study, 100

dependent variable, 98

dichotomize, 102

differential misclassification, 118

discussion, 130

dose response, 128

double-blind study, 123

ecological fallacy, 98

ecological study, 98

exclusion criteria, 130

experimental study, 122

exposure, 98

Review Questions

1. Do you think these cohorts continue to have important biological and risk information to provide regarding our current exposures to X-rays (for example, the thymus cohorts described in the Rochester Radiation Cohort discussion)? Keep in mind that we still use medical X-rays (annual mammograms, as an example), but the dose now used is quite a bit smaller.

2. For each of the following study descriptions, identify the type of study design used.

   Ecological study   Cross-sectional study   Cohort study
   Case–control study   Randomized trial   Community trial

   a. A research team is interested in whether warfarin (a medication to prevent blood from clotting) reduces the risk of stroke. They ask warfarin's manufacturer for the number of annual warfarin prescriptions in the United

States from 1990 to 2000 and use data from death certificates to assess the numbers of deaths due to stroke in the United States during the same time period. The resulting graph showed that the number of annual warfarin prescriptions increased in the United States from 1990 to 2000 and stroke mortality in the United States declined from 1990 to 2000.

b. A group of researchers is interested in quantifying the relationship between smoking and throat cancer, and they also hope to identify other risk factors for throat cancer. They design a study of 375 people sampled in the following way: 125 people who have been diagnosed with throat cancer and 250 people who have not been diagnosed with throat cancer were selected from hospital records. Among other exposures, these individuals were asked about their smoking history.

c. In 1747, James Lind conducted a study to evaluate several treatments for scurvy aboard a ship named the *Salisbury*. To find the most effective treatment for the disease, he chose twelve sailors with scurvy who were as similar as possible and divided them at random into six groups of two. He gave each pair of sailors a different treatment and followed them over several days to assess whether the sailors' conditions improved.

3. We design a study to investigate whether heavy alcohol consumption during college is related to mental health diagnoses later in life. We recruit one hundred college students who drink heavily and one hundred college students who do not drink heavily, follow them over twenty years, and look at incident mental health problems. Among heavy alcohol drinkers, twenty-two report mental health diagnoses after twenty years, and among the non-heavy drinker group, seventeen later report mental health diagnoses.

a. What is the study design used in this example?

b. What is the correct measure of association between heavy alcohol consumption during college and mental health diagnoses later in life?

4. In a study of tuna consumption and mercury poisoning, we find that as people consume more canned tuna, the likelihood they have mercury poisoning increases:

Average Servings of Canned Tuna per Week	Diagnosed Mercury Poisoning (*n*)	No Mercury Poisoning (*n*)	Relative Risk (RR) for Mercury Poisoning
0	1	5,150	1.0 (Reference group)
1–2	3	5,240	
3–5	5	5,100	
>5	16	5,120	

a. This provides evidence for which aspect of causal inference?

b. Fill in the remaining relative risk measurements in the last column of the table.

5. We are designing a study to quantify the risk of diabetes among people who are obese (body mass index [BMI] > 30) compared to people who are neither overweight nor obese (BMI < 25). Family history is known to be an important risk factor for diabetes. What would we call family history in this study?

6. In a cohort study of regular physical activity and incident diabetes in older adults, the researchers report the following data. Researchers used medical records and baseline examinations to assure all study participants were free of diabetes at the start of the study. Previous studies have found that regular exercise among older adults is protective against diabetes.

	Incident Diabetes	No Incident Diabetes
Adults who meet physical activity recommendations	50	50
Adults who do not meet physical activity recommendations	75	25

a. Calculate the appropriate measure of association between regular physical activity and incident diabetes in this study.

b. Interpret the measure of association you calculated in part (a).

c. Assess the five aspects of causal inference for this study using the information provided.

References

1. Kelsey JL, Whittemore AS, Evans AS, Thompson WD. *Methods in Observational Epidemiology*. 2nd ed. New York: Oxford University Press; 1986.

2. Koepsell TD, Weiss, NS. *Epidemiologic Methods*. New York: Oxford University Press; 2003.

3. Hennekens CH, Buring JE. *Epidemiology in Medicine*. Boston, Mass.: Little, Brown, and Co.; 1987.

4. Friedman GD. *Primer of Epidemiology*. 4th ed. New York: McGraw Hill; 1994.

5. Schlesselman JJ. *Case Control Studies: Design, Conduct, and Analysis*. New York: Oxford University Press; 1982.

6. Rothman KJ, Greenland S. *Modern Epidemiology*. 2nd ed. Philadelphia, Pa.: Lippincott-Raven; 1998.

7. Gail HG, Benichou J, eds. *Encyclopedia of Epidemiologic Methods.* New York: John Wiley; 2000.

8. Oleckno WA. *Essential Epidemiology.* Long Grove, Ill.: Waveland Press Inc.; 2002.

9. Selvin HC. Durkheim's suicide and problems of empirical research. *Am J Sociol.* 1958;63(6):607–619.

10. Blakely TA, Woodward AJ. Ecological effects in multi-level studies. *J Epidemiol Community Health.* 2000;54(5):367–374.

11. Greenland S, Robins J. Invited commentary: Ecological studies–biases, misconceptions, and counterexamples. *Am J Epidemiol.* 1994;139(8):747–760.

12. Piantadosi S. Invited commentary: Ecological biases. *Am J Epidemiol.* 1994;139(8): 761–764.

13. Schwartz S. The fallacy of the ecological fallacy: The potential miscues of a concept and the consequences. *Am J Public Health.* 1994;84(5):819–824.

14. Susser M. The logic in ecological: I. The logic of analysis. *Am J Public Health.* 1994; 84(5):825–829.

15. Susser M. The logic in ecological: II. The logic of design. *Am J Public Health.* 1994; 84(5):825–829.

16. Selove R, Andresen EM. *Early Onset of Mobility Impairment as a Significant Risk Factor for Adult Unemployment.* Saint Louis, Mo.: School of Public Health, Saint Louis University; 2000.

17. Samet JM, Muñoz A. Perspective: Cohort studies. *Epidemiol Rev.* 1998;20(1): 135–136.

18. Checkoway H, Pearce NE, Crawford Brown DJ. *Research Methods in Occupational Epidemiology.* New York: Oxford University Press; 1989.

19. DeFries Bouldin EL, Andresen EM. Caregiver health. In: J. C. Cavanaugh and D. K. Cavanaugh (eds.). *Aging in America: Psychological, Physical, and Social Issues.* Westport, Conn.: Greenwood Publishing Group; 2010 (in press).

20. Simonsick EM, Newman AB, Nevitt MC, et al. Measuring higher level physical function in well-functioning older adults: Expanding familiar approaches in the Health ABC study. *J Gerontol A Biol Sci Med Sci.* 2001;56(10):M644–M649.

21. Taaffe DR, Simonsick EM, Visser M, et al. Lower extremity physical performance and hip bone mineral density in elderly black and white men and women: Cross-sectional associations in the Health ABC Study. *J Gerontol A Biol Sci Med Sci.* 2003;58(10):M934–M942.

22. WHI Study Group. Design of the Women's Health Initiative Clinical Trial and Observational Study. *Control Clin Trials* 1988;19(1):61–109.

23. Kannel WB. Some lessons in cardiovascular epidemiology from Framingham. *Am J Cardiol.* 1976;37(2):269–282.

24. Lenfant C, Stone E, Castelli W. Celebrating 40 years of the Framingham Heart Study. *J Sch Health.* 1987;57(7):279–281.

25. Splansky GL, Corey D, Yang Q, et al. The Third Generation Cohort of the National Heart, Lung, and Blood Institute's Framingham Heart Study: Design, recruitment, and initial examination. *Am J Epidemiol.* 2007;165(11):1328–1135.

26. Andresen, EM, Hildreth NG. On epidemiology and the obligation to notify study subjects. *Letter Epidemiology Monitor.* 1992;13(4):4,6.

27. Hildreth NG, Shore RE, Dvoretsky PM. The risk of breast cancer after irradiation of the thymus in infancy. *New Engl J Med.* 1989;321(19):1281–1284.

28. Shore R, Hempelmann LH, Kowaluk E, et al. Breast neoplasms in women treated with x-rays for acute postpartum mastitis. *J Natl Cancer Inst.* 1977;59(3):813–822.

29. Shore RE, Hildreth N, Dvoretsky P, Pasternack B, Andresen E. Benign thyroid adenomas among persons X irradiated in infancy for enlarged thymus glands. *Radiat Res.* 1993;134(2):217–223.

30. Shore RE, Hildreth N, Dvoretsky P, Andresen E, Moseson M, Pasternack B. Thyroid cancer among persons given X-ray treatment in infancy for enlarged thymus glands. *Am J Epidemiol.* 1993;137(10):1068, 1080.

31. Andresen EM, Machuga CR, Van Booven ME, Egel J, Chibnall JT, Tait R. Effects and costs of tracing strategies on noresponse bias in a survey of workers with low-back injury. *Public Opin Q.* 2008;72(1):40–54.

32. Koo MM, Rohan TE. Use of World Wide Web-based directories for tracing subjects in epidemiologic studies. *Am J Epidemiol.* 2000;152(9):889–894.

33. Centers for Disease Control and Prevention (CDC). National Death Index page. Available at: www.cdc.gov/nchs/ndi.htm. Accessed Oct. 21, 2009.

34. Fillenbaum GG, Burchett BM, Blazer DG. Identifying a national death index match. *Am J Epidemiol.* 2009;170(4):515–518.

35. Rich Edwards JW, Corsano KA, Stampfer MJ. Test of the National Death Index and Equifax nationwide death search. *Am J Epidemiol.* 1994;140(11):1016–1019.

36. Hildreth NG, Shore RE, Hempelman LH, Rosenstein M. Risk of extrathyroid tumors following radiation treatment in infancy for thymic enlargement. *Radiat Res.* 1985;102(3):378–391.

37. Thompson WD. Statistical analysis of case-control studies. *Epidemiol Rev.* 1994;16(1):33–50.

38. Porta M, ed. *A Dictionary of Epidemiology.* 5th ed. New York: Oxford University Press; 2008.

39. Armstrong BK, White E, Saracci R. *Principles of Exposure Measurement in Epidemiology.* Monographs in Epidemiology and Biostatistics, vol. 21. New York: Oxford University Press; 1992.

40. Silverman DT, Hoover RN, Swanson GM. Artificial sweeteners and lower urinary tract cancer: Hospital vs. population controls. *Am J Epidemiol.* 1983;117(3):326–334.

41. Greenland S, Thomas DC. On the need for the rare disease assumption in case-control studies. *Am J Epidemiol.* 1982;116(3):547–553.

42. Piantadosi S. *Clinical Trials. A Methodologic Perspective.* Hoboken, N.J.: John Wiley; 2005.

43. Rossignol A. *Principles and Practice of Epidemiology: An Engaged Approach.* New York: McGraw Hill; 2005.

44. Savitz DA. *Interpreting Epidemiologic Evidence.* New York: Oxford University Press; 2003.

45. Rothman KJ, ed. *Causal Inference.* Chestnut Hill, Mass.: Epidemiologic Resources Inc.; 1988.

46. Herbst AL, Ulfelder H, Poskanzer DC. Adenocarcinoma of the vagina. Association of maternal stilbestrol therapy with tumor appearance in young women. *New Engl J Med.* 1971;284(15):878–881.

47. Veurink M, Koster M, Berg LT. The history of DES, lessons to be learned. *Pharm World Sci.* 2005;27(3):139–143.

48. Bonomi AE, Anderson ML, Reid RJ, Rivara FP, Carrell D, Thompson RS. Medical and psychosocial diagnoses in women with a history of intimate partner violence. *Arch Intern Med.* 2009;169(18):1692–1697.

49. Martin SL, Rentz ED, Chan RL, et al. Physical and sexual violence among North Carolina women: Associations with physical health, mental health, and functional impairment. *Women's Health Issues.* 2008;18(2):130–140.

50. Duffey KJ, Gordon-Larsen P, Ayala GX, Popkin BM. Birthplace is associated with more adverse dietary profiles for US-born than for foreign-born Latino adults. *J Nutr.* 2008;138(12):2428–2435.

51. Moore LV, Diez Roux AV, Brines S. Comparing perception-based and geographic information system (GIS)-based characterizations of the local food environment. *J Urban Health.* 2008;85(2):206–216.

52. Beral V. Mortality among oral-contraceptive users. Royal College of General Practitioners' Oral Contraception Study. *Lancet.* 1977;2(8041):727–731.

53. Mann JI, Inman WH. Oral contraceptives and death from myocardial infarction. *Br Med J.* 1975;2(5965):245–248.

CHAPTER 6

BIOSTATISTICS

Babette A. Brumback, PhD

LEARNING OBJECTIVES

- Discover the field of biostatistics and learn about its history.
- Become familiar with two case studies involving biostatistical analyses of epidemiological data.
- Recognize sources of bias in the collection and analysis of epidemiological data.
- Become familiar with a few basic descriptive statistical methods, both numerical and graphical.
- Learn basic statistical concepts such as probability, sample, population, simple random sampling, statistic, sampling distribution, *p* values, confidence intervals, and statistical significance.
- Interpret logistic regression analyses that adjust for confounding of an odds ratio.
- Apply what you have learned about biostatistics to the investigation of the two case studies.

Biostatistics is the theoretical, methodological, and applied science of collecting, organizing, summarizing, presenting, analyzing, and interpreting data for the purpose of advancing health science and health policy (see Chapter 14 for more on health policy). Biostatistics has its beginnings as early as 1662, when John Graunt investigated death records of London parishes in an attempt to answer questions such as, What percentage of children die before six years of age[1]? In 1854, John Snow famously plotted households with deaths due to cholera on a graph of the London water supply and then correctly interpreted these data to claim a causal connection. The source of water predicted who died of cholera (see more about this historical event in Chapter 1). The fields of biostatistics and statistics are very closely related, primarily differing in *purpose*. Both experienced tremendous theoretical advances in the early twentieth century due to the pioneering efforts of K. Pearson, W. Gosset, R.A. Fisher, J. Neyman, and E.S. Pearson. In the mid-twentieth century, the field of biostatistics began to grow due to the new presence of biostatisticians at the U.S. National Institutes of Health[2], training grants for young people to study biostatistics at universities, and the inclusion of departments of biostatistics within schools of public health. Today, biostatisticians routinely make use of ever more powerful computers and statistical software to analyze large datasets that were, until recently, impossible to handle. There continues to be a shortage of biostatisticians and job opportunities are many; a recent survey ranked mathematicians, actuaries, and statisticians (including biostatisticians) as having the three best jobs in the country when rated on stress, physical demands, hiring outlook, compensation, and work environment[3].

In this chapter we will introduce you to biostatistics through two case studies of biostatistical analyses of epidemiological data. Students are often drawn to study biostatistics when they first need to analyze or interpret data in order to address an intriguing and important scientific question. We will use the case studies to describe sources of bias in collection and analysis of epidemiological data, to illustrate some basic descriptive statistical methods, to introduce basic biostatistical concepts, and to demonstrate the use of regression analysis to adjust for one of the most important sources of bias, that of confounding (see Chapter 3 for more information about public health data).

Two Case Studies

One of the most important principles of biostatistics is the necessity of a clearly posed scientific question to guide meaningful data collection and analysis. Sometimes we are limited in our ability to address the question due to practical constraints or barriers to data collection, such as ethical constraints preventing us from forcing people to participate in observational studies or barring us from undertaking some kinds of randomized clinical trials (see Chapter 5 for more detail on study designs). Furthermore, health researchers and policy makers may be limited by the biostatistical techniques familiar to them. Therefore, it is common and desirable for public health researchers to develop a collaborative relationship with biostatisticians, who make it their business to learn, research, develop, and apply a large variety of statistical techniques appropriate for health data. Additionally, biostatisticians will rank among the best critics of published data analyses due to their highly trained analytical minds and their constant exposure to a myriad of research designs and analytical strategies for investigating a wide spectrum of health questions.

Case Study A

Does a Reduction in Sodium Intake Prevent Cardiovascular Disease?

In the February 6, 2009, issue of the *New York Times*, an op-ed article entitled "A Pinch of Science," written by a scientist named Michael Alderman[4], questioned a recent campaign by the New York City Department of Health and Mental Hygiene "to persuade the makers of processed food to reduce its salt content by more than 40 percent over the next 10 years." Alderman argued that if such a large reduction were actually achieved, people in the United States would be consuming less sodium than people in most other developed countries and that this might have unintended harmful consequences. He also pointed out that although it is commonly presumed that increased salt intake raises blood pressure, in some people there is no effect and in others blood pressure actually falls. And although it is fairly well established that increased sodium intake increases blood pressure on average, it is a matter of controversy whether reducing salt intake will ultimately prevent heart attacks and strokes and thus improve health or extend life[5,6].

We followed up on this article by researching the health literature for studies on the connection between sodium intake and cardiovascular disease. In this chapter, we will focus on three such studies: (1) an observational study by He et al.[7] published in the *Journal of the American Medical Association* analyzing data from participants enrolled from 1971 to 1975 in the first National Health and Nutrition Examination Survey (NHANES) Epidemiologic Follow-Up Study; (2) an observational study by Cohen et al.[8] published in the *American Journal of Medicine* analyzing data from participants enrolled from 1976 to 1980 in the second NHANES cohort study (Alderman is a coauthor of this study); and (3) a long-term follow-up study by Cook et al.[9] published in the *British Medical Journal* analyzing data from randomized clinical trial participants enrolled from 1987 to 1992 in the first and second Trial of Hypertension Prevention (TOHP).

The results are conflicting. The He study concludes that higher sodium intake is associated with *increased* risk of cardiovascular disease mortality in overweight persons. The Cohen study concludes that higher sodium intake is associated with *decreased* risk of cardiovascular disease mortality. The Cook study concludes that higher sodium intake is associated with *increased* risk of cardiovascular disease morbidity and mortality. Due to its position as the *gold standard* of evidence-based research, the randomized clinical trial would typically weigh heavily in health policy decisions such as the one undertaken by the New York City Department of Health and Mental Hygiene. However, in the next section, we will show that all three studies are prone to sources of bias common among epidemiological studies, whether randomized or not. As described in Chapter 5,

bias is a systematic difference in the results of a study from what in fact is occurring[10].

Case Study B

Does Treatment with Zidovudine Increase Short-Term CD4 Counts in a Cohort of HIV-Positive Men?

Acquired immunodeficiency syndrome (AIDS) was first described in 1981; by March 1983, the Centers for Disease Control and Prevention had received reports of more than 1,200 cases, about 75 percent of which had occurred in homosexual men. In mid-1983, the Multicenter AIDS Cohort Study (MACS) was conceived to try to better understand the early course of disease, to explore possible protective factors for infection by the human immunodeficiency virus (HIV), and to formulate possible prevention and/or early therapy trials. Nearly 5,000 homosexual men from four cities (Los Angeles, Chicago, Baltimore/ Washington, D.C., and Pittsburgh) volunteered for semiannual interviews, physical examinations, and laboratory testing[11]. Zidovudine (also known as azidothymidine, or AZT) was one of the earliest therapies found in randomized clinical trials to be somewhat efficacious in treating AIDS and in increasing CD4 cell counts, a marker of immune system health, in asymptomatic HIV infection[12,13]. In 1991, an analysis of HIV-positive MACS participants showed that pre-AIDS zidovudine was associated with a reduction in the rate of progression to AIDS[14].

The MACS **data** are publicly available for a small fee and are subject to no sharing restrictions (see www.statepi.jhsph.edu/macs/pdt.html for information on obtaining the dataset). Participants were tested biannually over a period of time. We obtained MACS data and restricted the **cohort** to 812 participants who were positive for HIV as of visit number 9, who had never used zidovudine, and who had valid CD4 count measurements for visits 9 and 10. Visit 9 occurred in or around 1988 and was selected because zidovudine had been available for long enough that several study participants were starting to use it. Visit 10 occurred approximately six months afterward. Ninety-nine of the participants started zidovudine therapy between visits 9 and 10. In this chapter, we use these data to answer the following question: did initiation of zidovudine between visits 9 and 10 increase the odds of a CD4 count above 250 at visit 10? To answer this question, we will **dichotomize** the participants, or split them into two groups, according to whether their visit-10 CD4 count was greater than 250 (CD4 outcome = 0) or less than 250 (CD4 outcome = 1). Later in the chapter, we will show you how to use logistic regression to adjust for **confounding bias** in the analysis of whether zidovudine use reduces odds of a low CD4 outcome.

Biases in Collecting and Analyzing Epidemiological Data

The collection and analysis of epidemiological data invariably introduces some biases into the attempt to answer a scientific question. For example, in a randomized clinical trial, participants are typically not randomly selected from the population of interest, but rather they are a *convenience* sample of people who will agree to enroll and to sign an informed consent form. Furthermore, enrolled participants often do not follow the treatment protocol as written, and if the follow-up time is lengthy, several will typically drop out of the study, rendering their outcomes unobservable and unanalyzable. In this context alone, we already have three examples of sources of bias in collecting epidemiological data. The first, **selection bias**, is bias that results when the sampled participants are not a representative probability sample of the population of interest. A **probability sample** is one in which the chance of selecting any given subset of the population is known. The simplest form of a probability sample is a **simple random sample**, in which any subset of size n has an equal chance of being selected from a population of size N. Intuitively, a simple random sample will be a **representative sample** of the population because it does not increase the chance that any one group will be included; for example, it is not over-representing older people, or healthier people, or men. Researchers are often left with no option but to use a convenience sample, which is not a probability sample, let alone a representative sample. However, it is commonplace to *assume* that the theoretical properties of biostatistical methods developed for simple random samples pertain to the convenience sample. This assumption can be dangerous, and it is rarely correct, but in some circumstances it may be a reasonable approximation. In other circumstances, researchers might render conclusions about a **hypothetical population**, as if the convenience sample had been obtained from the hypothetical population using a simple random sample. The problem with this approach is that the researcher may not understand the nature of the hypothetical population very well at all. For example, the TOHP follow-up trial studied participants in the two prior TOHP I and TOHP II clinical trials. As with most clinical trials, these participants were partly selected based on the inclusion/exclusion restrictions of the protocol (for example, age thirty to fifty-four, mean diastolic blood pressure of 80–89 mm Hg without antihypertensive medication, etc.) but also based on their willingness to enter the trial. Thus the hypothetical population is defined not only by inclusion/exclusion restrictions but also by willingness to enter the trial, a vague characteristic. Finally, because the participants are not a random sample of people who are willing to enter the trial but rather a convenience sample of people who happened to successfully volunteer, the researchers may not have accounted for other characteristics of the group of participants, such as their health status or their distance to clinic sites.

The second source of bias in the randomized clinical trial context is that of **measurement error**; that is, some participants are documented to be following the treatment protocol, but they are not, in fact, following it. For example, a participant may have discontinued treatment after a short period due to adverse side effects or may have switched to an alternative treatment. When these participants are analyzed as if they were following the treatment protocol, the analysis is biased due to measurement error. More generally, measurement error ensues when a recorded measure is not completely correct. In case study A, sodium intake for the two observational studies is measured using a self-reported 24-hour recall questionnaire; however, the measurement is interpreted to represent general level of sodium intake over a long period of time. Clearly, this interpretation is incorrect, and thus the data on sodium intake are subject to measurement error. Related to this, another known source of bias is called **recall bias**, in which participants cannot correctly recall the answer to one or more survey questions. Recall bias is a special case of measurement error, as is **interviewer bias**, which is due to improper data collection methods used by a survey interviewer, such as asking a question while displaying an obvious opinion or prejudice as to the desirable answer. To avoid this bias, interviewers should be trained well and have good communication skills.

The third source of bias that plagues many randomized clinical trials is bias due to **missing data**. A participant in the trial will have missing outcome data if he or she drops out of the study before the outcome is measured. Sporadic missing data can also occur at any time in the study if the participant refuses to answer a question (participants often refuse to answer questions about their income for example), data on a participant are lost, or the participant is too sick to attend a scheduled laboratory or clinical visit. Many standard methods of statistical analysis simply ignore participants for whom some data are missing; these methods are called **complete-case analyses**. In general, these methods are biased, and assistance of a biostatistician should be sought in using more advanced methods that attempt to adjust for bias due to missing data. For example, suppose that the randomized trial is designed to compare a new treatment to a standard treatment, and the health status outcome is more often missing in people who were taking the new treatment because it had adverse effects that caused them to be very ill and drop out of the study. Here, in a complete-case analysis, the new treatment will appear to be better than it really is because the people excluded from the analysis in the new treatment group would all have had poor outcomes. In this example, we can see that a complete-case analysis effectively imposes selection bias by dropping some participants from the sample. A biostatistician can aid in implementing statistical analyses that adjust for this selection bias.

One important source of bias in observational studies that does not hamper ordinary clinical trials is bias due to confounding. Confounding of an exposure or treatment effect can occur when participants who happen to be exposed or treated are not comparable with participants who happen to be unexposed or untreated due to a fundamental difference that may also affect the outcome. In case study A, the observational studies of sodium intake each began with a nationally representative probability sample, because that is how NHANES is conducted[15]. However, people in the sample are not randomized to various dosages of sodium intake; rather, they have chosen to eat a given quantity of salty foods to suit their taste or health beliefs. Therefore, the people on high-sodium diets are not necessarily comparable to the people on low-sodium diets; perhaps the study respondents on high-sodium diets tend to be predisposed to cardiovascular disease for other reasons, whereas those on low sodium diets do not have this tendency. In this case, sodium intake will appear to cause cardio-vascular disease, even in the very circumstance in which it has no effect what-soever. In case study B, there is likely to be what is often termed **confounding by indication**; that is, participants on zidovudine are likely to be those who were *indicated* for it due to low CD4 counts, presence of opportunistic infections, or other symptoms of HIV illness. Thus the health status of these individuals tends to be compromised compared with those who do not take zidovudine. In particular, the CD4 counts prior to zidovudine initiation will likely be lower in the zidovudine group than in the control group. Therefore, CD4 counts just subsequent to zidovudine initiation will likely be lower in the zidovudine group, even if zidovudine itself has no effect. The bias in the simple, unadjusted com-parison of CD4 counts across the zidovudine group and the control group (those who did not initiate zidovudine between visits 9 and 10) thus causes zidovudine to appear harmful, when, in fact, it may even be helpful. Later in the chapter, we will use logistic regression to adjust for confounding of this comparison by CD4 count at visit 9.

Confounding is considered to be such an insidious form of bias that random-ized clinical trials are recognized as the gold standard for evidence-based research, despite their own limitations, which we have only partly summarized here; that is, methods for adjusting for confounding bias are considered to be inadequate relative to the validity of results from randomized clinical trials. **Validity** refers to a lack of bias in data or results[10, p. 251]. This is because the leftover confounding, or **residual confounding**, is seldom thought to be readily apparent and hence is not amenable to further adjustment. In short, consumers of health advice based on either observational studies or randomized clinical trials should be wary. In fact, one good reason for citizens to learn more about biostatistics is to be able to read and understand the statistical methods used for health study design and analysis, as well as their limitations due to various sources of bias, including but not limited to those we have just described. Citizens who are more informed about biostatistical methods will, arguably, be better equipped to gauge relative health hazards and benefits and make better personal choices (see more about health behavior in Chapter 11).

Health scientists plan to collect as much data as possible in their research study design in order to adjust for various sources of bias. For example, data on important confounders such as age, gender, and health status are necessary in order to adjust for confounding bias due to these factors. When the data used for bias adjustment are collected as part of the research study, the bias adjustment is termed *internal adjustment*. However, it is often impossible to collect all the data that would be required for full bias adjustment. In these cases, knowledge or opinions or data gathered outside of the research study can be used for *external bias adjustment*. One method of external bias adjustment is that of a **sensitivity analysis**, in which data pertaining to the bias are fabricated and the analysis is redone. Often, the sensitivity analysis is repeated for several different suspected types of bias to investigate the sensitivity of results to various unmeasured sources of bias. We will illustrate this method in the next section in the context of case study A.

Basic Descriptive Statistical Methods

In all data analyses, the first and most important step is to fully describe the data collected. Data description can be numerical, such as presentation of **frequencies** (numbers of people within certain categories), **means** (averages), or **odds ratios** (refer back to Chapter 5 for a complete discussion), or graphical, such as the histograms we will present for case study B. Data description can focus on one measurement at a time, which is called a **univariate** description (because a measurement is sometimes termed a *variable*), or on two measurements at a time (**bivariate** description), or on many measurements at a time (**multivariate** description).

We will illustrate some of the basic descriptive statistical methods for the two case studies. For case study A, Table 6.1 presents descriptive statistics showing some of the results of the sodium reduction TOHP follow-up study extracted from Cook et al.[9], Table 6.2. Participants (3,126 people) were randomized into one of two intervention groups: a **treatment group** (1,518 people) given an intervention designed to reduce sodium intake and a **control group** (1,608

Table 6.1 Descriptive Statistics for the TOHP Follow-up Study

Disease (D)	I = 1 (Treatment)			Response (R)	I = 0 (Control)	
	R = 1	R = 0			R = 1	R = 0
D = 1	88	?		**D = 1**	112	?
D = 0	1,081	?		**D = 0**	1,134	?
Totals	1,169	349			1,246	362
Proportions	88/1,169 = 0.075	?			112/1,246 = 0.090	?

Table 6.2 Analytic 2 × 2 Table for TOHP Follow-up Study

	Cardiovascular Event or Death (D = 1)	No Cardiovascular Event or Death (D = 0)
Intervention (I = 1)	88 (a)	1,081 (b)
Control (I = 0)	112 (c)	1,134 (d)

people) designed for its participants to receive usual medical care. Several of these participants were lost to follow-up, meaning that the outcome, or presence of cardiovascular disease or mortality years later, was not obtained. The measurements, often termed **variables** due to the algebraic notation, we will concern ourselves with are intervention group ($I = 1$ for treatment and $I = 0$ for control); response ($R = 1$ for an outcome that was obtained and $R = 0$ for a participant who was lost to follow-up); and the outcome, cardiovascular disease or mortality ($D = 1$ for a responding participant with cardiovascular disease or who died, and $D = 0$ for the other responding participants).

Table 6.1 presents multivariate descriptive statistics, focusing on the joint relationship between the measurements I, R, and D. From the table, we see that the percentage of cardiovascular events in the treatment group is 7.5% versus 9.0% in the control group, if we focus only on the responders (those with $R = 1$). Some further calculation shows us that the proportion responding is 1,169/ (349 + 1,169) = 0.77 in the treatment group and 1,246/(1,246 + 362) = 0.77 in the control group. Thus the proportion responding is similar in the two groups. If we assume that the nonresponders (those with $R = 0$) are similar to the responders in terms of their rates of cardiovascular events, then we would conclude that those randomized to the treatment group had a lower cardiovascular event rate than those randomized to the control group and that the intervention to reduce sodium intake appears to prevent cardiovascular disease. The odds ratio is 0.82, which quantifies the **preventive effect** of the treatment, the amount by which the intervention reduces the odds of the outcome.

Table 6.3 Sensitivity Analysis in Terms of Descriptive Statistics for the TOHP Follow-up Study

Disease (D)	$I = 1$ (Treatment)			$I = 0$ (Control)	
	$R = 1$ (Response (R))	$R = 0$		$R = 1$	$R = 0$
$D = 1$	88	49	$D = 1$	112	9
$D = 0$	1,081	300	$D = 0$	1,134	353
Totals	1,169	349		1,246	362
Proportions	88/1,169 = 0.075	49/349 = 0.140		112/1,246 = 0.090	9/362 = 0.025
Overall proportion	137/1,518 = 0.090			121/1,608 = 0.075	

$$OR = ad/bc = (88*1,134)/(1,081*112) = 0.8242$$

However, it may be that the nonresponders are quite different from the responders in terms of their rate of cardiovascular events. Thus the complete-case analysis above (in which we used data only from responders or those with complete data and ignored data from nonresponders) may be biased due to missing data from the nonresponders. A simple sensitivity analysis depicted in Table 6.3 shows that this bias could conceivably have had the effect of exactly *reversing* the correct conclusion: we see that if the event rate in the nonresponders in the treatment group were 49/349 = 0.14, and if in the nonresponders it were 9/362 = 0.025, then the comparison of the overall event rate in the treatment group would then be 9% and in the control group 7.5%. The odds ratio would then be 1.22, the reciprocal of the previous result. It is the responsibility of the scientists to design and present results of plausible sensitivity analyses, but not everyone has the same vision of what is plausible or not. If a scientist thought it plausible that 14% of the nonresponders in the treatment group had an event whereas only 2.5% of the nonresponders in the control group had such an event, then that scientist would think it plausible that the treatment appears to harm patients in terms of causing cardiovascular disease.

Perhaps the largest source of bias in the TOHP follow-up study is measurement error. Participants in the treatment group were taught to reduce sodium intake, but it is unknown whether they maintained such a diet over the several years of the follow-up period. Furthermore, some participants in the control group may have reduced the sodium in their own diets. Possibly just being in the study, coupled with news and medical advice on sodium intake, would prompt participants to change their diets. Thus, analyzing participants according to intervention group may give a biased impression of the effect of a reduction of sodium intake on cardiovascular outcome due to measurement error. It is the responsibility of the scientists reporting the study results to discuss the plausible direction of this bias.

Case study B gives us another opportunity to illustrate basic descriptive statistics in action. Previously, we mentioned the possibility that study participants who were on the HIV treatment zidovudine had lower CD4 counts at the pretreatment visit (sometimes called the **baseline** visit) than those not on zidovudine. The histograms displayed in Figure 6.1 confirm this. A **histogram**, which is similar to a bar chart, portrays the distribution of measurements within

FIGURE 6.1 Histograms of Baseline CD4 Count in the Non-Zidovudine Group (Top) and in the Zidovudine Group (Bottom)

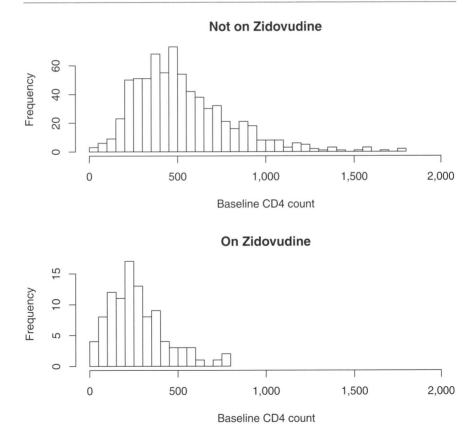

the sample. Each bar represents the frequency of sampled participants within each range (shown in Figure 6.1) of the measurements. We observe that there are ten bars between 0 and 500; thus, each range is of size 50. We see, for example, that of those who do not initiate zidovudine between visits 9 and 10, over 60 people have CD4 counts between 450 and 500 at visit 9, whereas of those who do initiate the treatment, fewer than 5 have CD4 counts between 450 and 500 at baseline. To account for there being more persons not on zidovudine than on zidovudine, we could instead present *relative* frequencies on the *y* axis rather than frequencies; that is, we could divide the frequencies by the total number of people in each group. However, the histograms we have drawn show us clearly that in the zidovudine group the bulk of the sampled people have CD4 counts below 500, whereas in the not-on-zidovudine group a sizeable proportion have CD4 counts above 500. Thus, as we anticipated, there is confounding by indication in this case study.

The histogram is helpful and conveys a lot of information at once, but sometimes a numerical description is helpful as well. It is typical to accompany a histogram with a **five-number summary**, which conveys the quintiles of the distribution. The five quintiles list the five **percentiles**: 0th percentile (also known as the **minimum**), 25th percentile, 50th percentile (also known as the **median**), 75th percentile, and 100th percentile (also known as the **maximum**.) Recall that the 25th percentile is the measurement below which 25% of the sample has scored, and so forth for the other percentiles. For the group that is not on zidovudine, the five-number summary is 3, 343, 474, 675, and 1,771; thus half of that group have baseline CD4 counts lower than 474. For the group that is on zidovudine, the five-number summary is 12, 174, 245, 358, and 781; thus half of that group have baseline CD4 counts lower than 245—further confirmation that the measurements are lower in the group on zidovudine.

Other descriptive statistics that are useful for our example are the sample means and proportions or percentages. About 12% of the entire group is in the subgroup on zidovudine versus about 88% not on zidovudine. The sample mean baseline CD4 count, the average for the study participants, is 273 for the subgroup on zidovudine and 529 for the subgroup not on zidovudine. We see that the sample means convey information similar to that which the sample medians reported previously. We also notice that the sample means are higher than the sample medians. This is due to the shape of the histograms: the histograms are not bell-shaped (also referred to as normal) curves, but rather have a longer tail to the right. These higher measurements in the right-hand tails cause the means to be higher than the medians.

Basic Biostatistical Concepts

We have already encountered some basic biostatistical concepts in our discussion of the two case study examples and in our discussion of various forms of bias. Some formal definitions can be helpful, however. For example, **probability** quantifies chance on a scale from 0 to 1, with 0 indicating no chance and 1 indicating certainty. A probability is thus a proportion, and it can be thought of as representing the long-run relative frequency of a chance event. For example, the probability of heads on a fair coin toss is 0.5; this means that if we repeatedly toss the coin in an independent fashion (so that one toss is not related to the next), the proportion of heads (the number of times the coin shows heads divided by the number of tosses) will tend toward 0.5 or 50%. Probability is sometimes called **risk**; for example, perhaps the risk for members of a certain population developing cardiovascular disease within a defined period of time is 9%. That is, if we take a random member of that population, there is a 9% probability that he or she will develop cardiovascular disease. If we sample more and more members of that population at random, the proportion developing cardiovascular disease will tend toward 0.09.

The goal of applied statistics can be **descriptive**, as we saw in the previous section, in which we used numerical and graphical techniques to describe the sample, or **inferential**, meaning that we use a random sample to draw conclusions, or make inferences about, an entire population. For example, suppose that, in case study A, the TOHP study responders represented a simple random sample of the general population of the United States. In that case, one might draw the conclusion that the effect of treatment to encourage sodium intake reduction would decrease the risk of cardiovascular disease and mortality during the follow-up time period from 9% to 7.5% *in the United States population* and not just in the sampled study participants. Thus we would use the study sample to draw an inference about the entire United States population. The sample proportions 0.09 and 0.075 are known as statistics. A **statistic** is simply a quantity computable from the data collected on the sample. When the sample is a probability sample, in other words, a random sample, any statistic computed from the data would vary from one possible sample to another.

For example, in one sample, the risk of cardiovascular disease in untreated individuals might be 9.0%, but in another sample it may be 9.4%, and in yet another, 8.8%. Similarly, the odds ratio we observed in the sample of responders was 0.82 (indicating protection or prevention effect). In another sample, it might be 0.74 and in yet another, 0.99. The variability of a statistic (for example, the odds ratio) is known as its **sampling variability**. Sampling variability refers to the spread of the distribution of the statistic for repeated samples, that is, the spread of its **sampling distribution**. In the case of the TOPH study, 1,169 U.S. residents were randomized to the treatment and 1,246 randomized to the control group. In those particular residents, in other words, in our sample, the odds ratio was 0.82. One summary of the spread of the sampling distribution for this statistic is a 95% confidence interval. A 95% **confidence interval** is a random interval, computed based on the random sample, which has a 95% probability of including the population odds ratio. The **population odds ratio** is the odds ratio we would compute if we had randomized the *entire* U.S. population to the two intervention groups. It is a single, nonrandom, number. The 95% confidence interval for our population odds ratio is (0.62, 1.10). All the values of the population odds ratio within this confidence interval are considered plausible; thus, the population odds ratio might plausibly be greater than 1, or less than 1. The data from the study are not conclusive for deciding whether the treatment prevents or causes cardiovascular disease.

Sometimes we are interested in testing a statistical hypothesis, such as: the population odds ratio is equal to 1, meaning that there is no association in the population between the intervention and the cardiovascular outcome. The result of such a test is summarized by what is known as a p value. A p **value** is the probability that the sample statistic will be as far or farther away from the hypothesized value on repeated sampling. In our example, the p value is 0.19. The sample statistic odds ratio is 0.82, which is somewhat far from 1 (or 1.0, meaning the groups are equally likely to have the outcome). However, there is a 19% chance that repeated sample statistics would be as far away from 1. The measure of distance in this case is not simple: we actually measure the distance from 0.82 to 1.0 on a *log-transformed* scale. Thus there is a 19% chance that repeated sample statistics would be either below 0.82 or above 1.22; these two numbers are not symmetric about 1.0 due to the log-transformed scale. A common threshold for deciding whether to reject the hypothesis is 5%; thus p values below 5% would lead us to reject the hypothesis and conclude that the population odds ratio is not equal to 1. A frustrating feature of hypothesis testing is that one cannot ever conclude that the hypothesis is true: we are only allowed to conclude that it is false or that it may or may not be true. In our example, the p value of 19% is greater than the threshold of 5%, thus we cannot reject the hypothesis. We are left in a state of limbo and uncertainty. We cannot say for certain that the hypothesis is true, that is, that the true odds ratio is 1, because the 95% confidence interval tells us that numbers between 0.62 and 1.10 are all plausible. Were the p value, instead, less than 5%, we would be able to conclude that the odds ratio of 0.82 was **statistically significant**. This would mean that it is not less than 1 due to chance, that is, due to random sampling, and that we can conclude that the population odds ratio is indeed less than 1. However, because our p value is 19%, we can only conclude that the odds ratio of 0.82 is *not statistically significant* and that it may be less than 1 due to chance variability.

Using Regression Analysis to Adjust for Confounding

The investigators in the TOHP study in case study A did not stop with the odds ratio of 0.82 and the p value of 19%. Instead, they used regression to adjust the measure of effect for precision variables such as age, race, and gender. Because the intervention was a randomized trial, we would conclude there is not a large amount of confounding. However, the risk of a cardiovascular event in the control group might vary across age, race, and/or gender groups. This leads to excess sampling variability, which can be reduced using regression analysis to adjust for precision variables. When the TOHP investigators adjusted for precision variables, they found that treatment was statistically significantly associated with reduced incidence of cardiovascular disease outcomes.

Another reason to use regression analysis is to adjust for confounding variables. In observational studies, such as case studies A and B, it is necessary to adjust for confounding bias when reporting a treatment effect because the treatment has not been randomized. In case study A, some of the confounding variables adjusted for were age, race, sex, baseline blood pressure, and body mass index (a measure of obesity). Note that the same variable, age, can be treated as a precision variable in one study but as a confounding variable in another.

In this section, we will use logistic regression analysis with case study B to adjust for confounding by indication of the odds ratio, which measures the association between zidovudine and CD4 count at visit 10. We will consider only one confounding variable, CD4 count at visit 9, because it is arguably the most important confounder in this analysis.

A **logistic regression model** is a statistical model of the form:

$$\log[P(E,C)/(1-P(E,C))] = \alpha + \beta E + \gamma C \qquad (1)$$

where, in our example, $P(E,C)$ is the probability of the outcome event under the conditions of E and C, E is a dichotomized exposure or treatment of interest ($E = 1$ for treatment, $E = 0$ otherwise), and C is a confounder (such as CD4 count at visit 9.) One can also use the model without C, as

$$\log[P(E)/(1-P(E))] = \alpha + \theta E \qquad (2)$$

In model (2), the coefficient θ can be shown to represent the log odds ratio for the association between E and the outcome, because for $E = 1$, $\alpha + \theta = \log[P(1)/(1 - P(1))]$ is the odds of the outcome given exposure, and for $E = 0$, $\alpha = \log[P(0)/(1 - P(0))]$ is the odds of the outcome given no exposure. Simple algebra yields $\theta = \log[P(1)/(1 - P(1))] - \log[P(0)/(1 - P(0))]$, and thus θ is the log odds ratio. Hence, a logistic regression model such as (2) can be used to calculate odds ratios.

A logistic regression model such as (1) can be used to calculate the odds ratio for the association between E and the outcome for individuals with the same value of C. That is, suppose we consider only individuals with a CD4 count of, say, $C = k$ (k could equal 200, 500, or some other fixed value) at visit 9. Then again, simple algebra yields that the coefficient $\beta = \log[P(1,k)/(1 - P(1,k))] - \log[P(0,k)/(1 - P(0,k))]$, and thus β is also a log odds ratio, but for individuals with the same value of C. We can thus use model (1) to adjust for confounding bias by computing not the overall odds ratio $\exp(\theta)$ (often termed the **crude odds ratio** because it is unadjusted), but the **adjusted odds ratio** $\exp(\beta)$, which controls for confounding bias by gauging the association between E and the outcome for individuals with the same value of the confounder. The idea is to measure the effect of E on the outcome, *all else being equal*.

We used the free Centers for Disease Control and Prevention software Epi Info, downloadable at www.cdc.gov/epiinfo/, to conduct logistic regression analyses using the MACS data. Recall that the outcome event is a CD4 count at visit 10 that is less than 250, and the exposure, or treatment, is zidovudine use between visits 9 and 10 ($E = 1$ for zidovudine use, $E = 0$ for no zidovudine use). For model (2), we estimated the crude odds ratio $\exp(\theta)$ at 5.10 with a 95% confidence interval of (3.28, 7.96). The p value is less than 0.0001. Hence, the crude odds ratio is statistically significant, and we can conclude that the population crude odds ratio is greater than 1, indicating that zidovudine use between visits 9 and 10 is associated with a CD4 count below 250 at visit 10.

Could zidovudine use be causing CD4 counts at subsequent visits to be below 250? Possibly. Or perhaps our estimate suffers from confounding bias. Thus we next used model (1) and estimated the adjusted odds ratio $\exp(\beta)$ at 0.95, with a 95% confidence interval of (0.52, 1.75). The p value is 0.88. Hence the adjusted odds ratio is not statistically significant, and we cannot conclude that the population adjusted odds ratio is less than 1. However, we also cannot conclude that the population adjusted odds ratio is greater than 1, and so our adjusted analysis leads us to believe that zidovudine use is not necessarily causing subsequent CD4 counts to be below 250. Rather, our initial result was confounded.

Revisiting the Two Case Studies

You may have noticed that for each of the case studies, our answer to the scientific question is we still do not know. Further research is necessary to discover the answers, if in fact they are discoverable. It is possible that, due to logistics such as measurement error of sodium intake and the long duration of the required follow-up period, we will never know the answer to the question in case study A. For case study B, clinical trials and larger observational studies have documented that zidovudine use does in fact increase CD4 counts[12,13,16]. Our adjusted analysis estimated the odds ratio at 0.95, which represents an association of zidovudine use with subsequent CD4 counts above 250, but it was *not* statistically significant. Perhaps if we had a larger sample, we would have observed a statistically significant result. It is a fact of biostatistics that ever larger samples tend to lead to statistical significance, eventually. Given this fact, it is important to judge not only whether a result is statistically significant but whether it is *practically* significant. Is an odds ratio of 0.95 practically significant, when compared with an odds ratio of 1.0? That depends on subject matter considerations; it is not strictly speaking a biostatistical question. It is also a difficult question because an odds ratio of 0.95 might represent the change in risks from 0.20 to 0.21, or from 0.020 to 0.021, for example. The former change may or may not be thought to have practical significance, depending on the severity of the disease, but the latter is unlikely to have practical significance. Issues in causal inference, adding to statistical inference, are discussed in Chapter 5.

Nevertheless, without knowledge of biostatistics, you would not be able to make much sense of the scientific health evidence presented for either of our two questions. Some investigations return an answer of *yes*, others *no*, and still others *we do not know*, but nearly all investigations rely on biostatistics.

Summary

This chapter has introduced you to the exciting field of biostatistics and demonstrated its relevance to research and policy in the health sciences by way of two case studies. We have taught you to begin to recognize various forms of bias in epidemiological data analysis because bias is the primary threat to the validity of epidemiological conclusions. Bias may arise because of the way a sample is selected; selection bias results when the sampled participants are not a representative probability sample of the population of interest. We discussed different types of samples, including convenience and simple random samples. Measurement error can lead to bias, for example, when study participants are incorrectly classified as being exposed when they did not follow the treatment protocol. Recall bias and interviewer bias are also types of measurement error that can lead to inaccurate conclusions. We have introduced you to some basic descriptive statistical techniques, including numerical descriptions using frequencies (numbers of people within certain categories), means (averages), or odds ratios (the odds of an outcome in the exposed group compared to the unexposed group), and graphical presentations using histograms (for case study B). We also covered some basic biostatistical concepts. We discussed the concept of probability, the proportion (ranging from 0 to 1) that represents the relative frequency of a chance event, which is sometimes called risk. We also described the meaning and use of confidence intervals and p values related to odds ratios. Finally, we have given you a quick tutorial on the use of regression analysis to adjust for confounding bias. Regression analysis provides an odds ratio to measure the effect of an exposure on the outcome of interest. Odds ratios may be crude measures or they may be adjusted for confounding variables.

The field of biostatistics is quite broad, and we have only begun to introduce you to it. There are so many biostatistical methods in common use, and still others being invented all the time, that a full study of biostatistics can take longer than one lifetime. We hope this chapter will lead you to an appreciation of the field of biostatistics and a desire for more understanding of and proficiency with the biostatistical tools that are used by virtually all researchers and policy makers in the health sciences. Who knows, perhaps one day you will become a biostatistician!

Key Terms

adjusted odds ratio, 154

baseline, 149

bias, 142

bivariate, 146

cohort, 142

complete-case analysis, 144

confidence interval, 152

confounding bias, 142

confounding by indication, 145

control group, 146

crude odds ratio, 154

data, 142

descriptive, 151

dichotomize, 142

Review Questions

1. Describe sources of bias that can hinder the interpretation of randomized clinical trials.
2. Describe sources of bias that can hinder the interpretation of observational studies.
3. If you read the two medical articles associated with the observational studies of case study A, you find that both studies began with representative random samples of the U.S. population. However, the Cohen et al.[8] study excluded 2,096 out of 9,250 (23%) participants due to medical and other reasons, whereas He et al.[7] excluded 4,922 out of 14,407 (34%) participants. Do you think this differential exclusion rate might have caused selection bias? Could it possibly account for the discrepancy in study results (which go in opposite directions)?
4. Reconstruct the missing data in Table 6.1 to redo Table 6.3 such that the overall proportions are equal to 0.09 in each of the intervention groups.
5. Referring to Figure 6.1, which group has a higher proportion of people with baseline CD4 counts greater than 1,000: the group on zidovudine or the group not on zidovudine?
6. When using biostatistics for the purpose of inference, do we make inferences from the population to the sample or from the sample to the population? Discuss.

7. Download Epi Info and the MACS dataset (the MACS dataset is available at this textbook's Web site) and conduct the two logistic regression analyses for yourself. Do you get the same answers?

References

1. Gehan EA, Lemak NA. *Statistics in Medical Research: Developments in Clinical Trials.* New York: Plenum Medical Book Company; 1994.
2. National Institutes of Health. NIH History. Available at: www.nih.gov/about/history.htm. Accessed May 9, 2010.
3. Streiber A. Careercast Web site. JobsRated.com: A comprehensive ranking of 200 different jobs. Available at: www.careercast.com/jobs/content/JobsRated_Top200Jobs. Accessed May 9, 2010.
4. Alderman M. A pinch of science [op-ed contribution]. *The New York Times.* February 6, 2009. Available at: http://www.nytimes.com/2009/02/06/opinion/06alderman.html. Accessed May 24, 2010.
5. Centers for Disease Control and Prevention (CDC). Salt Web page. Most Americans should consume less sodium. 2009. Available at: www.cdc.gov/dhdsp/library/sodium.htm. Accessed May 9, 2010.
6. Centers for Disease Control and Prevention (CDC). Application of lower sodium intake recommendations to adults—United States, 1999–2006. *MMWR.* 2009;58:281–283.
7. He J, Ogden LG, Vuppurturi S, Bazzano LA, Loria C, Whelton PK. (1999). Dietary sodium intake and subsequent risk of cardiovascular disease in overweight adults. *J Am Med Assoc.* 1999;282:2027–2034.
8. Cohen HW, Hailpern SM, Fang J, Alderman MH. (2006). Sodium intake and mortality in the NHANES II follow-up study. *Am J Med.* 2006;119:275.e7–275.e14.
9. Cook NR, Cutler JA, Obarzanek E, et al. (2007). Long term effects of dietary sodium reduction on cardiovascular disease outcomes: Observational follow-up of the trials of hypertension prevention (TOHP). *Br Med J.* 2007;334:885.
10. Porta M, ed. *A Dictionary of Epidemiology.* 5th ed. New York: Oxford University Press; 2008.
11. Kaslow, RA, Ostrow DG, Detels R, Phair JP, Polk BF, Rinaldo CR Jr. The multicenter AIDS cohort study: Rationale, organization, and selected characteristics of the participants. *Am J Epidemiol.* 1987;126:310–318.
12. Fischl MA, Richman DD, Grieco MH, et al. The efficacy of azidothymidine (AZT) in the treatment of patients with AIDS and AIDS-related complex. *N Engl J Med.* 1987;317:185–191.
13. Volberding PA, Lagakos SW, Koch MA, et al. Zidovudine in asymptomatic human immunodeficiency virus infection: A controlled trial in persons with fewer than 500 CD4-positive cells per cubic millimeter. *N Engl J Med.* 1990;322:941–949.

14. Graham NMH, Zeger SL, Park, LP, et al. Effect of zidovudine and *Pneumocystis carinii* pneumonia prophylaxis on progression of HIV-1 infection to AIDS. *Lancet.* 1991;338:265.

15. National Center for Health Statistics. National Health and Nutrition Examination Survey. Available at: www.cdc.gov/nchs/nhanes.htm. Accessed May 9, 2010.

16. Hernan MA, Brumback BA, Robins JM. Estimating the causal effect of zidovudine on CD4 count with a marginal structural model for repeated measures. *Stat Med.* 2002;21:1689–1709.

CHAPTER 7

PHARMACOEPIDEMIOLOGY

Almut G. Winterstein, PhD

LEARNING OBJECTIVES

- Outline the development of drug safety and pharmacoepidemiological research in the United States.
- Describe key areas of inquiry in pharmacoepidemiology.
- Explain key methodological challenges, including sample size requirements for the discovery of rare drug effects, exposure definition and misclassification, determination of proximity, and confounding.

This chapter will describe the use of epidemiology in assessing and understanding the effects of pharmaceutical drugs on human health. Many of the study designs and methods described in previous chapters can be used in the field of pharmacoepidemiology, but there are also unique challenges and terminology to learn. This chapter will begin with a more complete description of the field, followed by a brief history of pharmacoepidemiology, including the role of the Food and Drug Administration and the drug approval process in the United States. We will then discuss the core areas of discovery in pharmacoepidemiology. The chapter will conclude with a brief introduction of some of the key methodological challenges in pharmacoepidemiology.

What Is Pharmacoepidemiology?

Pharmacoepidemiology has been defined as the application of epidemiological reasoning, methods, and knowledge to the study of the uses and effects of drugs in human populations[1]. Evaluating causal relationships between *exposure* (drugs) and *outcomes* (clinical or other effects on human well-being) is grounded in pharmacology. Pharmacology in turn encompasses two disciplines, **pharmacokinetics**, the science of how drugs are absorbed, distributed, metabolized, and excreted by the body (what the *body* does to the drug), and **pharmacodynamics**, how drugs act through receptors or other mechanisms in the body (what the *drug* does to the body)[2]. Both scientific disciplines are needed to predict and explain how drugs have positive or negative effects on patient health. Although some or most of these effects are explained in preclinical and small-scale clinical trials prior to drug approval, a substantial body of evidence accumulates after a drug has been approved and is used by larger populations with more diverse characteristics and under less controlled conditions. The exploration of these effects, the *population-based* evaluation of drug effects, is the core area of discovery in pharmacoepidemiology. Because population-based evaluation studies take place in real life, with health care providers and patients making decisions about drug use or nonuse rather than following a stringent study protocol, pharmacoepidemiology offers some of the greatest methodological challenges in clinical research. However, its ability to ascertain information on drug effects in millions of people positions it as an indispensable discipline in clinical science.

History of Pharmacoepidemiology

Pharmacoepidemiology evolved with the increasing concern about adverse drug effects. Today it is inconceivable that in the past drugs were marketed without proof of efficacy or safety. Visit a pharmacy museum and you will discover heroin cough syrup or digoxin (a medication for heart failure that can be lethal if not dosed very carefully) tablets sold over-the-counter, illustrating the lack of regulation at the beginning of the twentieth century. Concerns manifested when, in the 1930s, a druggist sold a cough syrup with the active ingredient, sulfanilamide, accidentally dissolved in glycol (anti-freeze), killing more than one hundred people[3]. The Federal Food, Drug, and Cosmetic Act of 1938, requiring preclinical (animal) toxicity testing, was introduced shortly thereafter.

It took several decades until the next great regulatory step toward drug safety and efficacy was made, the **Kefauver-Harris Amendment**. This amendment was preceded by several drug disasters, including the discovery of chloramphenicol-induced blood dyscrasias (abnormalities) and the detrimental birth defects caused by thalidomide, a drug that had been praised as a mild and harmless sleep agent.[4] (For a great review of the thalidomide case see also Seidman and colleagues[5].) The Kefauver-Harris Amendment not only strengthened the requirements for premarketing safety studies but also asked for proof of efficacy before a drug can be marketed in the United States. Some of the key events in the twentieth century that characterize the evolution of drug safety are as follows:

- 1906: Pure Food and Drug Act

- 1937: Sulfanilamide disaster

- 1938: Food, Drug, and Cosmetic Act

- 1952: American Medical Association (AMA) Council on Pharmacy and Chemistry first registry of adverse drug effects (ADE)

- 1960: Food and Drug Administration (FDA) hospital-based ADE reporting system (Johns Hopkins, Boston Collaborative Drug Surveillance Program, and Shands at University of Florida)

- 1961: Thalidomide disaster (not marketed in United States)

- 1962: Kefauver-Harris Amendment to Food, Drug, and Cosmetic Act

The last three decades of the twentieth century were characterized by increasing data on adverse drug events, some with severe consequences and impact on large populations. Examples include subacute myelo-optic neuropathy (SMON) caused, presumably, by clioquinol, which was marketed for mild diarrhea; clear cell adenocarcinoma in females who were exposed to diethylstilbestrol in utero (before birth)[6]; and blood dyscrasia caused by phenylbutazone[7]. The increase in adverse drug events was a result of the increasing variety and use of medications as well as a continuously improving surveillance system that was better at detecting patterns and establishing linkages between adverse outcomes and drug exposures. The 1970s and 1980s saw the first population-based safety studies, predominantly based on retrospective analysis of Medicaid claims data. This field has expanded tremendously during the early twenty-first century, not only in the number of individuals that are represented in such data but also in the breadth and depth of data that can be accessed electronically.

Drug Approval and Safety Systems

The United States drug approval process governed by the current version of the Food, Drug and Cosmetic Act largely follows the original requirements established by the Kefauver-Harris Amendment and is divided into several phases. The first is a **preclinical phase** in which efficacy and safety are established

FIGURE 7.1 The Food and Drug Administration (FDA) Drug Development Process

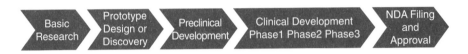

in animal models. Next, there are three **clinical phases** (i.e., conducted in humans). The first includes studies in healthy volunteers (phase 1); the second includes a small number of patients (usually less than one hundred) with the disease, symptom, or risk factor the medication is supposed to treat or prevent (phase 2); and the third clinical phase includes a larger number of patients (about one hundred to one thousand) with the condition of interest (phase 3). Acceptable data on preclinical and clinical phases suggesting a greater benefit than harm are required before a drug is approved by the Food and Drug Administration (FDA)[8]. All of these studies are considered **premarketing**, meaning that they occurred before a drug was approved by the FDA and allowed to be marketed to the general public. Later we will discuss **postmarketing** studies, those studies conducted once a drug is FDA-approved and publicly available.

The drug development and approval process depicted in Figure 7.1 is exemplified by the following timeline[9]. Paclitaxel, a core treatment for ovarian cancer, was isolated from the Pacific yew tree in 1971. In 1977 preclinical studies were started to explore potential antineoplastic (anti-cancer) effects, resulting in an **investigational new drug (IND) application** to the FDA in 1983. An IND application is the formal request for authorization to use an investigational drug in humans. Phase 1 studies began in 1984, followed by phase 2 in 1986, and phase 3 studies in 1990. Finally, the **new drug application (NDA)**, the vehicle through which drug sponsors formally propose that the FDA approve a new drug for sale and marketing in the United States, was submitted in July 1992 and approved by the FDA in December of the same year. More than twenty years passed between the discovery of the chemical substance and the appearance of the approved drug on the market. Fast approval tracks are available in special circumstances such as the development of medications for the treatment of AIDS.

It is important to note that the number of patients who have been exposed to a new drug before it is approved has not exceeded a few thousand. In addition, these patients are commonly healthier than the broad population who may use the drug after approval. Shortcomings of premarketing studies, including those just stated, are that subjects:

- are too few (small study samples);

- are too healthy (free of comorbidities, and subjects have only the disease the drug is supposed to treat);

- have no concomitant use of medications (to avoid interactions with the study drug);

- are too middle-aged (children and elderly patients who may be more frail are not enrolled);

- are too controlled (drug use and patient health is monitored closely as part of trial protocol); and

- are too narrowly defined (patients are recruited by a few study centers, have little sociodemographic diversity).

The focus on a very narrowly defined, well-controlled, and quite homogenous patient sample is scientifically warranted because it allows estimation of the best drug effect under ideal conditions, the drug efficacy. It is therefore not surprising that side effects often are not detected; they might be rare (not detectable in the small samples of premarketing studies) or manifest only in certain predisposed patients who were not included in the clinical trials. If safety concerns arise during the premarketing trials that do not warrant that a beneficial agent be withheld from the public but should be investigated further, the FDA can require postmarketing studies (phase 4 studies). Approval is then contingent upon completion of such studies by the manufacturer within a defined time period (but the drug can be sold and marketed before the study is completed). Unfortunately, the FDA used to have no regulatory power to act if phase 4 studies were not completed, which has resulted in many delays and heavy debate in recent years[10]. The Food and Drug Administration Amendment Act (FDAAA) has established some ability to enforce the requirements for phase 4 studies, but the effect of this change remains to be seen.

In contrast to premarketing studies, which are typically designed as randomized trials, phase 4 studies can be randomized or observational (see Chapter 5 for details about study design). For example, it would be ethically impossible to recruit and randomize pregnant women to explore potential teratogenic (causing birth defects) effects of a new drug. However, some pregnant women will be intentionally or unintentionally exposed to a new drug in real life, and drug effects can then be studied with retrospective observational designs.

Even if phase 4 studies are not required, the FDA will ask the manufacturer to establish an active surveillance system to monitor side effects after a new drug is marketed. This system draws on spontaneous reports of side effects by patients or health care providers either to the manufacturer or directly to the FDA. Although spontaneous reports cannot establish causality between the drug and a suspected side effect (each report is a single case study), they can provide important signals that can be evaluated in subsequent studies. The effectiveness of spontaneous reporting systems is, of course, dependent on individuals' ability to recognize relationships between drugs and patient signs or symptoms and the realization that these should be reported. The vigilance of a physician in New Zealand who observed similarities between birth defects of the offspring of several of his patients and noticed the commonality in exposure to thalidomide accelerated the withdrawal of thalidomide through his case report, but many other drug safety problems have gone unnoticed or unreported.

In summary, the U.S. regulatory mechanisms used to ascertain drug safety information are the following:

- preclinical trials
- premarketing clinical trials (phases 1–3)
- postmarketing studies (phase 4)
- spontaneous reporting

This brief review may already demonstrate that the current drug approval and vigilance system is not optimal to ensure that drugs are safe. In fact, between 1975 and 2000 a total of nineteen drugs were withdrawn from the market because of safety problems that had been unknown or considered minor at the time of approval[11].

The most large-scale safety problem in the history of drugs, the withdrawal of rofecoxib (Vioxx®) in 2005, occurred after the increased risk of cardiac events was discovered by chance[12]. Rofecoxib, a pain medication, had been approved without requirement for phase 4 studies. Although the premarketing studies suggested mild increases in blood pressure among patients taking rofecoxib, effects had been considered negligible. No alert was published by the FDA indicating a large number of spontaneous reports of cardiac side effects after approval. Concern arose from a postmarketing clinical study that had been designed by the manufacturer to prove the superiority of rofecoxib over traditional painkillers in terms of reduced gastrointestinal side effects. Analysis of cardiac events in the two comparison groups suggested a larger risk for myocardial infarction (heart attack) in patients exposed to rofecoxib when compared to naproxen (e.g., Aleve®, manufactured by Bayer Healthcare). Subsequent retrospective

Table 7.1 Case–control Study Results Comparing the Risk for Myocardial Infarction or Sudden Cardiac Death in Patients Exposed to Rofecoxib or Ibuprofen to Remote Use of Pain Medications

	Cases	Controls	Unadjusted Odds Ratio (95% CI)	Adjusted Odds Ratio (95% CI)	p
Remote use	4,658	18,720	1.00	1.00	
Ibuprofen	670	2,573	1.07 (0.98–1.18)	1.06 (0.96–1.17)	0.27
Rofecoxib (all doses)	68	196	1.39 (1.05–1.83)	1.34 (0.98–1.82)	0.066
Rofecoxib ≤25 mg	58	188	1.23 (0.92–1.66)	1.23 (0.89–1.71)	0.21
Rofecoxib >25 mg	10	8	5.03 (1.98–12.76)	3.00 (1.09–8.31)	0.03

CI, confidence interval; p, probability.
Source: Reference 14.

observational studies and the early termination of a long-term study evaluating potential benefit of rofecoxib in preventing certain types of colon cancer confirmed the concern and resulted in drug withdrawal. Thus, the detection of this safety problem occurred by accident (because the manufacturer was motivated by potential marketing advantages) and not as part of an effective safety surveillance mechanism surrounding new medications. Observational studies were further able to clarify the concern in a very expeditious manner because pharmacoepidemiologists used retrospective data from a large population, allowing immediate investigation of tens of thousands of exposed patients (Table 7.1)[13].

Core Areas of Discovery in Pharmacoepidemiology

The shortcomings of the drug approval and postmarketing surveillance system identified above explain the need for phase 4 population-based studies and thus the position of pharmacoepidemiology in clinical science. If you have followed the previous paragraphs, you will be able to identify drug safety studies as the core area of discovery in pharmacoepidemiology. Pharmacoepidemiological phase 4 studies can address whether drugs have different effects in subpopulations or how drug effects are altered when used concomitantly with other medications. They can also investigate whether drugs have additional positive effects, which can lead to applications to the FDA for additional indications. In addition to real-life drug safety, two additional areas of inquiry are equally important, **effectiveness studies** and **drug utilization studies**.

The term *effectiveness* is used to distinguish the real-life drug effect from efficacy, the drug effect that has been quantified under controlled conditions and that often describes the most optimal effect that can be expected. At the time of approval, it is not clear whether drug efficacy is generalizable to the whole population who ends up using a certain medication.

Effectiveness can be estimated against a placebo, a biologically inactive substance, but because effectiveness is usually determined in observational studies, comparators including other medications, other treatment options, or no therapy are mostly used. Effectiveness studies compare health outcomes in patients who used a certain medication to health outcomes in patients with the same indication who did not use the medication (not because of the study protocol but because physicians, patients, or other factors determined exposure). An indication is a condition that makes a certain treatment or procedure advisable. For example, a research team at the University of Florida evaluated the effectiveness of palivizumab, a monoclonal antibody with FDA approval for the prevention of certain respiratory viral infections in infants. The drug had shown variable efficacy in different clinical trial populations, leaving questions about its overall effectiveness in real life and specifics on factors that modify efficacy. The need for monthly physician office visits to administer injections raised further questions regarding whether patients would adhere to such a schedule and how nonadherence would affect drug benefit. Thus we compared infection rates in children with and without palivizumab use, considering that the decision to prescribe or receive the prophylactic medication may very well be related to a higher background risk for infections (see discussion on confounding below).

One type of effectiveness evaluation that is currently heavily promoted is comparative effectiveness research. The goal of **comparative effectiveness research** is not the quantification of a drug effect (drug versus no drug) but rather the comparison of two treatment options against each other (drug versus drug). In identifying the best treatment option, comparative effectiveness research fills another gap left unanswered by premarketing studies, which are usually placebo-controlled: whether a new drug is truly superior to an established treatment. Several benefits arise from this information: first, common belief that "newer is better" can be balanced against solid evidence. Second, the fact that a medication with years of marketing history has an inevitably more complete safety profile than a newly approved medication can be considered in light of potential treatment benefits (or lack thereof). And finally, the incremental health gain associated with the superior medication can be compared to the incremental cost (i.e., the difference in cost of the two treatment options) for cost-effective decision making (see Chapter 15 on issues of health care cost in the United States).

Comparative effectiveness studies have a counterpart in **comparative safety studies** in which the safety of two treatment options is compared. Although safety studies are commonly understood to support a decision to remove a medication from the market, milder safety concerns that do not justify withdrawal are also relevant. For example, research had suggested that serious cardiac side effects of short-term use of central nervous system stimulants for the treatment of attention deficit/hyperactivity disorder (ADHD) seem to be rare, but many questions such as consequences of long-term use or safety in predisposed populations (with increased cardiac risk) remained unanswered. Consequently, pharmacoepidemiologists designed a study to compare the risk for milder cardiac symptoms in users of the two most prevalent stimulants, methylphenidate and amphetamines[15].

Drug utilization studies, finally, quantify use of certain medications over time, place, or in certain populations. They may also evaluate what factors determine what, or even if, pharmacological treatment is initiated, switched, or discontinued. For example, interest in pediatric psychopharmacotherapy resulted in several research questions about use of central nervous system stimulants, a drug class including, for example, methylphenidate (Ritalin, manufactured by Novartis) for ADHD. The data show changes in the use and initiation of stimulants during 1995 to 2005, indicating a continuing (and perhaps alarming) growth[16]. Researchers also described patient and provider characteristics that influenced the initiation of stimulants in newly diagnosed children and evaluated how similar factors were related to early treatment discontinuation. For example, youths in rural areas tended to be more likely to receive drug therapy than those in urban areas, even if adjusted for the complexity or severity of disease[17]. Although these findings do not directly deliver clinical information about drug action, they reveal potential disparities or problems in clinical care.

Methodological Challenges in Pharmacoepidemiology

This book has introduced challenges in observational research in Chapter 5, and all these challenges are important in pharmacoepidemiology, as well. Four key challenges are briefly discussed below in the context of pharmacoepidemiological studies:

1. Sample size and data requirements to detect rare drug effects

2. Data ascertainment and definition of drug exposure and misclassification

3. Determination of proximity

4. Confounding

Sample Size Requirements for the Discovery of Rare Drug Effects

Because pharmacoepidemiology has a strong safety focus, the ability to discover rare drug effects is one of the key challenges in respective studies. Not considering ethical or economic constraints, some safety issues cannot be addressed by experimental designs because of simple sample size limitations. For example, in investigating the risk for cardiac sudden death in stimulant users and considering the low baseline risk for such an outcome in an adolescent population, we estimated that one would need approximately two million person-years of follow-up to detect a doubling in risk. One could argue that effects of such rare frequency do not warrant further study or changes in clinical care, but thresholds for serious effects such as death are debatable.

There is to this author's knowledge no prospective study of any drug safety concern that has actively collected data for a sample of such a size. Only retrospective analysis of data collected for clinical or administrative purposes will provide such access, and even these sources have limitations. This is the major explanation for why pharmacoepidemiological study units are centered around large health databases, either in countries with centralized health care systems or third-party payers with good electronic record systems. Active pharmacoepidemiological research units located in Europe and Canada use, for example, National Health Service (NHS) data or the General Practitioner Research Database (GPRD) in the United Kingdom or the Saskatchewan provincial national health care database in Canada. In the United States, academic centers use health care payment data such as Medicaid or Medicare part D claims or group model health maintenance organization (HMO) claims and electronic medical records such as Kaiser Permanente or Group Health of Puget Sound.

Definition of Drug Exposure and Misclassification

The Kaiser Family Foundation reports that a total of 3.6 billion prescription drugs were filled in U.S. pharmacies in 2008[18]. These drugs can be categorized in pharmacological classes, doses, and dosage forms, each with a different pharmacological profile and ten-digit code, the National Drug Code (NDC) maintained by the FDA. There are a number of drug references that offer classification systems that assign each NDC code to broader pharmacological or chemical classes, but careful review of such approaches is important. Some drugs may have multiple indications and appear in multiple categories, and other drugs are combined products with multiple ingredients. To complicate matters, exposure is typically not one-dimensional (yes/no). Drug use can be interrupted, drugs can be switched or discontinued, or several drugs can be used concurrently. Concurrent use of multiple drugs can in turn have synergistic therapeutic effects, meaning that the drug effects can be potentiated when used concomitantly, or drug combinations can increase the risk of side effects. Finally, common methods to ascertain information on exposure are flawed. Prescribing records don't reflect whether patients truly filled their prescriptions, pharmacy dispensing records don't consider whether patients administered their medication, and patient report may not be reliable.

Failure to properly define exposure can result in severe bias. For example, misclassification of patients as being exposed to the study medication who in reality decided not to take the medication will result in a study medication group that is composed of a mix of exposed and unexposed subjects. Thus outcomes in this pseudo-exposed group and the unexposed group will start to look more similar, and the estimate of drug effects will be biased toward the null hypothesis (no effect). Comprehensive ascertainment and validation of exposure information, careful definition of exposed periods, and consideration in design or analysis when exposure is interrupted or discontinued are therefore critical.

Determination of Proximity

The challenges described above can be potentiated when the pharmacological mechanism of a drug effect is not completely clear. Establishment of a causal association between exposure and outcomes requires a temporal relationship, in other words, that exposure comes first and the effect develops thereafter (see also Chapter 5). Another important criterion for causality is proximity, which means that the outcome has to occur soon enough after exposure. *Thereafter* defines a time frame that is long enough for the effect of exposure to develop and short enough for the exposure effect to last. In terms of study design, *thereafter* defines the length of follow-up time that needs to be chosen to determine a certain drug effect. For example, if a drug effect takes some time to manifest, a follow-up time that is too short will not capture the drug effect and will produce a biased result. Understanding of the pharmacological mechanism to quantify such a *latent* or *induction period* is critical. Likewise, if a drug effect is not permanent, a follow-up time that extends beyond the manifestation period of this drug effect may erroneously find no difference between the exposed and unexposed group. Flexible analysis and study designs such as survival analysis, in which the hazard for a certain outcome can be plotted over time, are superior in these circumstances, but a good understanding of the pharmacological mechanism should drive any decisions about the follow-up period.

For example, aminoglycoside antibiotics are known to cause renal problems. Manifestation of renal problems does not happen immediately but rather over a period of several days. (Even if the medication was discontinued in the meantime, adverse renal effects can be observed after several days). Thus studies aimed at assessing the degree of renal damage caused by aminoglycosides that do not allow sufficient follow-up time for manifestation will underestimate the risk. On the other hand, renal problems are typically fully reversible when aminoglycosides are discontinued. Thus, studies that evaluate renal status after a time period that is too removed from the time of exposure will underestimate the problem as well.

Confounding

Confounding represents a significant bias for most observational studies, but it presents a particularly complex challenge in pharmacoepidemiology. Confounding describes a circumstance in which the exposed and unexposed groups show differences in a certain characteristic that is also a direct risk factor for the outcome of interest. Figure 7.2 denotes the relationship between the confounder, exposure, and outcome. Note that there is an association (not necessarily causal) between the confounder and exposure and a causal association between the confounder and the outcome. In terms of pharmacoepidemiology, prescribers or patients choose to use a certain drug for a certain reason, and this reason may very well be directly related to the outcome and thus advantage or disadvantage the exposed when compared to the unexposed. Three specific types of confounding are common and difficult to address in pharmacoepidemiology: confounding by indication, confounding by severity, and confounding by time.

Confounding by Indication

Confounding by indication describes a situation in which a drug is chosen based on a patient's predisposition for the outcome of interest. A common

FIGURE 7.2 Causal or Not Causal Relationships in Confounding

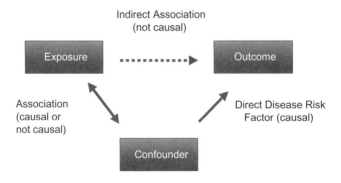

example is the effect of COX-2 inhibitors, a newer class of pain killers with a lower rate of gastrointestinal (GI) side effects compared to traditional pain killers in terms of gastric ulcers or hemorrhage. Because prescribers know about the superiority of COX-2 inhibitors related to GI side effects, they prefer these over traditional pain killers in patients with a history of GI problems. Thus patients at higher risk for recurrent GI problems will be more likely to receive COX-2 inhibitors, and direct (unadjusted) comparisons with traditional pain killers will bias the results, that is, the GI "protective" effect of COX-2 inhibitors may be entirely masked.

Confounding by Severity

Confounding by severity also describes a situation in which a patient will preferably use a medication due to a certain risk that is a direct risk factor for the outcome. In this scenario, the confounder is the severity of the disease the drug is supposed to treat. A common example is when a new drug is perceived as superior to the traditional treatment and is used in circumstances for which the traditional treatment option failed to produce the desired result. This will result in sicker patients in the new drug group when compared to the traditional drug group, a significant disadvantage for the new drug that will lead to biased results.

Confounding by Time

Similar to confounding by severity, **confounding by time** is linked to changes in the underlying disease and the preference for certain treatments. It describes a scenario in which disease progression (or the treatment effect) over time results in preferential drug use. The comparison groups may be well balanced at the beginning of the study, but differential treatment effects may result in treatment adjustments or changes. If this happens, these treatment changes are directly related to the effects of the initial treatment and adjustments for confounding become extremely difficult. In fact, traditional methods such as multivariate models cannot be used to adjust for this type of confounding. An example is the practical response (in terms of treatment choices) in blood pressure control. Typically, a patient will be started on a single blood pressure medication, and the treatment regimen will be modified based on the response. If the blood pressure is not controlled, treatment will be changed. Even if the initial choice of the blood pressure treatment were completely at random, the response to treatment and the subsequent medication choices are not. More difficult to control patients will end up with more effective, higher doses, or multiple drugs, resulting in time-modified confounding.

Summary

Pharmacoepidemiology contributes a critical piece of evidence regarding the use and effects of medications. The increasing focus on drug safety and comparative effectiveness has amplified the need for phase 4 studies and the position of pharmacoepidemiology within drug research. The complexity of drug use poses unique challenges resulting in a wide array of methodological approaches that have been developed, in part, specifically for pharmacoepidemiological research. Sound understanding of both the pharmacology of drug action as well as understanding of sociobehavioral and clinical parameters surrounding prescriber and patient decisions are needed to disentangle drug effects from confounders and other biases.

Key Terms

clinical phase, 164

comparative effectiveness research, 168

comparative safety studies, 169

confounding by indication, 172

confounding by severity, 173

confounding by time, 173

drug utilization studies, 167

effectiveness studies, 167

investigational new drug (IND) application, 164

Kefauver-Harris Amendment, 162

new drug application (NDA), 164

pharmacodynamics, 162

pharmacoepidemiology, 161

pharmacokinetics, 162

postmarketing, 164

preclinical phase, 163

premarketing, 164

Review Questions

1. Describe the various approaches that are in place to govern drug safety in the United States.
2. What are the shortcomings of phase 1 to 3 clinical trials to identify drug safety problems?
3. Consider a study that bases ascertainment of drug exposure on physician records of prescriptions. It is unclear whether patients decided to fill these prescriptions, and even if they did fill them, whether they decided to take the medication. Thus patients who are identified as being exposed to the medication may in fact be unexposed. How does such a misclassification affect the

internal study validity, and if it does introduce bias, how does it change the results?

4. Consider an observational study that compares the effectiveness of a new drug marketed to treat heart failure against the traditionally used treatment regimen. Because the new drug has to be given intravenously, physicians have continued to use the traditional regimen but have started to use the new drug in patients with extremely severe forms of heart failure. What challenges does this scenario pose?

5. Explain how you would determine the follow-up time needed to ascertain whether chronic exposure to antipsychotic medications increases the risk for cardiac events.

References

1. Porta M, Hartzema AG, Tilson HH. The contribution of epidemiology to the study of drug uses and effects. In: Hartzema AG, Porta M, Tilson HH. *Pharmacoepidemiology–An Introduction*. 3rd ed. 1998. Cinicinnati, Ohio: Harvey Whitney Books Company; 1998.

2. Buxton ILO. Pharmacokinetics and pharmacodynamics: The dynamics of drug absorption, distribution, action, and elimination: Introduction. In: Brunton LL, Lazo JS, Parker KL. *Goodman & Gilman's The Pharmacological Basis of Therapeutics* 11th ed. McGraw-Hill's AccessPharmacy. Available at http://www.accessmedicine.com/resourceTOC.aspx?resourceID=28. Accessed October 26, 2009.

3. Geiling EMK, Cannon PR. Pathogenic effects of elixir of sulfanilamide poisoning. *JAMA*. 1938;111:919–26.

4. Lenz W. Malformations caused by drugs in pregnancy. *Am J Dis Child*. 1966;112:99–106.

5. Seidman LA, Warren N. Frances Kelsey and thalidomide in the U.S.: A case study relating to pharmaceutical regulations. *Amer Biol Teacher*. 2002;64:495–500.

6. Herbst AL, Ulfelder H, Poskanzer DC. Adenocarcinoma of the vagina: Association of maternal stilbestrol therapy with tumor appearance in young women. *N Engl J Med*. 1971;284:878–881.

7. Inman WHW. Study of fatal bone marrow depression with special reference to phenylbutazone and oxyphenbutazone. *BMJ*. 1977;1:500–505.

8. Department of Health and Human Services, Food and Drug Administration, Center for Drug Evaluation and Research. *2007 Center for Drug Evaluation and Research update—improving public health through human drugs*. Available at: www.fda.gov/downloads/AboutFDA/CentersOffices/CDER/WhatWeDo/UCM121704.pdf. Accessed July 22, 2009.

9. FDA Consumer Special Report. *From test tube to patients: New drug development in the United States*. 2nd ed. Washington, D.C.: Department of Health and Human

Services, Food and Drug Administration; 1995. Available online at Google books: http://books.google.com/books?id=90vY9523zi8C&pg=PA29&lpg=PA29 &dq=fda+testtube+NDA&source=bl&ots=rUQ7Llez5-&sig=VFHXhf6dLxvYVV pQVRlWRaLCDM&hl=en&ei=ejqUSujODpqQtger3bVC&sa=X&oi=book_ result&ct=result&resnum=2#v=onepage&q=&f=false. Accessed August 24, 2009.

10. Crosse, M. *Drug safety: Further actions needed to improve FDA's postmarket decision-making process.* Washington, D.C.: U.S. Government Accountability Office; May 2009. Available at: www.gao.gov/new.items/d07856t.pdf. Accessed October 26, 2009.

11. Lasser KE, Allen PD, Woolhandler SJ, et al. Timing of new black box warnings and withdrawals for prescription medications. *JAMA.* 2002;287:2215–2220.

12. Kweder, S. *Vioxx and drug safety.* FDA Web site. November 18, 2004. Available at: www.fda.gov/NewsEvents/Testimony/ucm113235.htm. Accessed August 24, 2009.

13. Graham DJ, Campen D, Hui R, et al. Risk of myocardial infarction and sudden cardiac death in patients with cyclo-oxygenase 2 selective and non-selective non-steroidal anti-inflammatory drugs: Nested case-control study. *Lancet.* 2005;365: 475–481.

14. *Ibid.*

15. Winterstein AG, Gerhard T, Shuster J, Saidi A. Cardiac safety of methylphenidate versus amphetamine salts in the treatment of attention-deficit/hyperactivity disorder. *Pediatrics.* 2009;124:e75–80.

16. Winterstein AG, Gerhard T, Shuster J, et al. Utilization of pharmacological treatment in youths with attention-deficit/hyperactivity disorder in Florida Medicaid 1995–2004. *Ann Pharmacother.* 2008;42:24–31.

17. Chen CY, Gerhard T, Winterstein AG. Determinants of initial pharmacological treatments for youths with attention-deficit/hyperactivity disorder. *J Child Adolesc Psychopharmacol.* 2009;19:187–195.

18. Kaiser Family Foundation. *StateHealthFacts.org Web page.* Available at: http:// statehealthfacts.org/profileind.jsp?ind=265&cat=5&rgn=1#at. Accessed October 26, 2009.

CHAPTER 8

INFECTIOUS DISEASE EPIDEMIOLOGY

Cindy Prins, PhD, MPH, CIC

LEARNING OBJECTIVES

- Identify the steps involved in investigating an infectious disease outbreak.
- Describe different types of vaccines.
- Name several diseases that can be prevented by vaccination.
- Recognize the factors that can contribute to emerging infections.

Infectious disease epidemiology focuses on the distribution, spread, and control of infectious diseases. These may include diseases such as smallpox, which can be traced back to 1200–1000 years BC, and more recent emerging infections such as avian influenza. This chapter will describe the history of infectious disease epidemiology, introduce methods used to investigate and mitigate infectious disease outbreaks, explain vaccination and vaccine-preventable diseases, and outline efforts to eradicate certain infectious diseases. As described in Chapter 1, modern nations such as the United States have undergone a transition such that chronic diseases are more common than infectious diseases. However, infectious diseases still account for a substantial amount of the effort expended in public health, and they predominate in developing nations.

History of Infectious Disease Epidemiology

In Chapters 1 and 4, the story of John Snow, considered to be the father of modern epidemiology, was presented. But infectious disease epidemiology dates back much further than London's cholera outbreak of 1854 that Snow mapped. The Greek physician Hippocrates, who lived from 460 BC to 377 BC, described symptoms of disease and categorized infectious disease occurrences as **endemic** (always present within a population) or **epidemic** (not always present within a population, but occasionally affecting a large part of the population). In the mid-sixteenth century, the Italian scientist Girolamo Fracastoro proposed that infectious diseases were caused by particles that spread through the air or from person to person, either directly or through contaminated surfaces. Fracastoro likely did not understand that the particles he referred to were actually **microbes**, minute living organisms, and it was not until over one hundred years later that the Dutch scientist Antoine Van Leeuwenhoek was able to use microscopes to see microbes. Louis Pasteur, a French scientist, demonstrated that microbes were abundant in the environment and proposed that microbes could be the cause of infectious diseases. In the late nineteenth century, German microbiologist Robert Koch proved this connection between microbes and infectious diseases. Koch hypothesized that if a microbe was responsible for a certain disease, then we should be able to isolate the microbe from the diseased individual, grow it in the laboratory, and then use it to infect a healthy individual. The microbe should then cause the same disease in that healthy individual and be reisolated from that individual. This theory was proven and came to be known as **Koch's postulates** (Figure 8.1). Numerous other people, both scientists and nonscientists, made crucial contributions throughout history to the understanding and prevention of infectious diseases. Early infectious disease epidemiology has given way to modern methods of determining how to recognize, control, and ultimately prevent outbreaks of infectious diseases.

Infectious Disease Epidemiology Methods

Chapters 4 and 5 introduced methods of epidemiological investigation and study design. Infectious disease epidemiology uses most of the same methods as other types of epidemiology, but there are some terms and techniques that are specific to the investigation of infectious diseases. In infectious disease epidemiology, a **case** is defined as a person who has clinical signs of an infection. The case may show outward physical signs of infection such as fever, cough, and diarrhea, or may have laboratory results that indicate infection despite the absence of symptoms (also called an **inapparent infection**). An **outbreak** of infectious disease occurs when the number of actual cases is higher than the number of expected cases. The actual and expected number of cases may be determined by using data obtained from government agencies, hospitals, school records, syndromic surveillance systems, or even by determining whether sales of antibiotics or over-the-

FIGURE 8.1 Koch's Postulates

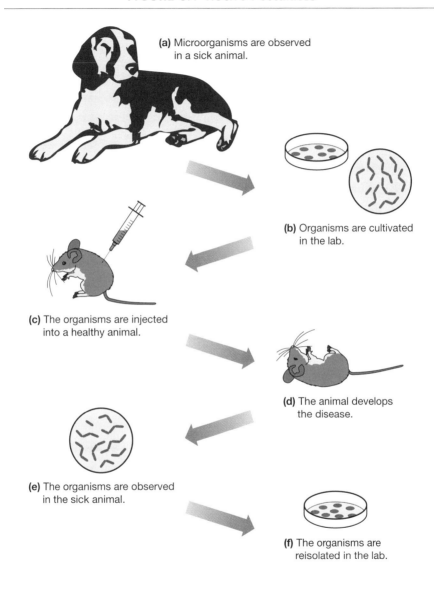

(a) Microorganisms are observed in a sick animal.

(b) Organisms are cultivated in the lab.

(c) The organisms are injected into a healthy animal.

(d) The animal develops the disease.

(e) The organisms are observed in the sick animal.

(f) The organisms are reisolated in the lab.

counter remedies have increased. Chapter 3 describes surveillance data systems in more detail. The calculation of an attack rate is valuable when determining the severity of an outbreak. The formula for calculating the **attack rate** is

$$\text{Attack rate} = \frac{\text{Number of cases}}{\text{number of susceptible people}}$$

It is important to count only susceptible people in the denominator, because people who have been vaccinated against a disease or who were not exposed to the disease will not get it. If those people are included in the denominator, then a lower attack rate will be calculated and the outbreak may not be detected. Once it has been established that an outbreak has occurred, it is crucial to identify people who may have come into contact with an infected person. This is done through a process known as **contact tracing**, which allows epidemiologists to fully investigate and describe the outbreak and to intervene to stop the spread of infection. In the **chain of infection** (Figure 8.2), it is necessary to have a source of the infection, a host for the infection, and a method for carrying the infection from the source to the host. **Sources of infection** may include other people who are infected; animals or insects known as **vectors**, which carry the organism; and an inanimate source such as food or the environment. A **host** is any being that is capable of being infected with the organism that carries the disease. The specific methods of getting the infection from the source to the host vary widely among microbes, but there are three general methods for linking a source and a host. One is **contact transmission**, which is either direct or indirect. Direct contact occurs when the source touches the host and transmits infection. Indirect contact occurs when the source touches an object that then comes into contact with the host. Another method of transmission is **airborne transmission**, in which the source releases the microbe into the air, usually by breathing, coughing, or spitting, and the host comes in contact with it. A vector, described above, usually transmits infection by biting the host.

FIGURE 8.2 Diagram of the Chain of Infection

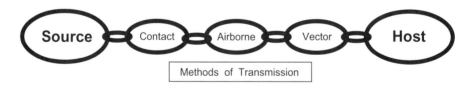

Once it has been established that an outbreak is occurring, it must be described with regard to person, place, and time. These methods of **descriptive epidemiology** are also discussed in Chapter 5. A description of **person** would include demographics such as sex, age, and any other characteristics relevant to the investigation. A description of **place** may make use of a map to determine the geographical area in which the outbreak is occurring or describe the type of place, for example, a day care center or classrooms in a school. An epidemic can be described in terms of **time** by creating an **epidemic curve** (Figure 8.3). This is a graph of the number of infections per unit of time and can be used to

FIGURE 8.3 Epidemic Curves Illustrating a Point Source Outbreak, a Common Source Outbreak, and a Propagated Outbreak

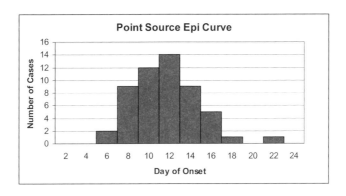

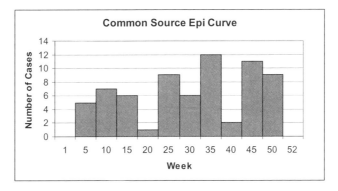

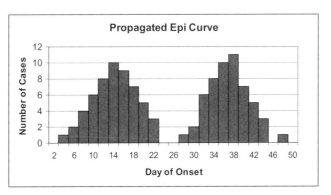

determine whether all the cases were exposed to a single source at a single time (a **point source**), whether the cases were exposed to a single source over a period of time (a **continuous source**), and whether the spread of the infection is from person to person (**propagated**). The elements of time in an epidemic also might include looking at what season is involved (for example, some viruses are more common in fall and winter) or other temporal clues.

Throughout the investigation of an infectious disease outbreak, efforts should be made to control the spread of the disease and to prevent the outbreak from occurring in the future. This effort may be aided by the development and evaluation of a **hypothesis**, or testable theory of the source of the outbreak. The final step of an investigation of an infectious disease outbreak is often overlooked but is crucial to the prevention of future outbreaks from similar sources or situations. This step is to report the findings of the investigation and to share those findings with any groups that may be affected by the results of the investigation.

Today's scientific advances prevent many of the infectious disease outbreaks that have taken place over the past several hundred years. One major advance is the practice of vaccination.

Vaccines and Vaccine-Preventable Diseases

Vaccination is a process that takes advantage of the body's ability to recognize and attack foreign materials inside it and to create a memory of the method of attack, thereby recognizing the foreign object again in the future. When a bacterium or a virus invades the body, antibodies are produced that may specifically recognize the invading microbe. The next time the body encounters that microbe it can destroy it quickly and thus prevent the person from developing an infection. For example, most people who have had chickenpox only develop the disease once. They may be exposed to the disease again, and the virus may enter their bodies, but the antibodies that developed during the first infection prevent the virus from copying itself enough to cause a second bout of chickenpox. Vaccination works in a similar way, except the process prevents a person from developing the initial disease.

Types of Vaccines

There are several types of vaccines that can be categorized by the form of the bacterium or virus used in them. A **live vaccine**, such as the smallpox vaccine, contains a live (infectious) microbe that is similar enough to the disease-causing microbe that it allows the body to later recognize the disease microbe as foreign but not cause disease in the person vaccinated. A **live attenuated vaccine** also uses an infectious microbe, but in this case the microbe has been altered in the laboratory to allow the immune system to recognize it as foreign but to prevent it from causing the disease during vaccination. Examples of live attenuated vaccines are the **intranasal** (sprayed in the nose) influenza vaccine; the measles, mumps, and rubella vaccine (MMR); the chickenpox vaccine; and the oral poliovirus vaccine.

Another type of vaccine is the **inactivated vaccine**. In this case, the disease-causing organism is not infectious, but enough of the organism is present in the vaccine to elicit an immune response. Examples of inactivated vaccines are the **intramuscular** influenza vaccine (administered into the arm muscle), hepatitis A and B vaccines, the human papillomavirus (HPV) vaccine, the rabies vaccine, and the tetanus vaccine. Finally, there are **component vaccines**, which are made up of only the parts of the microbe that the immune system will react to. Examples of component vaccines are the pneumococcal vaccine, the meningococcal vaccine, and the *Haemophilus influenzae* type B vaccine.

Side Effects and Fear of Vaccination

Vaccines have played a major role in the reduction of infectious diseases and the increase in the health of the population, but sometimes they can have side effects. Careful testing of the vaccine before licensing and diligent screening of the individual being vaccinated can reduce the likelihood of adverse vaccine-related events. All potential human vaccines must first be tested in a laboratory setting in a process called preclinical evaluation. The vaccine is then tested on volunteers during the clinical evaluation, which includes three phases of clinical trials to determine whether the vaccine is safe and effective. Finally, the safety and effectiveness data are assessed by the Food and Drug Administration (FDA). The FDA makes the final decision regarding whether the vaccine will be approved, how it should be used, and who should receive it. In general, people who are allergic to any of the vaccine components are advised not to get that vaccine. For example, the influenza vaccine is produced using chicken eggs, so if a person has a severe egg allergy, he or she should not receive the vaccine. Some vaccines are contraindicated for people with weakened immune systems, particularly those vaccines made with live virus, such as the oral polio vaccine.

Despite the low occurrence of serious postvaccination events there has been a trend in recent years to be more fearful of vaccination than the risk warrants and to avoid vaccination altogether. Vaccination is protective for a community in part because when most of the people in the community are vaccinated, the organism has much less of a chance of being carried to and infecting those in the community who are not immune. This concept is known as **herd immunity** or **community immunity**, and it allows the entire community to be protected from a disease. If numerous people within a community refuse vaccination, then there is a much higher likelihood that an outbreak will occur among the nonvaccinated members. Clusters of measles and mumps outbreaks have been reported in recent years stemming from the refusal by some parents to allow their children to receive the MMR vaccine because of perceived risk of the child developing autism after vaccination[1]. This association has been studied, and several publications conclude that there is no link between the MMR vaccine and increasing rates of autism, but fear of the vaccine persists[2]. Vaccination has been credited with saving millions of lives, and it is likely that the success of vaccination in preventing disease contributes to the reluctance of some people to be vaccinated. The current perception that the vaccine is more harmful than the illness itself may arise from present-day experience: people have not seen nor experienced the dangers and side effects of infection from these vaccine-preventable diseases. Over the past fifty years, vaccines have reduced the number of illnesses and deaths due to measles, mumps, rubella, polio, tetanus, pertussis, and scores of other infections. The specific example of the reduction in polio cases in the United States relative to the availability of vaccines appears in Figure 8.4.

FIGURE 8.4 Cases of Polio before and after Introduction of the Inactivated and Live Oral Polio Vaccines, United States 1950–2007

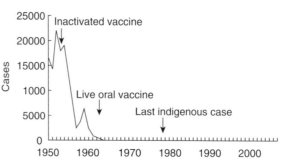

Source: Reference 3.

Disease Eradication

Vaccination has also been responsible for the elimination of one illness completely. The story of the **eradication** of smallpox demonstrates the power of vaccination over a virus that existed for thousands of years.

Smallpox Infection

Smallpox, a disease caused by Variola virus, is transmitted through respiratory secretions and contact with the virus. After an **incubation period**, the time between exposure to the virus and the appearance of symptoms, of seven to seventeen days, the infected person develops fever, headache, malaise, and aches. This is known as the **prodromal stage** of the illness and lasts approximately two days. After this, a rash develops in the mouth and throat and then spreads to the face, arms, and legs. The rash then moves to the hands and feet and the torso. Finally, the rash changes to fluid-filled vesicles, which contain virus, that scab over after about two weeks (Figure 8.5). The infected person is

FIGURE 8.5 Smallpox Pustules on a Child

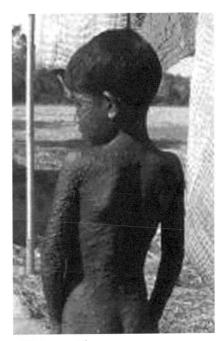

Source: CDC Public Health Image Library.

contagious until all of the scabs have fallen off. The development of the vesicles and scabs usually results in scarring on the person's skin, which visibly distinguishes them as a smallpox survivor.

History of Smallpox

Reliable written accounts of smallpox infection exist from at least the fourth century AD, but there is evidence that the disease was present well before that time. Several Egyptian mummies dating back to 1200–1100 BC have been noted to have lesions consistent with smallpox infection, and the disease is believed to have been the cause of their deaths[4]. By the fifth century AD, smallpox epidemics occurred in Asia, India, and Europe. In Africa, smallpox devastated communities that had never been affected by the disease before it was brought in by ships supplying European settlements in the fifteenth century. In turn, settlers from Europe and slave ships from Africa brought the disease to colonial America. Although some colonists had already been infected with smallpox and developed immunity to the disease, the Native American population of North America was not immune and was devastated by smallpox. Colonists sometimes took advantage of the susceptibility of the Native American population and helped to spread the disease among them. There is speculation that in the eighteenth century smallpox was used as a bioweapon against the Native American population by giving them blankets inoculated with the virus[5]. It would be impossible to account for the full number of deaths caused by smallpox worldwide throughout history, but regional epidemics provide a picture of the ability of the disease to devastate populations. In London there were 36,000 deaths attributable to smallpox from 1780 to 1800[6]. In Quebec City, Canada, an outbreak at the start of the eighteenth century is believed to have killed 25 percent of the population. By the late eighteenth century, smallpox is believed to have killed approximately 400,000 people in Europe yearly. Notable deaths due to smallpox include Ramses V of Egypt in 1157 BC, Queen Mary II of England in 1694, and King Louis XV of France in 1774.

Control of Smallpox Infection

One of the early methods used to protect against naturally acquired smallpox infections was the practice of **variolation** (also referred to as **inoculation**). This practice can be traced to China in 1000 AD and likely also took place in India around the same time. Variolation involved inoculating variola virus from the smallpox scabs of one person into the skin or nose of a nonimmune person. This usually resulted in a less severe smallpox infection with less scarring and a lower mortality rate than naturally acquired smallpox, but still left the person with immunity against the smallpox virus. The practice of variolation spread from India to Asia to Central Europe. In Turkey, Lady Mary Wortey Montague, a British aristocrat living in Constantinople with her ambassador husband and two children, adopted the practice of variolation[4]. In 1715, Lady Montague became infected with smallpox; her brother had died from the disease at the age of twenty. Determined to protect her children from smallpox, Lady Montague had her five-year-old son inoculated against smallpox in Turkey. The family returned to London in 1721, where she had her daughter inoculated in the presence of notable physicians. This action is credited with promoting the wide adoption of variolation in England in the eighteenth century, and the practice then spread to the British colonies in North America. Despite the success of variolation, the practice did have some drawbacks. The mortality rate for variolation was about 0.5 percent to 2 percent, which is lower than the 30 percent mortality rate for naturally acquired smallpox but still high enough to discourage some people from the practice. In addition, variolation of the skin carried a risk of bacterial infection from the incision that was made to introduce the virus into the system, and often people who underwent variolation had a mild illness that allowed them to remain mobile and then spread the disease to others who were not immune. In the late eighteenth century, thanks to the observations of British physician Edward Jenner who himself underwent variolation in 1756 as a boy, the process of variolation began to be replaced with a safer method of protecting people against smallpox called *vaccination.*

It was known in the British countryside at this time that milkmaids were prone to an infection acquired from cows, called cowpox, which resulted in lesions on the hands that resembled smallpox. In contrast to smallpox, cowpox infection was minor, it did not spread from human to human, and it seemed to protect the milkmaids against smallpox infection. Edward Jenner hypothesized that variolation with cowpox virus would protect against infection with smallpox. His opportunity to test this hypothesis came in 1796, when a milkmaid named Sarah Nelmes developed cowpox virus. Jenner isolated the material in the pustules on her hand and used it to inoculate eight-year old James Phipps, who had never had smallpox disease or undergone variolation (Figure 8.6). When Phipps was later variolated with smallpox virus, he did not develop the disease, supporting Jenner's hypothesis that cowpox infection could protect against smallpox infection. Jenner published his findings and named his protective method *Variolae vaccinae*, deriving *vaccinae* from the Latin term for "cow," *vaca*. The term *vaccination*, now widely used, arose from this practice.

Eradication of Smallpox

Jenner's vaccination gained popularity and was used worldwide to protect against smallpox infection. Originally, the virus was passed from person to person

FIGURE 8.6 Artist's Depiction of Edward Jenner Inoculating James Phipps with Cowpox Virus Isolated from Sarah Nelmes's Hand

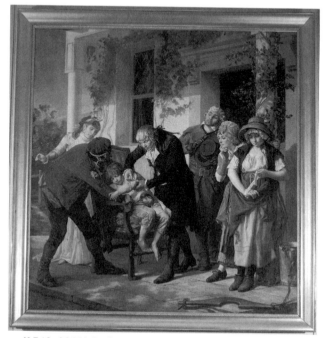

Edward Jenner (1749–1823) Performing the First Vaccination Against Smallpox in 1796, by Gaston Melingue (1840–1914). Used by permission from the Bridgeman Art Library.

through vaccine chains consisting of unvaccinated people, sometimes orphans, who were successively vaccinated to maintain the supply of virus. This arm-to-arm vaccination method was used to transport vaccine throughout the world. In the early twentieth century, vaccine production occurred in factories, and the vaccine strain itself changed from cowpox virus to *Vaccinia* virus, a virus of unknown origin that became the modern smallpox vaccine. Smallpox was eradicated in North America by 1952 and in Europe by 1953. But in India and in many African countries smallpox was still endemic. In 1959 it was proposed that the World Health Organization (WHO) should undertake the smallpox eradication program with the goal of making it the first infectious disease to be eradicated by humans. Smallpox was an excellent candidate for eradication because the vaccine was highly effective in preventing disease and could survive without refrigeration, and vaccination left a scar as proof that a person was immune. In addition, the smallpox virus does not mutate frequently, so repeated vaccination was not necessary. Eradication efforts were hampered initially by lack of funding and low interest in smallpox as a target disease for eradication. Eradication efforts were stepped up in 1967, and the success of the program was supported by an increase in vaccine production and better methods of vaccination. Less than two hundred years after the discovery of Jenner's smallpox vaccine, the last naturally occurring smallpox infection was identified in a village in Somalia in a man named Ali Maow Maalin (Figure 8.7) in 1977.

The final chapter in the eradication of smallpox was to be the destruction of all smallpox laboratory strains, initially set to occur in 1993 and then delayed until 1995, and then delayed again until 1999. After that time, perceived threat of the use of smallpox as a bioterrorist weapon again caused a delay in destruction of virus stocks. As of 2010, smallpox is still being studied in laboratories and debate continues on whether and when the virus stocks should be destroyed.

FIGURE 8.7 Ali Maow Maalin, the Last Person to Have Naturally Acquired Smallpox

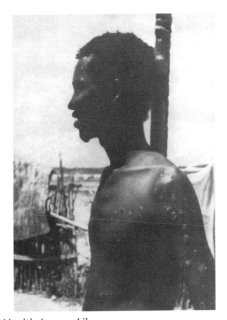

Source: CDC Public Health Image Library.

Polio Eradication

The success of the global smallpox eradication program encouraged the eradication efforts of other viruses, including **poliovirus** (polio). Poliovirus causes poliomyelitis, a disease with no symptoms (inapparent infection) in approximately 95 percent of those infected but can cause flaccid paralysis in about 1 percent of infected people[3]. The virus is shed in the stool of infected people and is transmitted through the **fecal-oral route**. It was first described by British physician Michael Underwood in 1789 but was not a disease of major significance until the early twentieth century. At its peak in the early 1950s poliovirus was responsible for more than twenty-one thousand cases of paralysis in the United States. In an unprecedented public campaign to support research to develop a vaccine against poliovirus, the National Foundation for Infantile Paralysis was established in 1938 (this organization is now known as the March of Dimes). In 1955, Jonas Salk developed an oral polio vaccine that contained live attenuated poliovirus. This was followed in 1963 by Albert Sabin's inactivated oral polio vaccine (Figure 8.8).

Both vaccines have been effective in vastly reducing the number of poliovirus infections worldwide; the Western Hemisphere was declared free of polio in 1994, and Europe was declared free of polio in 2002[7,8]. In other areas of the

FIGURE 8.8 A Child Receiving Oral Polio Vaccination

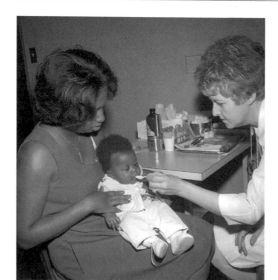

Source: CDC Public Health Image Library.

world, poliovirus eradication has so far not been achieved. There is evidence that people in different regions of the world respond differently to the oral polio vaccine, the vaccine used most frequently in developing countries because it is easy to transport and administer. In some countries multiple doses are required to achieve immunity. Poliovirus still exists in nature as well, most likely in sewer systems of developing countries. In 1988 a poliovirus eradication plan was initiated by the WHO, United Nations Children's Fund (UNICEF), and the Centers for Disease Control and Prevention (CDC) with the initial goal of eradication of poliovirus in nature by the year 2000. Unfortunately, this effort has proven to be more difficult than anticipated. Recently, there have also been difficulties with the vaccination program in Nigeria due to rumors that the virus contains HIV and will reduce the fertility of the recipient[9]. Recent conflicts in African countries also have prevented vaccination programs from being carried out. However, the goal of worldwide poliovirus eradication, while delayed, is still at the forefront of worldwide disease control efforts.

Dracunculiasis Eradication

Smallpox and polio eradication efforts rely on vaccination to prevent disease, but **dracunculiasis**, or guinea worm disease, is entirely preventable by non-vaccine interventions. Guinea worm disease is contracted when a person drinks stagnant water contaminated with the larvae of the guinea worm or walks unprotected in infected waterways. The disease is caused by a parasite called *Dracunculiasis medinensis*, which can invade the intestinal wall and migrate to the body's extremities (Figure 8.9).

The female guinea worms can grow up to 3 feet in length, and after ten to fourteen months the infected person develops a blistered area on the skin where the guinea worm will emerge. This painful area is soothed by immersion in water, which triggers emergence of the guinea worm larvae into the water and starts the cycle of infection again. Although infected people are generally not symptomatic until shortly before emergence of the worm, the emergence itself is associated with pain and swelling. The worm emergence can often result in secondary bacterial infection in the area that can incapacitate the infected person for weeks or months. Infection with guinea worm does not produce any immunity, so a person may be infected many times during his or her life. Although descriptions of guinea worm disease are dreadful, the disease is actually easily eradicated by simple interventions. The flea that carries the guinea worm larvae is large enough that it may be filtered out of drinking water using an inexpensive mesh or cloth filter. Water pumps also can also filter the water as it is being dispensed so no further filtration is necessary after collecting the water. To help

FIGURE 8.9 Dracunculiasis Life Cycle

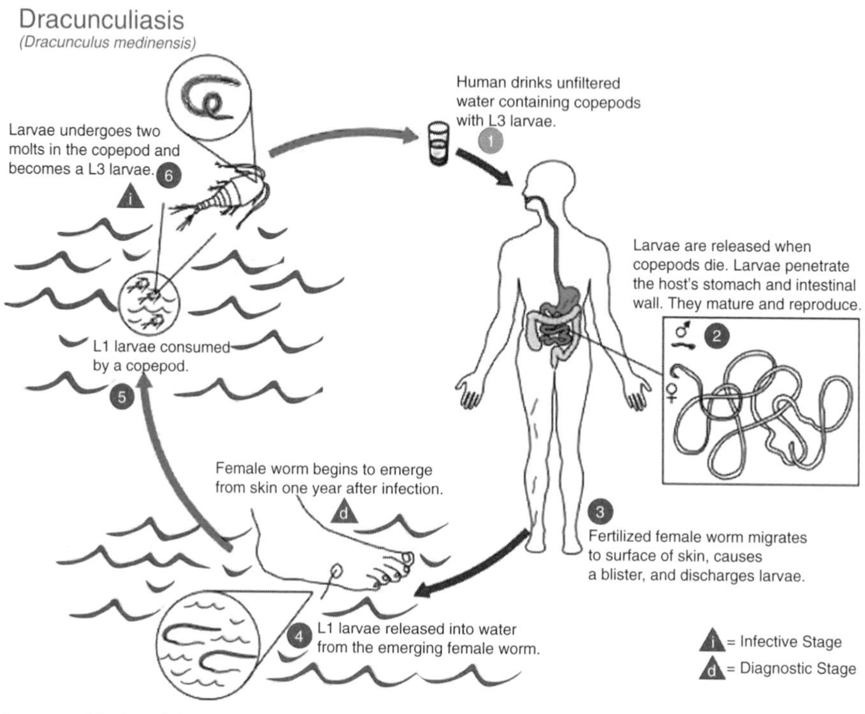

Source: CDC Public Health Image Library.

prevent the contamination of drinking water with guinea worm larvae, people from whom the worm is emerging can practice controlled immersion, in which they immerse the affected area in a bucket of water rather than in the source of drinking water. These simple efforts have reduced the prevalence of guinea worm from twenty countries in 1986 to only six countries in 2008.

Emerging and Reemerging Infectious Diseases

Despite the advances made in preventing and treating infectious diseases, emerging and reemerging pathogens create new challenges in fighting infections. In 1981, the first cases of **human immunodeficiency virus (HIV)** and **acquired immune deficiency syndrome (AIDS)** were described when a cluster of rare lung infections in homosexual men was identified. This emergence and spread of HIV is one factor that has contributed to the reemergence of **tuberculosis (TB)** in regions such as the United States. Rates of TB infection, which had been in decline since 1953, began to increase steadily in 1986[10]. Other factors contributing to the reemergence of TB are higher rates of immigration of people from countries where TB is not well controlled and diminished surveillance and recognition of the disease due to the history of declining rates. TB is discussed in greater detail in Chapter 13.

TB is recognized as being a disease that has reemerged, but some infectious diseases are emerging for the first time as a public health threat. In 2002, a new form of a coronavirus emerged, causing a disease called **severe acute respiratory syndrome (SARS)**[11]. Coronaviruses had been known previously to cause disease in humans and other mammals, but the 2002 outbreak was unique due to the new form of the virus, and the speed with which it spread resulted in a pandemic. The first case of SARS was identified in China, but the virus, which spread through respiratory and contact transmission, eventually infected people in other parts of Asia and in Europe, North America, and South America. During the SARS outbreak of 2003, over 8,000 people became infected with the virus; 774 of those people died. The SARS outbreak was significant for the speed with which it spread globally and the actions taken to prevent further spread of infection. Modern air travel played a major role in transporting the virus from the initial outbreak in China to other areas of the world. This outbreak saw the rise of thermal scanners used at airports to check passengers for fevers, home quarantine of people known or suspected to be infected with the virus, and elevated infection control measures in hospitals to protect health care workers from infection. As of this writing, there have been no new SARS cases in the world, indicating that the virus, for now, is under control. But the lessons from the SARS outbreak have recently been put to use in controlling a new emerging infectious disease called the H1N1 influenza virus, or swine flu.

Different forms of influenza have existed for centuries and have caused epidemics throughout history. In the early twenty-first century, the focus of infection prevention has been the H5N1 influenza virus, commonly known as bird flu. Preparations for a pandemic of H5N1 were put into place in the spring of 2009; however, the H1N1 swine flu emerged as the next pandemic threat. This outbreak originated in Mexico and quickly spread to the United States through travelers who carried the virus across borders. The H1N1 flu differed from the usual seasonal influenza because no vaccine existed for it, and people under the age of sixty-five generally had not been exposed to this strain of influenza. This meant that a large portion of the population was susceptible to the virus. In addition to people with underlying illnesses that normally make them more prone to develop severe illness when infected with influenza viruses, pregnant women had much greater morbidity and mortality due to H1N1 than with other influenza strains. Control efforts initially included emphasizing hand washing and the use of alcohol gels to clean hands, temporarily closing schools with high numbers of infected students, using anti-influenza drugs to prevent those who had close contact with infected people from becoming infected, and emphasizing that people should stay home and avoid social situations when experiencing flu symptoms. In October of 2009, a vaccine specific for the H1N1 swine flu was approved and large-scale vaccination of the public took place. Between April and November of 2009, an estimated 47 million cases of H1N1 occurred in the United States, of which 213,000 people were hospitalized and nearly 10,000 people died[12].

Summary

Efforts to control infectious diseases have been part of the past, are part of the present, and will no doubt be part of the future of public health. In this chapter the statistical methods of studying infectious diseases were introduced and the biological methods of preventing diseases were discussed. The success stories of smallpox eradication and control of polio and dracunculiasis provide insight into methods that may be used in the future to reduce, control, and eventually eliminate the threat of both known and potentially emerging infectious diseases.

Key Terms

acquired immune deficiency syndrome (AIDS), 192

airborne transmission, 180

attack rate, 179

case, 178

chain of infection, 180

community immunity, 184

component vaccines, 183

contact tracing, 180

contact transmission, 180

continuous source, 182

descriptive epidemiology, 180

dracunculiasis, 191

endemic, 178

epidemic, 178

epidemic curve, 180

eradication, 185

fecal-oral route of transmission, 190

herd immunity, 184

host, 180

human immunodeficiency virus (HIV), 192

hypothesis, 182

inactivated vaccine, 183

inapparent infection, 178

incubation period, 185

inoculation, 186

intramuscular, 183

intranasal, 183

Koch's postulates, 178

live attenuated vaccine, 183

Review Questions

1. Several guests who attended a wedding developed symptoms of food poisoning the following day. An epidemiological investigation indicates that the chicken entree was the source. Of the 125 guests who attended the wedding, 82 ate the chicken entree, and 67 of those guests became ill.
   a. What was the attack rate of this illness?
   b. Which epidemic curve would be used to describe this outbreak?
2. Although a tuberculosis vaccine (called BCG) exists, it is not widely used in the United States. Why is that the case? (A good source of information on this subject is the CDC's Web site at www.CDC.gov.)
3. List some of the challenges involved in the efforts to eradicate poliovirus.
4. The final goal of the smallpox eradication program was to destroy all frozen laboratory stocks of the smallpox virus, but this action has been delayed because of fears of reemergence of the disease through bioterrorism. Do you believe that the stocks should be destroyed? Why or why not?

References

1. Grigg MA, Brzezny AL, Dawson J, et al. Update: Measles—United States, January–July 2008. *MMWR*. 2008;57(33):893–896.
2. Hornig M, Briese T, Buie T, et al. Lack of association between measles virus vaccine and autism with enteropathy: A case-control study. *PLoS One*. 2008;3(9):e3140.
3. Atkinson W, Wolfe S, Hamborsky J, McIntyre L, eds. *Epidemiology and Prevention of Vaccine-Preventable Diseases*. Washington, D.C.: Public Health Foundation; 2009.
4. Barquet N, Domingo P. Smallpox: The triumph over the most terrible of the ministers of death. *Ann Int Med*. 1997;127(8):635–642.
5. D'Errico P. *Jeffrey Amherst and smallpox blankets*. Available at: www.umass.edu/legal/derrico/amherst/lord_jeff.html. Accessed May 9, 2010.
6. Fenner F, Henderson DA, Arita I, et al. *Smallpox and Its Eradication*. Geneva, Switzerland: World Health Organization; 1988.

7. DeJesus N. Epidemics to eradication: The modern history of poliomyelitis. *Virol J.* 2007;4:70.

8. Dutta A. Epidemiology of poliomyelitis—options and update. *Vaccine.* 2008;26: 5767–5773.

9. Rey M, Girard MP. The global eradication of poliomyelitis: Progress and problems. *Comp Immuno Microbiol Infect Dis.* 2008;31:317–325.

10. Murray, JF. A century of tuberculosis. *Am J Respir Crit Care Med.* 2004;169: 1181–1186.

11. CDC Web site. *Basic Information About SARS.* Fact sheet. Available at: www.cdc.gov/ ncidod/sars/factsheet.htm. Accessed May 9, 2010.

12. CDC Web site. Estimates of 2009 H1N1 influenza cases, hospitalizations and deaths in the United States, April–November 14, 2009. Available at: www.cdc.gov/h1n1flu/ estimates_2009_h1n1.htm. Accessed May 9, 2010.

CHAPTER 9

ENVIRONMENTAL PUBLIC HEALTH

Lisa Conti, DVM, MPH, DACVPM, CEHP
Greg Kearney, DrPH, MPH, RS
Sandra Whitehead, MPA
Kendra Goff, PhD
Alan Becker, PhD, MPH

LEARNING OBJECTIVES

- Understand the elements of environmental public health practice.
- Understand the use of environmental epidemiology in public health.
- Describe disease processes that result from environmental exposures.

Environmental public health (EPH) is concerned with preventing diseases of environmental origin. These diseases can arise from exposures to infectious pathogens in food, water, air, animals (zoonoses), or vectors (such as mosquitoes, lice, and ticks); toxicants (including pesticides, heavy metals, carbon monoxide, airborne particulates); excess radiation; or lack of physical exercise (for example, resulting from a poorly built environment). Recall from Chapter 2 the ten essential public health services that fit into the three core functions (Figure 2.1). These ten services can be modified to apply specifically to environmental health, as seen in Public Health Connections 9.1.

EPH prevention and control programs are focused on the population's health rather than on individual disease care. Moreover, EPH is seen as a critical factor in a "one health" concept of the inextricable linkages of human, animal, and environmental health[2]. Understanding *one health* and our ability to

PUBLIC HEALTH CONNECTIONS 9.1

TEN ESSENTIAL ENVIRONMENTAL PUBLIC HEALTH SERVICES

1. **Monitor** environmental and health status to identify and solve community environmental health problems.

2. **Diagnose and investigate** environmental health problems and health hazards in the community.

3. **Inform, educate, and empower** people regarding environmental health issues.

4. **Mobilize** community partnerships and actions to identify and solve environmental health problems.

5. **Develop policies and plans** that support individual and community environmental health efforts.

6. **Enforce** laws and regulations that protect environmental health and ensure safety.

7. **Link** people to needed environmental health services and assure the provision of environmental health services when otherwise unavailable.

8. **Assure** a competent environmental health care workforce.

9. **Evaluate** effectiveness, accessibility, and quality of personal and population-based environmental health services.

10. **Research** for new insights and innovative solutions to environmental health problems and issues.

Adapted from Public Health in America statement[1]

effectively use to advantage the human–animal–environment interface is now a new dictum for health professionals.

Environmental Public Health: History and Progression

As described in Chapter 1, early societies learned that basic sanitation—clean water and removal of waste and vermin—was critical to population health. In

Greek mythology, the gods tasked Apollo's son Asclepius and his two daughters, Hygeia and Panacea, to care for the population of Greek mortals. Whereas Apollo was more directly associated with healing, Hygeia championed the prevention of disease and the use of basic sanitation practices as the beginning of wellness ("cleanliness is next to godliness"). Panacea cured individuals who were already sick, one at a time. Humans remained healthier when they followed Hygeian principles, creating a healthy environment and preventing disease.

Today, we see how altering our environment in an unsustainable way has impacted climate change and humankind's morbidity and mortality. For example, sprawling communities centered on automobile travel lead to issues such as traffic injury, air pollution, and lack of exercise manifesting as asthma, hypertension, and stress-related illness[3]. Moreover, failing to design communities in a way that promotes neighborhood interaction reduces community resilience. This is most noticeable following a disaster such as a hurricane, when environmental public health plays a profound role in restoring clean water, removing waste, and controlling vermin.

PUBLIC HEALTH CONNECTIONS 9.2
ENVIRONMENTAL HEALTH PROGRAMS

Environmental public health protects human health from environmental hazards and threats. Drinking water quality, food safety, and sewage treatment and disposal are the most commonly thought-of programs in environmental health, but this worldwide profession includes a wide variety of programs.

The term **environment** encompasses personal, occupational, global and natural environment (such as land, water, air, etc.). The aim of environmental health services is to protect and enhance environmental quality for all people.

Every kind of chemical, biological, physical, and other related factors that can have an impact on the behavior of a human being and harm his or her health are considered to be potentially dangerous and are concerns of environmental health.

No matter where in the world or which programs are being regulated and enforced, environmental health programs have one thing in common: they are all about prevention and creating health-supportive environments. Keeping people healthy is far less expensive than healing an ill population.

Source: Reference 4.

Environmental public health professionals are from various backgrounds, including but not limited to biology, chemistry, geology, hydrology, human and veterinary medicine, land use planning, toxicology, health physics, education, and epidemiology. Environmental public health professionals are policy makers, health educators, facility inspectors, and first responders. The ten essential environmental public health services provide the fundamental framework for the profession's performance standards by describing the environmental public health activities that should be undertaken in all communities[1].

To assess and quantify environmental risks to health, EPH uses **environmental epidemiology** as a critical tool for surveillance, scientific evaluation, and risk communication for adverse health outcomes. The health and environmental data gathered and information used forms the foundation for setting policy and practice. The International Society for Environmental Epidemiology (ISEE) has adopted the following definition: "Environmental epidemiology is the study of the effect on human health of physical, biologic, and chemical factors in the external environment, broadly conceived. By examining specific populations or communities exposed to different ambient environments, it seeks to clarify the relationship between physical, biologic, or chemical factors and human health."[5]

Preventing Infectious Diseases of Environmental Origin

An infectious disease is an illness stemming from an organism's exposure to pathogens such as viruses, bacteria, fungi, protozoa, multicellular parasites, and aberrant proteins known as prions. These pathogens may be able to cause disease in animals or plants. Infectious pathologies are usually qualified as contagious or communicable diseases due to the potential of transmission from one person or species to another[6]. Epidemiologists classify infectious diseases in a population as being **sporadic** (occasional occurrence), **endemic** (regular cases often occurring in a region), **epidemic** (an unusually high number of cases in a region), or **pandemic** (a global epidemic).

There are many ways that infectious diseases can be transmitted to a host, as described in Chapter 8. Environmental epidemiologists describe how infectious disease agents spread to humans by classifying them as having either direct or indirect transmission. As the name implies, **direct transmission** occurs when there is physical contact with an infected person or animal; in other words, when an infected host transmits an infectious agent directly to another. Typically, direct transmission occurs through touching, kissing, biting, or sexual contact. **Indirect transmission** occurs when there is no direct contact with an infected source. In this case, a susceptible host can be infected via food, water,

FIGURE 9.1 Relationship Between Host, Environment, and Interaction in Infectious Disease

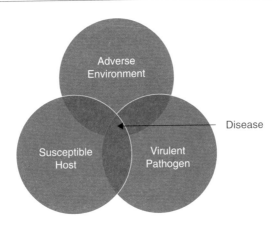

or inanimate objects such as toys, soiled clothes, or even a computer keyboard. Vector-borne and airborne transmissions are two forms of indirect transmission of infectious disease.

Vector-borne diseases include those transmitted by flies, ticks, mosquitoes, and lice. The mosquito is responsible for the most common vector-borne diseases, including malaria, West Nile virus, and dengue and yellow fevers. In 2002, malaria was the fourth leading cause of death in children in developing countries, responsible for 11 percent of all childhood mortality[7]. The female mosquito transfers pathogens in her saliva when taking a blood meal from a host. Public health messages to prevent mosquito-borne diseases are aimed at avoiding mosquito bites: repair window and door screens, wear long pants and long-sleeved shirts, and use insect repellents such as DEET according to the manufacturer's specifications.

Changing patterns of individual and global economic behavior have complicated the public health control of food and waterborne diseases in recent years and have accentuated the need for an improved public health infrastructure to detect illness. Florida has a unique structure in place for food and waterborne disease surveillance and investigation using nine regional food and waterborne illness epidemiologists to assist the state's sixty-seven county health departments in the investigation of these outbreaks. In Florida's system, the counties maintain food and waterborne illness complaint logs and perform outbreak investigations using a regional epidemiological team composed of an environmental health professional, a nurse, and an epidemiologist (see Public Health Connections 9.3). The regional epidemiology team provides technical assistance in outbreak

PUBLIC HEALTH CONNECTIONS 9.3

CASE STUDY: NORWALK VIRUS AT A CATERED WEDDING RECEPTION

On August 29, 2000, the Escambia County Health Department (ECHD) received a complaint that a group of people had fallen ill after eating a catered meal at a wedding reception in Pensacola, Florida, three days earlier. Approximately fifty-five people had attended this event at a private residence. The bride's mother, who had hired the caterer, provided a list of all attendees.

Case histories for the attendees were obtained through questionnaires administered over the telephone. Stool samples were collected for viral analysis. In all, fifty case histories and nine viral stool samples were collected. Thirty wedding guests experienced illness (60 percent); primary symptoms were diarrhea, vomiting, abdominal cramps, and fever. Investigation of the caterer's facility revealed that the food had been prepared in a private home and the caterer was unlicensed and unregulated. The caterer's young child and the caterer both had experienced diarrheal illness three to five days prior to the wedding reception. The 60 percent attack rate among the attendees of this wedding reception indicated that there was a point–source common exposure among the ill people. The food-specific attack rate correlated to those who consumed food from tables containing cheeses, citrus punch, and chicken salad. Additionally, seven of twenty-one stool samples from attendees, the caterer, and the caterer's child tested positive for Norwalk-like virus, type G2. Poor personal hygiene and/or unsanitized food preparation surfaces and equipment in an unlicensed catering facility resulted in this Norwalk-like viral outbreak[8].

investigations, report writing, and assistance in questionnaire development and statistical analysis. Regional epidemiologists also play a role in helping to train county health department staff in a variety of aspects of outbreak investigations. The statewide food and waterborne disease coordinator synthesizes annual and quarterly statewide data and provides information to other state and federal agencies during outbreak investigations.

Zoonotic diseases are caused by microorganisms of animal origin that can be transmitted to humans. The World Health Organization (WHO) recognizes over two hundred zoonotic diseases involving all types of agents, including bacteria, parasites, viruses, and novel agents such as prions. Zoonotic diseases have gained increasing attention due to widespread international travel and extensive food exportation. Over two thirds of the emerging pathogens, including severe acute respiratory syndrome (SARS) and monkeypox, are considered zoonoses. WHO has established a Global Early Warning System for Major Animal Diseases (GLEWS), conceived with the aim of predicting and responding to animal diseases, including zoonoses, worldwide. Some of the top priority zoonotic diseases include the following:

- Anthrax

- Bovine spongiform encephalopathy (BSE)

- Brucellosis (*Brucella melitensis*)

- Crimean-Congo hemorrhagic fever

- Ebola virus

- Foodborne diseases

- Highly pathogenic avian influenza (HPAI)

- Japanese encephalitis

- Marburg hemorrhagic fever

- New World screwworm

- Nipah virus

- Old World screwworm

- Q fever

- Rabies

- Rift Valley fever

- Sheep pox/goat pox

- Tularemia

- Venezuelan equine encephalomyelitis

- West Nile virus

Rabies is a serious infectious viral disease that affects the nervous system of animals and humans. Humans contract rabies primarily through the bite of an infected animal (see Public Health Connections 9.4). In the United States, bat rabies variants have been the most common source for human rabies cases in recent years[9].

FIGURE 9.2 Map Showing the Location and Source of Various Emerging or Reemerging Infectious Zoonotic Diseases Worldwide. Credit: Data compiled by Thomas P. Monath, MD

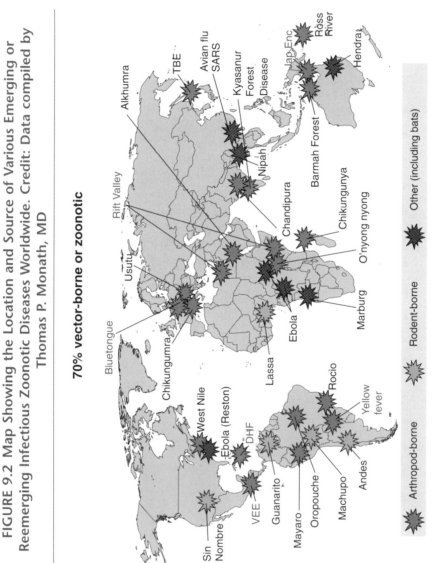

70% vector-borne or zoonotic

Arthropod-borne   Rodent-borne   Other (including bats)

PUBLIC HEALTH CONNECTIONS 9.4

CASE STUDY: RABIES EXPOSURE

In October 2007, a forty-six-year-old man was hospitalized with fever and progressive respiratory failure. Because rabies was suspected, his family was interviewed about his exposure to animals. He had handled a bat in August, and reported a needle-prick sensation before releasing it. The patient died and rabies was confirmed. This case demonstrates several points:

- The man's infection with rabies was most likely the result of a bat bite.
- Bats are not typically tame enough to handle unless they are ill or young. This strange behavior should lead to a strong suspicion of rabies and the bat should have been tested.
- Public health recommendations call for provision of antirabies treatment for a person bitten by a bat when the animal is not available for rabies testing.

Source: Reference 9.

Chronic Diseases and Environmental Health

Chronic diseases are those of slow progression or long duration. They rarely resolve spontaneously. According to WHO, chronic diseases account for seven of every ten deaths and affect the quality of life of 90 million Americans[10]. Although these diseases are among the most common and costly health problems, most are preventable, primarily through behavior modification[11].

A senior scholar at the Institute of Medicine (IOM) has estimated that the largest contributor to early deaths, accounting for 40%, is behavior. In addition, 30% of early deaths are attributable to genetics, 20% stem from the social and physical environments, and 10% are the result of

> Surrounding ourselves with cars, roads and ample parking—but neither sidewalks to walk on, nor destinations worth walking to—increases how much we drive, and decreases how much we walk. Still, many transportation planners interpret the decision to hop in a car as an expression of a deep-seated personal preference, rather than a choice that's powerfully influenced by the built environment.
>
> *Clark Williams-Derry*[13]

substandard medical care[12]. Yet, behavior and environment are intrinsically linked. Our **physical environment**, the objects we surround ourselves with and the places we make for ourselves, can have a potent influence both on what we do and on how we think.

There are many chronic diseases that have environmental contributors. Obesity, cancer, and asthma are three of the most common, and they will be discussed in more detail here.

Obesity

Obesity is usually defined by one's weight and height, combined into a measure known as body mass index (BMI). For adults, a BMI of higher than 30 is considered obese. This translates to being at least 20 percent above the weight recommended for one's height. Obesity and its associated health problems have a substantial economic impact on the U.S. health care system[14]. Medical costs associated with obesity involve direct and indirect costs[15,16]. Direct costs include preventive, diagnostic, and treatment services related to obesity. Indirect costs relate to morbidity and mortality costs. Morbidity costs consist of the value of lost income from decreased productivity, restricted activity, and absenteeism. Mortality costs are defined as the value of future income lost by premature death. The estimated annual cost of obesity is $147 billion and growing. This number translates to $1,250 per household, paid through taxes and rising health insurance costs[17].

Recall from Chapter 4 the growing prevalence of obesity in the United States (see Figure 4.1). In 2008, obesity prevalence was equal to or greater than 25 percent in thirty-two states; six of these states had prevalence above 30 percent[14]. Only Colorado had an obesity prevalence of less than 20 percent. The current trend toward obesity and its costs involve many different factors but can primarily be traced to environmental and behavioral issues. These include the way we plan human habitats for cars instead of people, resulting in physical inactivity. According to the United States Surgeon General, 60 percent of adults do not meet recommended levels of physical activity and 25 percent are completely sedentary[14]. Sedentary lifestyles are estimated to contribute to as many as 255,000 preventable deaths each year[18].

An emerging body of evidence shows that transportation and land use patterns can influence people's decisions to be physically active or not[19]. Community design characteristics such as the provision of biking and walking trails and access to public transit increase the likelihood of pursuing exercise and decrease the dependence on vehicles[20]. Instead of designing our communities to encourage physical activity, we have been shaping our built environment to encourage

PUBLIC HEALTH CONNECTIONS 9.5

CASE STUDY: WABASSO COMMUNITY IN INDIAN RIVER COUNTY, FLORIDA

The Florida Department of Health's Division of Environmental Health has provided seed money to local health departments to begin projects known as Protocol for Assessing Community Excellence in Environmental Health (PACE EH; see www.doh.state.fl.us/environment/programs/PACE-EH/PACE-EH.htm). These programs connect a staff member from the county health department with leaders of an underserved community to form a committee of residents who identify their most urgent environmental public health needs.

In the Wabasso community, one of the top issues identified was barriers to exercise, such as an absence of parks, street lights, walking trails, and sidewalks. Through the PACE EH process, residents were empowered to contact their local decision makers to effect changes in their neighborhoods. They were ultimately successful in their efforts, and over two years Indian River County funded a walking trail, sidewalks, and street lights. The direct result of these modifications is that residents are exercising more.

getting into and staying in our cars. In the suburban United States, you can do most everything from your car, from ordering a latte to getting married. In sprawling suburban and urban communities where few other travel options are available, cars are now used for 80 percent of trips less than 1 mile in length[21]. The ease of using the automobile and poor community planning (for example, schools being located far from neighborhoods and few attractive, accessible places to exercise) contribute to physical inactivity, which leads to obesity.

Neighborhood characteristics associated with higher levels of physical activity include high density, mixed-use development, good public transportation, and proximity to destinations (see Public Health Connections 9.5). In addition, bicycle and pedestrian facilities, good street connectivity, the presence of parks and open space, and a feeling of safety can all promote more exercise[22–24].

Cancer

Cancer is a generic term for a large group of diseases that can affect any part of the body; other terms used to denote cancer are *malignant tumors* and *neoplasms*. One defining feature of cancer is the rapid creation of abnormal cells that grow beyond their usual boundaries. These cells can then invade adjoining parts of the body or spread to other organs (metastasize). Cancer is a leading cause of death worldwide, accounting for 7.4 million deaths in 2004 (around 13 percent of all deaths)[25]. The most frequent types of cancers found globally include lung, stomach, liver, colorectal, esophagus, and prostate among men and breast, lung, stomach, colorectal, and cervical among women.

Cancer may occur because of genetic factors or environmental exposures that alter or potentiate genes. The harmful health effects of environmental exposure depend on the dose, strength of the physical or chemical agent, and the length of exposure. It has been said that genetics loads the gun and environmental exposure pulls the trigger. Environmental causes of cancer include physical and chemical carcinogens such as components of tobacco smoke (such as benzene), ultraviolet and ionizing radiation, asbestos, aflatoxin (a food contaminant), and arsenic (a drinking water contaminant). Therefore, environmental pollution through chemicals or radionuclides in tobacco smoke, drinking water, air, and food may contribute to cancer. The estimates for cancer deaths attributable to tobacco have been consistently around 30 percent.

Determining whether an environmental chemical is associated with cancer can be researched in two ways: through human or other animal studies (in vivo) and through laboratory experiments (in vitro). Biennially, the National Toxicology Program within the Department of Health and Human Services (HHS) compiles the *Report on Carcinogens* that lists substances that are either known or suspected of causing human cancer[26]. The report also describes where these substances are found in our environment.

Human Studies

Human studies are used to determine with the most certainty whether a substance causes cancer. Most cancer-causing chemicals were first recognized in occupational settings. The workplace is unique because workers are often exposed to large amounts of chemicals. Benzene, asbestos, vinyl chloride, and arsenic are examples of toxic substances that are known human carcinogens.

Animal Studies

Some chemicals have been shown to cause cancer in animals. Rodents (mice and rats) are typically used to study whether environmental chemicals can cause cancer. The chemical exposures are usually at much higher levels than would occur among humans. Scientists reason that if no cancer is seen at an extremely high level of exposure, then the chemical most likely does not cause cancer at lower levels either. Animals may have responses to chemicals similar to humans, but most chemicals tested on animals alone are classified by the United States Environmental Protection Agency (EPA) as "possible or probable human carcinogens." Chloroform, dichlorodiphenyltrichloroethane (DDT), formaldehyde, and polychlorinated biphenyl (PCBs) are examples of such chemicals.

Changes to human cells exposed to chemicals in a laboratory can be used to determine whether a chemical is a carcinogen. These studies can be performed more easily than animal studies and can help reduce the number of animal cancer studies.

Individual Risk and Cancer

The risk of cancer after being exposed to a chemical depends upon many things: the amount of a chemical, the length of time exposed, the number of times exposed, and the route (oral, dermal, etc.) of contaminant exposure all determine an individual's risk. It may only take one molecule of a carcinogen to genetically alter a cell[27].

Often it seems there is a cluster of cancers in a particular community. Because one out of three people in the United States will develop some type of cancer in his or her lifetime, it may appear that people with cancer live in close proximity. The natural tendency is to blame something in the environment. However, this is rarely confirmed because cancer is common in our population, different types of cancer have different causes, and the cause for many cancers is not known. Because cancer's latency period is comparatively long, it is difficult to recreate exposures that occurred years or decades earlier. It is not unusual to have many cases of cancer in a single community, especially in an aging community. In fact, cancers often occur in clusters and are not evenly spread out in the population. This does not necessarily mean that they are related.

Controlling Cancer-Causing Chemicals

To minimize exposure to known cancer-causing chemicals, federal and state standards are set at precautionary levels. These standards help protect people from high levels of chemicals in the workplace and at home. They also protect our natural resources: water, plants, and air. There are over forty known or suspected carcinogens present in tobacco smoke. Progress has been made in controlling exposure to secondhand smoke in public buildings and on the job. More information is needed to determine safe levels of individual chemicals and combinations of chemicals.

Asthma

Asthma, a chronic disease that affects the lungs, is a leading cause of pediatric morbidity, emergency department visits, and hospitalization in the United States. The prevalence of asthma increased in the United States from 1980 to 1996 but

FIGURE 9.3 Estimated Rate of Emergency Department Visits with Asthma as the First Diagnosis by Age and Year

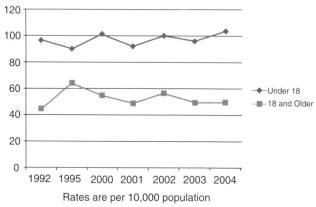

Rates are per 10,000 population

Source: National Hospital Ambulatory Medical Care Survey, 1992–2004, as reported in reference 28.

remained relatively constant from 1997 to 2004[28]. Common signs and symptoms include frequent episodic wheezing, shortness of breath, tightening of the chest, and coughing either at night or in the morning[29]. Although asthma medications are available, environmental triggers make it challenging for affected individuals to manage this disease. Some important environmental triggers are tobacco smoke, dust mites, outdoor pollution (particulate matter), cockroach allergens, pet dander, mold, and high humidity[28]. During an asthma attack, the airways constrict and become clogged with mucus, making it difficult to breathe. This air obstruction can cause shortness of breath and low blood oxygen, leading to hospitalization. Asthma attacks frequently occur when asthma is not managed and in the presence of environmental triggers. Figures 9.3 and 9.4 show the estimated rates of hospital emergency visits and discharges for people with asthma.

Preventing Adverse Chemical Exposure

Toxicants are chemicals that have an adverse impact on organisms, such as pesticides. A toxicant from a biological source is a **toxin** (for example, botulinum toxin). A developmental toxicant is called a **teratogen**. Toxicity can occur through many environmental media, including drinking, bathing, and recreational water; food; indoor and outdoor air (including things such as pesti-

FIGURE 9.4 Estimated Rate of Hospital Discharges with Asthma as the First Diagnosis by Age and Year

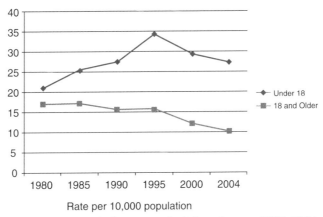

Rate per 10,000 population

Source: National Hospital Ambulatory Medical Care Survey, 1992–2004, as reported in reference 28.

cide drift); pharmaceuticals; and any number of other products we use in daily life. Public health seeks to provide sound policies and practices for case surveillance, risk assessment, and data analysis for the public and the scientific communities to prevent diseases related to chemical exposures. This section will cover examples of chemical exposure primarily related to air and water and also will provide information about how these exposures are measured and how guidelines for safe exposures are established. Table 9.1 lists some classic environmental exposures with adverse health effects.

Routes of exposure for toxicants include contact, inhalation, and ingestion pathways. The skin is the primary barrier to contact exposure, the lungs act as the barrier to inhaled toxicants, and the gastrointestinal tract protects against ingested compounds[30, pp. 2–3]. The route of exposure depends on the properties of the chemical. Large organic chemicals that are water soluble generally do not absorb well through the skin, lungs, or intestines unless there is damage to these organ systems. These compounds also do not readily absorb into cells or cross the blood–brain or placental barrier. However, small water-soluble compounds such as ethanol (alcohol) may be absorbed by simple diffusion through aqueous pores[31]. **Lead**, a water-soluble compound, also crosses the blood–brain barrier and the placental barrier.

Alcohol and lead both can act as teratogens, causing a variety of cognitive effects in children exposed to these compounds in utero, as noted in Table 9.1.

Table 9.1 Examples of Environmental Exposure and Adverse Health Effects

Chemical/Drug	Uses/Exposure	Adverse Effects
Thalidomide	Mild sedative (morning sickness)	Birth defect (phocomelia)
Diethylstilbestrol (DES)	Estrogen properties (prevent miscarriages)	Vaginal cancer (clear cell carcinoma)
Alcohol	Drinking alcohol during pregnancy	Mental retardation and learning disabilities
Cigarette smoke, radon gas, sunlight, air pollutants, high-fat diet	Everyday living	Various cancers
Soot from burning coal	Exposure through chimney sweeping	Scrotal cancer
Aflatoxins	Fungal toxins found in peanuts	Carcinogen
Asbestos, vinyl chloride, benzene, naphthylamine, hardwood dust	Occupational exposures	Various cancers
Lead	Lead-based paint, plumbing, lead-tainted toys	Neurological damage

The Centers for Disease Control and Prevention (CDC) advises women who are pregnant and women who are of childbearing age and not effectively using contraception to avoid all types of alcohol at all levels[32]. As mentioned, alcohol can cross the placental barrier (via the umbilical cord) and reach the developing child. This exposure can lead to one of the conditions within the **fetal alcohol spectrum disorders** (FASDs), including fetal alcohol syndrome (FAS) or potentially death. FASDs include specific facial features such as a smooth ridge between the nose and upper lip, a thin upper lip, and wide-set eyes; low birth weight and stunted growth in childhood; bone, heart, or kidney malformations; and problems with brain development leading to lower IQ, learning disabilities, behavior issues, and poor memory[32]. The CDC estimates that the prevalence of FAS at birth is 0.2–1.5 per 1,000 live births and projects that FASD prevalence at birth may be as much as three times higher than FAS alone[32]. Lead has many desirable properties that have contributed to its inclusion in a variety of products over time. Today, lead exposure is known to have harmful effects, especially among children, so its use has been limited where possible. Lead was a component of gasoline to increase octane until the Clean Air Act banned its inclusion in 1996 (though a phase-out began in 1973)[33]. Lead-based paint was banned for residential use in 1978; the Environmental Protection Agency (EPA) estimates that more than

80 percent of homes built in the United States before 1978 contain lead-based paint[33]. As a result, lead exposure continues among people who live in homes that still have lead paint on the walls. Over time, the paint chips and flakes, and children crawling on the floor indoors or playing in the dirt outside these homes may inadvertently ingest lead-based paint. This exposure can profoundly impact their cognitive development, leading to reduced IQ, learning disabilities, and trouble in school. As of 1990, children with blood lead levels of 10 milligrams per deciliter (mg/dL) or higher are classified as having lead poisoning and are at an increased risk of adverse outcomes associated with this exposure[34]. According to the CDC, around 250,000 children between the ages of one and five in the United States have blood lead levels that exceed this standard[35]. Childhood lead exposure raises the issue of **environmental justice**, or equitably distributing the risks associated with an environmental toxicant. Environmental injustices occur when economically disadvantaged populations are overrepresented in environmental contaminant exposures, leading to health disparities. Environmental justice is a concept related to social justice, one of the hallmarks of public health described in Chapter 1. Lead exposure is much more common among low-income, minority, and immigrant children in the United States than among higher income, White, non-Hispanic children. The number of children under the age of six in the United States who are tested for blood lead increased from about 1.6 million in 1997 to nearly 3.25 million in 2006. Over the same time period, the prevalence of elevated blood lead levels ($\geq$10 mg/dL) declined from more than 7.5 percent to less than 1.5 percent[36]. As of April 2010, the United States has new training and certification requirements for contractors and other renovators who work on homes, schools, or child care facilities built before 1978 to minimize lead contamination[37]. Lead paint removal can be very expensive and costly because the process requires that dust be minimized, contained, and properly disposed of and that workers be well protected and not track dust outside the work area. Both FASDs and childhood lead exposures are completely preventable and represent important public health issues.

Different individuals and different species develop disease at different chemical exposure levels because of varying susceptibility among individuals and genetic predispositions[38]. The **no observed adverse effect level** (NOAEL) is the highest dose at which no measurable or observable toxic or adverse effect is seen. The **lowest observed adverse effect level** (LOAEL) is the lowest dose at which an adverse effect occurs. The NOAEL or LOAEL is used to calculate the **risk reference dose** (RfD), a daily dose for humans that carries a low risk of harmful effects. Specifically, the RfD is the LOAEL or NOAEL divided by uncertainty factors[38]. These uncertainty factors include susceptibility in humans, extrapolating from animal data to human data. Additional uncertainty can be used for a steep dose-response curve and limited data. As discussed in Chapter 5, a **dose-response relationship** is one in which the severity of the toxic effect correlates with an increase in the level of the toxicant (exposure).

In addition to these interspecies factors, individual differences may contribute to exposure responses. The mapping of the human genome is a landmark accomplishment and is envisioned to change medicine for disease prevention and prediction. It is believed that genetic **polymorphisms** (genes expressing different phenotypes) cause a shift in the dose-response curve for various exposures (see Public Health Connections 9.6)[39]. Exposure assessment involves characterizing the type, duration, intensity, and timing of exposure, but consideration of the gene–environment interaction may also be important[39]. In addition to the genetic sequencing itself, the way that genes are physically packaged (around histones) can be altered as a result of chemical exposure, leading to changes in the way genes are expressed[39]. These changes can be inherited. Environmental epidemiology and toxicology research may someday be expanded to screen and discover genetic variability involving environmental chemicals and their metabolism.

PUBLIC HEALTH CONNECTIONS 9.6

PAROXONASE POLYMORPHISM IN ORGANOPHOSPHATE TOXICITY

Farmworkers routinely are exposed to organophosphates in agriculture. Polymorphisms in the *PON1* gene result in increased susceptibility to organophosphate toxicity and affect the metabolism of organophosphates such as chlorpyrifos, parathion, and diazinon[40]. Very severe symptoms can result from exposure to organophosphates, such as confusion, tremors, headache, salivation, lacrimation, urination, defecation, bradycardia, respiratory failure, and death. Pesticide companies generally test parent compounds that may be inherently weaker toxicants than the oxidized oxon analog, which is significantly more toxic and poses a greater risk to neurotoxicity. Huff and colleagues found that the oxon analog of chloropyrifos exhibited a thousand-fold inhibition of cholinesterase compared to the parent compound[41]. These analogs are produced endogenously through metabolism and climatic factors[42]. Oxon present in foliar residues range from 1 percent to 90 percent of all residues[43]. Age appears to be a factor affecting *PON1* activity and increased susceptibility to infants[44,45]. There is also concern that mothers with low *PON1* status may contribute to higher exposure levels of the pesticide to the fetus[39]. Environmental epidemiology studies are needed to verify the extent of the association between the *PON1* and adverse outcome among workers.

When evaluating a chemical, all animal studies, environmental studies, and human studies must be considered to create a strong body of evidence for adverse effects. Research animals, cell culture, and stem cells are used to study the acute and chronic effects of chemicals. These laboratory studies are typically based on the individual dose-response relationship. Field studies may be designed to measure toxicants in soil, water, vegetation, and air. **Biomonitoring**, the collection of biological samples from people, is used to help confirm chemical exposure.

Acute Chemical Exposure Surveillance

The World Health Organization (WHO) estimates that there are over 3 million cases of pesticide poisoning resulting in 220,000 deaths each year. Fumigants are readily absorbed through the lungs as a gas. In addition, pesticides may be absorbed through the skin during application or when harvesting crops sprayed with pesticides. Pesticides also can be absorbed in the gut after ingestion of fruits or vegetables contaminated with pesticide. Acute surveillance systems in the United States (see examples in Public Health Connections 9.7) include monitoring pesticide and chemical exposure by the CDC. The National Institute for Occupational Safety and Health (NIOSH) within CDC oversees the state-level Pesticide Poisoning Surveillance Program. Likewise, the Agency for Toxic Substances and Disease Registry (ATSDR) administers the Hazardous Substances Emergency Events Surveillance program. These programs are designed to monitor and assess acute toxicant releases so that appropriate public health decisions can be made. For example, a community may need to be evacuated to protect the public's health in the event of a chemical spill. In some cases, medical records and environmental samples may be collected to verify that an exposure has occurred. A confirmed exposure may result in regulatory investigations and corresponding corrective actions. Important considerations involve stakeholders, prevention outreach, and dissemination of information.

Rachel Carson's book, *Silent Spring*, indicted the misuse of pesticides and their effects on the environment and human health. After bald eagle, pelican, and falcon populations declined during the 1950s, high levels of 1,1-dichloro-2,2-bis(*p*-chlorophenyl)ethylene (DDE), a DDT metabolite, were shown to correspond with thinner egg shells that broke easily when the birds were nesting[46]. DDT was banned for agricultural use in the United States in 1972[47]; nevertheless, DDT and its metabolites (DDE and DDD) were detected in 94 percent of fish samples during the 1990s[47]. Eating fish is the major route of exposure for humans today. DDT has been shown to cause adverse effects on the liver[47], nervous system[48,49], reproductive system[50,51], adrenal gland[52], and thyroid[53].

PUBLIC HEALTH CONNECTIONS 9.7

EXAMPLES OF ACUTE EXPOSURE SURVEILLANCE

Aerial Pesticide Field Study

The Florida Department of Agriculture and Consumer Services monitors mosquito populations and public complaints to decide when to spray a low concentration of the organophosphate, **naled**, to control mosquitoes. The Florida Department of Health (DOH) Pesticide Surveillance Program collects information about pesticide exposure and health concerns. During the 2004 hurricane season, DOH in collaboration with the CDC conducted a field study following aerial naled spraying to determine whether residents in treated areas were exposed to the chemical. Environmental samples were not collected because naled rapidly breaks down in sunlight[54]. However, an analysis of human urine samples before and after aerial spraying showed no increase in metabolites from naled. In this population, two people had possible naled exposure: one a direct spray incident and the other a child with asthma who was exposed while waiting for a bus the morning after a spray. Recommendations from this analysis include notifying the public when a spray event will occur to reduce exposure (stay indoors)[55].

Carbon Monoxide Surveillance

During the 2005 hurricane season, DOH partnered with the Florida Poison Control Information Network (FPCIN) to monitor carbon monoxide (CO) exposures. CO is a concern in the aftermath of a hurricane because many people use generators in the absence of electricity. Without proper ventilation, CO poisoning is possible. In the process of reviewing the reports, DOH developed a classification for "probable" and "definite" cases. Over 126 hurricane-associated CO poisonings were classified using carboxyhemoglobin (COHb) as a biomarker[56]. Subsequent efforts by DOH resulted in the development of a more formal classification system, and CO poisoning is now a reportable condition. Armed with these data, DOH now targets prevention messages to reduce the CO exposure risk.

DDT also has been shown to cause liver cancer in laboratory animals, and the EPA, HSS, and WHO's International Agency for Research on Cancer (IARC) report that DDT can be reasonably thought to cause cancer in humans.

Chemical Exposure in Water

As evidenced by the efforts of the earliest societies and the experience of John Snow, safe, clean drinking water is an important part of daily life. Beyond

Table 9.2 Examples of MCLs for Selected Contaminants on the National Primary Drinking Water Regulations (NPDWR) List

Contaminant	MCL (mg/L)*	Long-term Effects (above MCL)	Common Source(s)	Public Health Goal (mg/L)*
Inorganic mercury	0.002	Kidney damage	Erosion of natural deposits: discharge from refineries and factories; runoff from landfills and croplands	0.002
Nitrate (measured as nitrogen) Nitrite (measured as nitrogen)	10 1	Blue baby syndrome (methemaglobinemia)	Runoff from fertilizer use, leaching from septic tank, sewage, erosion of natural deposits	10 1
PCBs	0.0005	Skin changes; thymus problems; immune deficiencies; reproductive or nervous system difficulties; increased risk of cancer	Runoff from landfills; Discharge of waste chemicals	0

*Units are in milligrams per liter (mg/L) unless otherwise noted. Milligrams per liter are equivalent to parts per million.
Source: Reference 57.

carrying infectious agents such as cholera or supporting the life cycle of vectors such as mosquitoes, water may contain chemicals and toxicants that are harmful to human health. In 1974 the U.S. Safe Drinking Water Act was the first legislation to address the problem. The act has been amended multiple times and is the backdrop for EPA regulations that govern water safety and quality[57]. The **maximum concentration level** (MCL) is defined as the highest level of a contaminant that is allowed in drinking water and is an enforceable standard of the EPA National Primary Drinking Water Regulations (NPDWR). Table 9.2 provides examples of MCLs.

Depending on its chemical and physical properties, a toxicant can be eliminated from the body unchanged following absorption, distributed throughout the body, biotransformed to a more or less toxic metabolite, and bioaccumulated in tissues. Lipid-soluble compounds readily absorb into cells and may result in bioaccumulation in various tissues such as the brain, fat, or bone. Some examples of chemicals that result in bioaccumulation include methyl mercury and PCBs, along with the previously described DDT.

Atmospheric mercury can circle the globe for years; precipitation brings it back to the earth, and it eventually ends up in a river or lake[58]. This mercury makes its way to the bottom of the water body where it is methylated by anaerobic bacteria into **methyl mercury**[59]. This mercury is lipid soluble, accumulating in large predator fish[60]. When people eat contaminated fish, up to 95 percent of the mercury is absorbed and distributed to all tissues in the body[61]. The first known widespread illness from methyl mercury occurred in Minamata Bay, Japan, from fish contaminated by wastewater mercury from an industrial plant. Severe neurological problems affected over ten thousand people: symptoms included paresthesia, impaired peripheral vision, slurred speech, unsteady gait, muscle weakness, irritability, memory loss, depression, and sleeping difficulties[62]. The early reports noted illness in the town's cats prior to signs of human disease.

Nitrate and nitrite are naturally occurring and are part of the nitrogen cycle. Microorganisms in the environment break down nitrate to nitrite from water, soil, and sewage. Other sources of nitrate contamination are organic, human, and animal. Because nitrite is easily oxidized to nitrate, **nitrate** is the compound mostly found in the environment[63]. Infants who consume water or other products that contain nitrate can develop methemoglobinemia (MetHb), or blue baby syndrome. Infants are at considerable risk because they have an incompletely developed ability to secrete gastric acid, higher levels of fetal hemoglobin, and enzymatic capacity to reduce MetHb. Most people are able to tolerate less than 10 percent MetHb[64].

Polychlorinated biphenyls (PCBs) were used as coolants and lubricants in electrical devices or appliances containing PCB capacitors, in old microscope oil, and in fluorescent lights. PCBs were banned in 1977 but are ubiquitous globally. These compounds are not naturally occurring but accumulate in fish and marine mammals and can also be found in meat and dairy products[65]. PCBs cause liver damage, anemia, acnelike skin condition, stomach injury, thyroid gland injury, immune depression, behavioral alterations, impaired reproduction, birth defects, and cancer[65]. Based on evidence from animal studies, HHS and IARC have determined that PCBs are probably carcinogenic in humans.

Chemical Exposure in Air

Humans are constantly surrounded by air; it touches our skin, enters our lungs, and even makes its way into our gastrointestinal tracts. Air is an important potential exposure medium for a variety of chemicals that may impact health.

In the United States, air quality standards focus on human health outcomes as well as the effects of air quality on agricultural products and on physical structures in the built environment[30, p. 81]. The primary air quality legislation in the United States is the Clean Air Act, originally passed in 1963 and modified substantially in 1970, 1977, and 1990[66]. It allows the EPA to set standards and limits on specific types of emissions, work to improve air quality and limit air pollution, and enforce its standards and regulations. Under the Clean Air Act, the EPA focuses on six **criteria air pollutants**, pollutants that are common in the United States, that negatively impact human health, and for which the EPA uses human or environmental health information to set acceptable levels[67]. These acceptable levels are known as the National Ambient Air Quality Standards (NAAQS). The criteria air pollutants are particulate matter, sulfur oxides, carbon monoxide, nitrogen oxides, lead, and ground-level ozone.

Particulate matter (PM) is the term used to describe small compounds and particles that are suspended in the air and can be drawn into the lungs. Particulate matter includes smoke, fine dust, and even droplets formed during industrial processes. It is a human health concern because it can be inhaled into various regions of the lungs with harmful effects. Particulate matter is often discussed in terms of the size of the particles in microns. Particulate matter $10\,\mu m$ (micrometers) in diameter (PM_{10}) is small enough to penetrate alveolar regions. $PM_{2.5}$ is even smaller; as of 1997 it is the standard size monitored by the EPA because of its demonstrated relationship to human health[68]. **Sulfur dioxide** from fuel combustion reacts with water vapor to produce sulfuric acid and sulfates that irritate the respiratory tract. **Carbon monoxide** (CO) from incomplete combustion binds to hemoglobin, causing hypoxia. Low levels of CO are believed to cause mental processes to slow. **Nitrogen oxide** (NO) can provoke shortness of breath or coughing, and children exposed to NO have an enhanced risk of respiratory problems. As described, lead (Pb) causes adverse impacts on mental and intellectual development in children and has been phased out of gasoline and paint[68]. **Ozone** (O_3) is known as a photochemical oxidant in the troposphere. O_3 reacts with volatile organic compounds to produce photochemical smog. Some cities post ozone alerts on newscasts or the radio to warn those with respiratory disease to stay indoors.

In addition to criteria air pollutants, the EPA also monitors toxic air pollutants, or **hazardous air pollutants** (HAPs), contaminants known to cause cancer or other serious health effects such as birth defects in humans or environmental damage[69]. There are 187 hazardous air pollutants, including metals such as lead and mercury; acrylamide, formed during high-temperature cooking and used in plastic production; formaldehyde, used in building materials such as pressed wood products and also a result of combustion and other processes;

and many others. As for criteria air pollutants, the EPA sets, monitors, and enforces restrictions on hazardous air pollutants through standards for industries, vehicles, and indoor settings.

Preventing Excess Radiation Exposure

Radiation is energy that travels in the form of waves or high-speed particles. According to the EPA, 80 percent of radiation sources are natural and 20 percent are synthetic (human-made)[70]. All humans are exposed to some form of radiation in their daily lives, for example, from solar radiation, watching television, using a computer monitor, or from a medical X-ray machine. Although excess radiation can be considered harmful, there are many benefits of radiation applications found in medicine, industry, and science.

There are two major types of radiation: nonionizing and ionizing radiation. What separates the two types is the ability to chemically move and change the structure of atoms. **Nonionizing radiation** is the weaker of the two types. It has the ability to move atoms around, but it does not have the ability to chemically change, or ionize, them. Visible light, microwave, and radio waves are examples of nonionizing radiation. Although this type of radiation is the weaker of the two, it still has the potential to induce or pose harm. Strong nonionizing radiation has a heating effect, which can burn and cause *erythema*, a redness of the skin such as sunburn, or *photokeratitis*, an inflammation of the cornea of the eye caused by an overexposure to ultraviolet B (UVB) light from the sun or artificial tanning device.

Ionizing radiation is energy in the form of waves or particles that has enough force to remove electrons from atoms. Like nonionizing radiation, it has the ability to move atoms around and most notably, chemically change the structure of them. This characteristic is what makes the ionizing form of radiation a threat to humans and the environment. The radiation symbol shown in Figure 9.5, is

FIGURE 9.5 Universal Symbol of Radiation Warning

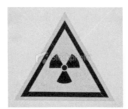

a universal sign used to identify or warn workers or people about the use of a radiation device.

Ionizing radiation consists of three major forms: alpha particles, beta particles, and gamma rays (see Public Health Connections 9.8). As shown in Figure 9.6, the characteristic difference between each subgroup of radiation is the ability to penetrate the skin or enter the human body.

PUBLIC HEALTH CONNECTIONS 9.8

IONIZING RADIATION

Alpha particles are energetic, positively charged particles consisting of two protons and two neutrons. Although alpha particles are energetic, they move slowly through the air; therefore, their penetrating power is low and they cannot pass through a sheet of paper or the outer dead layer of skin.

Beta particles are fast-moving electrons emitted from the nucleus during radioactive decay. They are more penetrating than alpha particles and can typically be stopped or blocked by a layer of clothing.

Gamma rays are a packet of electromagnetic energy: a photon. Gamma photons are the most energetic photons in the electromagnetic spectrum. Gamma rays (gamma photons) are emitted from the nucleus of some unstable (radioactive) atoms[70]. Gamma rays have the ability to pass through, or penetrate, the entire human body.

FIGURE 9.6 The Comparative Strength of Three Forms of Ionizing Radiation: Alpha Particles, Beta Particles, and Gamma Rays

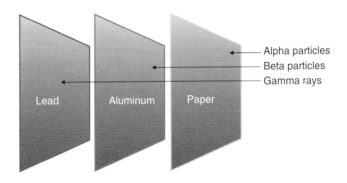

Radon and Public Health

Radon is a naturally occurring colorless, odorless, and tasteless radioactive gas. Radon is formed as a result of the natural decay of uranium throughout the earth's crust. As radon decays, it is released as tiny particles and rises up through the soil or rock to the surface of the earth. If these particles are inhaled over time, radon particles can alter the cells in the human lungs, causing lung cancer.

Radon represents a serious environmental health concern. It is the second leading cause of lung cancer in smokers (following smoking), and the number one cause of lung cancer in nonsmokers. Radon is responsible for about 21,000 lung cancer deaths every year, and about 2,900 of these deaths occur among people who have never smoked[71].

Radon gas is ubiquitous in the natural environment and found in some products developed by humans. However, it is not exposure to radon gas that actually leads to harm, but exposure to the decay products of radon, specifically those with short half-lives that emit alpha radiation. The alpha radiation particles can become attached to dust particles that may be breathed or inhaled by people exposed to the gas and become lodged in the respiratory tract. Radon offspring decaying in the lungs delivers radiation to the tissues. This dose, which is the energy of alpha particles absorbed by cells that line the lungs, is what gives rise to the potential for lung cancer associated with exposure to radon.

Because radon is a gas, it has the ability to seep up from underground and enter buildings through cracks in floors or walls; construction joints; or gaps in foundations around pipes, wires, or pumps. It is important to remember that, without ventilation or another way of dissipating, radon can build up and reach high levels in buildings. The EPA sets the U.S. standard for radon inside buildings and homes at 4 pCi/L (picocuries per liter). However, the EPA recently recommended that states with radon levels less than 4 pCi/L still pose a risk, especially for smokers. The only way to determine if radon is present is to use a radon test kit.

Radiation Misuse

Misuse of radiation can be disastrous and pose serious risks if exposure occurs. Examples include nuclear accidents such as the 1979 Three-Mile Island partial core meltdown; environmental radioactive pollution from past nuclear weapons testing; inappropriate nuclear waste disposal from transportation; and storage, loss, and abuse of radioactive sources. By effectively educating and raising the awareness of the risks posed by radiation and radon, environmental health and safety experts can protect the public's health.

Summary

Environmental public health practitioners are from various backgrounds and share a common goal of protecting communities from environmental causes of disease. Environmental epidemiology is a tool commonly used by environmental health practitioners to assess morbidity or mortality occurrence and trends. Analyses provide the scientific basis for policy decisions and for the evaluation of control measures. Exposures to infectious pathogens, hazardous chemicals, excess radiation, or environments that discourage physical activity can lead to acute and chronic diseases. In the United States, the Environmental Protection Agency and the Centers for Disease Control and Prevention play a key role in identifying and monitoring environmental health concerns, collecting data, and implementing guidelines and standards.

Key Terms

alpha particles, 221

asthma, 209

beta particles, 221

biomonitoring, 215

cancer, 207

carbon monoxide, 219

criteria air pollutants, 219

direct transmission, 200

dose-response relationship, 214

endemic, 200

environment, 199

environmental epidemiology, 200

environmental justice, 213

environmental public health (EPH), 197

epidemic, 200

fetal alcohol spectrum disorders, 212

gamma rays, 221

hazardous air pollutants, 219

indirect transmission, 200

ionizing radiation, 220

lead, 211

lowest observed adverse effect level, 213

maximum concentration level, 217

methyl mercury, 218

naled, 216

nitrate, 218

nitrogen oxide, 219

no observed adverse effect level, 213

nonionizing radiation, 220

obesity, 206

ozone, 219

pandemic, 200

particulate matter, 219

physical environment, 206

polychlorinated biphenyls, 218

polymorphisms, 214

radiation, 220

risk reference dose, 213

route of exposure, 211

sporadic, 200

sulfur dioxide, 219

teratogen, 210

toxicants, 210

toxin, 210

Review Questions

1. Review the state or local health department Web site and identify elements of the ten essential environmental public health services.
2. Select an emerging infectious disease of interest and determine what activities can be taken by the human health, veterinary, and environmental health sectors to collectively prevent the disease from spreading.
3. Determine what barriers in your neighborhood discourage physical activity.
4. Report on the concept of water solubility and lipid solubility and how this influences absorption of a chemical in the body or into cells.
5. Develop a surveillance system based on an issue of your choice.
6. What is bioaccumulation? Identify a compound that bioaccumulates in the food chain.
7. What is a maximum concentration level (MCL)? Look up the reference for EPA National Primary Drinking Water Regulations and describe another chemical not discussed in this chapter.
8. Describe the criteria air pollutants.
9. What are some things you can do to reduce ozone in the troposphere, especially on a hot day with air-quality warnings?
10. Describe how genomics will change how we study environmental health.
11. Discuss naturally occurring and anthropogenic sources of irradiation.

References

1. Public Health in America Web site. Vision statement. Public Health Functions Steering Committee. 1995. Available at: www.health.gov/phfunctions/public.htm. Accessed January 15, 2010.
2. One Health Initiative Web site. Available at: www.onehealthinitiative.com/index.php. Accessed January 15, 2010.
3. Rutt C, Dannenberg AL, Kochtitzky C. Using policy and built environment interventions to improve public health. *J Public Health Manag Prac.* 2008;14(3): 221–223.
4. Luther, C. What the heck is environmental health? *Volusia County Health Department Environmental Health Newsletter.* 2009;15(1):2.
5. Committee on Environmental Epidemiology, Board on Environmental Studies and Toxicology, Commission on Life Sciences. *Environmental Epidemiology.* Vol 1. *Public Health and Hazardous Wastes.* Washington, D.C.: National Research Council National Academy Press; 1991.

6. Saunders B. *Dorland's Illustrated Medical Dictionary*. Philadelphia, Pa.: Saunders and Co.; 2003.

7. Centers for Disease Control and Prevention. Malaria. Available at: www.cdc.gov/malaria. Accessed May 10, 2010.

8. Florida Department of Health. Food and waterborne illness surveillance and investigation annual report. 2000. Available at: www.doh.state.fl.us/environment/community/foodsurveillance/pdfs/annual2000.pdf. Accessed May 10, 2010.

9. Blanton JD, Palmer D, Christian KA, Rupprecht CE. Rabies surveillance in the United States during 2007. *JAVMA*. 2008;233(6):884–897. www.cdc.gov/rabies/docs/rabies_surveillance_us_2007.pdf. Accessed May 10, 2010.

10. World Health Organization. Preventing chronic diseases: A vital investment. Available at: www.who.int/chp/chronic_disease_report. Accessed February 14, 2010.

11. Florida Department of Health. Bureau of Chronic Disease Prevention and Health Promotion. Chronic disease definition. Available at: www.doh.state.fl.us/Family/chronicdisease/. Accessed February 21, 2010.

12. Institute of Medicine. Integrative Medicine and the Health of the Public: A summary of the February 2009 Summit. Washington, D.C.: The National Academies Press; 2009.

13. Williams-Derry C. Sightline Daily. Environment, attitudes and behavior. July 10, 2008. Available at: http://daily.sightline.org/daily_score/archive/2008/07/08/environments-and-attitudes. Accessed February 5, 2010.

14. U.S. Department of Health and Human Services. The Surgeon General's call to action to prevent and decrease overweight and obesity. Rockville, MD: U.S. Department of Health and Human Services, Public Health Service, Office of the Surgeon General; 2001.

15. Wolf AM, Colditz GA. Current estimates of the economic cost of obesity in the United States. *Obes Res.* 1998;6(2):97–106.

16. Wolf A. What is the economic case for treating obesity? *Obes Res.* 1998;6(suppl): 2S–7S.

17. Finkelstein EA, Fiebelkorn IC, Wang G. National medical spending attributable to overweight and obesity: How much, and who's paying? *Health Aff.* 2003;W3: 219–226.

18. Transportation Research Board and Institute of Medicine. *Does the Built Environment Influence Physical Activity? Examining the Evidence*. Special Report 282. Washington, D.C.: National Academy Press; 2005.

19. Frank L, Engelke P, Schmid T. *Health and Community Design: The Impact of the Built Environment on Physical Activity*. Washington, D.C.: Island Press; 2004.

20. Watson M, Dannenberg AL. Investment in safe routes to school projects: Public health benefits for the larger community. *Prev Chronic Dis.* 2008;5: A90.

21. Kraft M. Health effects of sprawl. Address to Women's Transportation Seminar, Robert Wood Johnson Foundation; October 30, 2002, Washington, D.C.

22. Frank LD, Schmid TL, Sallis JF, Chapman J, Saelens BE. Linking objectively measured physical activity with objectively measured urban form: Findings from SMARTRAQ. *Am J Prev Med*. 2005;28:117–125.

23. Saelens BE, Sallis JF, Frank LD. Environmental correlates of walking and cycling: Findings from the transportation, urban design and planning literatures. *Ann Behav Med*. 2003;25:80–91.

24. Hoehner CM, Brennan Ramierez LK, Elliott MB, Handy SL, Brownson RC. Perceived and objective environmental measures and physical activity among urban adults. *Am J Prev Med*. 2005;28:105–116.

25. World Health Organization. Preventing chronic diseases: A vital investment. WHOT Global Report. Available at: www.who.int/chp/chronic_disease_report. Accessed May 10, 2010.

26. U.S. Department of Health and Human Services, Public Health Services, National Toxicology Program. *Report on Carcinogens*. 11th ed. 2005. Available at: http://ntp-server.niehs.nih.gov/index.cfm?objectid=035E5806-F735-FE81-FF769DFE5509AF0A. Accessed February 11, 2010.

27. Pederson T. Dose-response assessment. Extoxnet, Oregon State University Web page. 1997. Available at: http://extoxnet.orst.edu/faqs/risk/dose.htm. Accessed February 11, 2010.

28. Moorman JE, Rudd RA, Johnson CA, et al. National surveillance for asthma—United States, 1980–2004. *MMWR*. 2007;56(SS08):1–14.

29. Centers for Disease Control and Prevention. Asthma. 2009. Available at: www.cdc.gov/asthma/. Accessed February 11, 2010.

30. Moeller DW. *Environmental Health*. Rev ed. Cambridge, Mass.: Harvard University Press; 1997.

31. Lehman-McKeeman LD. Principles of toxicology. In Klaassen C, ed. *Casarett and Doull's Toxicology*. 7th ed. New York: McGraw-Hill; 2008.

32. Centers for Disease Control and Prevention. Fetal alcohol spectrum disorders. Available at: www.cdc.gov/ncbddd/fasd/alcohol-use.html. Accessed February 21, 2010.

33. Environmental Protection Agency. Lead history. Available at: www.epa.gov/history/topics/lead/index.htm. Accessed February 21, 2010.

34. Centers for Disease Control and Prevention. Division of Laboratory Sciences: Lead. Available at: www.cdc.gov/nceh/lead.htm. Accessed February 21, 2010.

35. Centers for Disease Control and Prevention. Lead. Available at: www.cdc.gov/nceh/lead/. Accessed February 21, 2010.

36. Centers for Disease Control and Prevention. U.S. total blood lead surveillance report 1997–2006 (graph). Available at: www.cdc.gov/nceh/lead/data/State_Confirmed_ByYear_1997_2006Total.pdf. Accessed February 21, 2010.

37. Environmental Protection Agency. Lead in paint, dust, and soil: Renovation, repair, and painting. Available at: www.epa.gov/opptintr/lead/pubs/renovation.htm. Accessed February 21, 2010.

38. Eaton D, Gilbert S. Principles of toxicology. In: Klaassen C, ed. *Casarett and Doull's Toxicology*. 7th ed. New York: McGraw-Hill; 2008.

39. Battuello K, Furlong C, Fenke R, Austin M, Burke W. Paraoxonase polymorphisms and susceptibility to organophosphate pesticides. In: Khoury M, Little J, Burke W, eds. *Human Genome Epidemiology*. 1st ed. New York: Oxford University Press; 2004.

40. Atterberry TT, Burnett WT, Chambers JE. Age-related differences in parathion and chlorpyrifos toxicity in male rats: Target and non-target esterase sensitivity and cytochrome P450-mediated metabolism. *Toxicol Appl Pharmacol*. 1997;147: 411–418.

41. Huff RA, Corcoran JJ, Anderson JK. Chlorpyrifos oxon binds directly to muscarinic receptors and inhibits cAMP accumulation in rat striatum. *J Pharmacol Exp Ther*. 1994;269:329–335.

42. Environmental Protection Agency (EPA). U.S. Environmental Protection Agency Office of Pesticide Programs Web site. 2000. Available at: www.epa.gov/pesticides/reregistration/chlorpyrifos.htm. Accessed June 16, 2010.

43. Yuknavaage KL, Fenske RA, Kalman DA, Keifer MC, Furlong CE. Simulated dermal contamination with capillary samples and field cholinesterase biomonitoring. *J. Toxicol Environ Health*. 1997;51:35–55.

44. Augustinsson KB, Barr M. Age variation in plasma arylesterase activity in children. *Clin Chim Acta*. 1963;8:568–573.

45. Ecobichon DJ, Stephens DS. Perinatal development of human blood esterase. *Clin Pharmacol Ther*. 1973;14:41–47.

46. Peakall DB. Effect of DDT on calcium uptake and vitamin D metabolism in birds. *Nature*. 1969; 224(5225):1219–1220.

47. Agency for Toxic Substances and Disease Registry (ATSDR). Toxicology profile: For DDT, DDE, and DDD. Atlanta, Ga.: U.S. Department of Health and Human Services, Public Health Service; September 2002.

48. Joy RM. Chlorinated hydrocarbon insecticides. In: Ecobichon DJ, Joy RM, eds. *Pesticides and Neurological Diseases*. Boca Raton FL: CRC Press; 1982;91–150.

49. Woolley DE. Neurotoxicity of DDT and possible mechanisms of action. In: Prasad KN, Vernadakis A, eds. *Mechanisms of Actions of Neurotoxic Substances*. New York: Raven Press; 1982:95–141.

50. Leoni V, Fabiani L, Marinelli G. PCB and other organochlorines in blood of women with or without miscarriage: A hypothesis of correlation. *Ecotoxicol Environ Safety*. 1989;17:1–11.

51. Ron M, Cucos S, Rosenn B. Maternal and fetal serum levels of organo-chlorine compounds in cases of premature rupture of membranes. *Acta Obstet Gynecol Scand*. 1988;67:695–697.

52. Chowdhury A, Gautam A, Venkatakrishma-Bratt H. DDT induced structural changes in adrenal glands of rats. *Bull. Environ; Contam. Toxicol*. 1990;45: 193–196.

53. Rybakova MN. Effect of certain pesticides on the pituitary and its gonadotropic functions. *Gig Sanit.* 1968;33:27–31.

54. Kidd H, James DR, eds. *The Agrochemicals Handbook.* 3rd ed. Cambridge, UK: Royal Society of Chemistry Information Services; 1991.

55. Duprey Z, Rivers S, Luber G, et al. Community aerial mosquito control and naled exposure. *J Am Mosq Control Assoc.* 2008; 24(1):42–46.

56. Becker A, Jones J, Goodwin B, Mason T, Patel PS, Blackmore C. Florida Hazardous Substances Emergency Events Surveillance activities in classifying the severity of carbon monoxide exposures of the 2005 hurricane season. *Florida Environmental Health Association Journal.* 2006;(winter issue):20–25.

57. Environmental Protection Agency. National Primary Drinking Water Standards. Available at: www.epa.gov/safewater/consumer/pdf/mcl.pdf. Accessed July 29th, 2009.

58. Stephenson F. Florida's mercury menace. *Florida State University Research in Review.* 1997;8:10–21.

59. Gilmour CC, Riedel GS, Ederington MC, et al. Methylmercury concentrations and production rates across a trophic gradient in the northern Everglades. *Biogeochemistry.* 1998;40:327.

60. Fischer G, Rapsomanikis R, Andreae R. Accumulation of methylmercury and transformation of inorganic mercury by macrofungi. *Environ. Sci. Technol.* 1995; 29:993–999.

61. Hecky RE, Ramsey DJ, Bodaly RA, Strange E. In: Suzuki T, ed. *Advances in Mercury Toxicology.* New York: Plenum Press; 1991:33–52.

62. Kutsuna M (ed). *Minamata Disease: Study Group of Minamata Disease.* Kumamoto, Japan: Kumamoto University; 1968:1–4.

63. Agency for Toxic Substances and Disease Registry (ATSDR). Nitrate/nitrite toxicity. 2007. Available at: www.atsdr.cdc.gov/csem/nitrate/nitrate.html. Accessed July 29, 2009.

64. Ellenhorn MJ. Nitrate and nitrite toxicity. In: Schonwald S, Ordog G, Wasserberger J (eds). *Ellenhorn's Medical Toxicology.* 2nd ed. New York: Lippincott, Williams and Wilkins; 1997.

65. Agency for Toxic Substances and Disease Registry. Toxicology profile for PCBs. Atlanta, Ga.: U.S. Deparatment of Health and Human Services, Public Health Service; September 2000.

66. Environmental Protection Agency. Clean Air Act Web site. History of the Clean Air Act. Available at: www.epa.gov/air/caa/caa_history.html. Accessed February 21, 2010.

67. Environmental Protection Agency. The Plain English Guide to the Clean Air Act Web site. Cleaning up commonly found air pollutants. Available at: www.epa.gov/air/peg/cleanup.html. Accessed February 21, 2010.

68. Nadakavukaren A. *Our Global Environment: A Health Perspective.* 6th Ed. Long Grove, Ill: Waveland Press; 2008.

69. Environmental Protection Agency. Air toxics Web site. Available at: www.epa.gov/ttn/atw/index.html. Accessed February 21, 2010.

70. Environmental Protection Agency. Radiation protection. Available at: www.epa.gov/radiation/index.html. Accessed May 14, 2010.

71. Environmental Protection Agency. Radon. Available at: www.epa.gov/radon/. Accessed May 14, 2010.

CHAPTER 10

RISK AND EXPOSURE ASSESSMENT

Vito Ilacqua, PhD

LEARNING OBJECTIVES

- Define and describe risk and exposure in the context of public health.
- Describe the components of a risk assessment and exposure assessment.
- Identify the four major routes of exposure.
- Describe how risk is characterized.
- Understand how beliefs affect risk perceptions.

Legendary investor Warren Buffet has been quoted as saying, "Risk comes from not knowing what you're doing," implying that it can be reduced by adequate knowledge. In the context of environmental and public health, risk can also be reduced, or at least managed, through knowledge of its causes, mechanisms, and magnitude. To understand its nature, we must first understand its meaning: simply put, risk is a probability. In this case, it is the probability of an adverse health outcome to an individual or population from a specific cause. For example, we might hear that the risk of cancer from living near a nuclear power plant is no different from the risk of cancer in the general population or that the risk of lung cancer from a lifetime of smoking is far greater than the risk of lung cancer in the general population. The notion of risk is intuitive enough to be used even in everyday conversation, and yet it is quite problematic once we examine it closely. How do we assign a number to these probabilities? How do we use these numbers to make decisions? And what do they really mean for each of us?

This chapter presents an overview of the tools used to quantify risk. It also describes how risk information is used to manage threats (particularly those of an environmental nature), design regulations, and communicate with the general public.

Risk Assessment and Precautionary Principle

We are confronted by risk every time we do not know or understand the circumstances in which we find ourselves. In this respect, we always face some degree of risk when dealing with the future because it is intrinsically unknowable and beyond our control. There are two fundamental approaches to coping with unknown risks to public health. One approach is to gather information about the mechanisms by which undesirable effects occur so that the likelihood of their occurrence following a particular decision may be estimated. The other approach is to decide that potentially harmful situations are to be avoided as a matter of precaution, even (or especially) when insufficient information is available. The former approach is taken by **risk assessment**, an attempt to identify and quantify potential threats to public health. The latter approach is known as the **precautionary principle**, which in its best-known form states that even in the absence of full certainty about the extent and mechanisms of potential threats, actions should be taken to prevent serious and irrevocable damage.

These two approaches are often considered to be in opposition to each other, partly for political rather than scientific reasons. In the United States, risk assessment is the primary strategy, whereas the precautionary principle has found more ready acceptance in the European Union. In reality, and in practical applications, differences are much less dramatic than would appear when they are considered abstractly: both approaches are sensible, and public health is best served by using one to complement the other. The precautionary principle should not prevent investigation into the mechanisms of risk, the understanding of which is useful to limit harm to public health. A risk assessment, on the other hand, should not be used as a definitive indication that a particular course of action is safe for public health. Such confidence would ignore the numerous sources of uncertainty that are present in any risk assessment as well as the theoretical impossibility that anything is entirely safe and risk free.

Definition of Risk

Imagine someone is being rushed to the emergency room with acute poisoning symptoms. What factors would you guess impact the person's prognosis? Two factors you might think of are the type of poison and the amount received. In fact, these two factors determine the most general operational definition of risk:

$$Risk = Hazard \times Exposure$$

This fundamental equation remains true even in more subtle and complicated circumstances. In other words, the probability of an adverse outcome (**risk**) depends on both the intrinsic ability of the agent causing the risk to produce harm (**hazard**) and the quantity of that agent that contacts the person(s) involved (**exposure**). If both hazard and exposure are known, then calculating risk is a simple enough operation. The difficulty, of course, is to obtain reliable measurements of both hazard and exposure.

Misconceptions About Risk

Although we have defined what risk is, it is just as important to clarify what risk is not. In particular, a quantitative estimate of risk obtained according to the equation above is not to be interpreted or used as a prediction of the future. This may seem confusing, but there are very good reasons why assessing risk and predicting the future are entirely different endeavors.

The most important reasons a risk equation should not be used to predict the future have to do with the nature of probability (recall from Chapter 6 that risk is a probability). Imagine, for example, that the lifetime risk of cancer from benzo(a)pyrene (BaP) in the diet of a particular population is 1 in 1 million. This does *not* mean that if we examine 1 million people from that population, exactly 1 individual will be found with cancer resulting from BaP exposure. In fact, there is only a 36.8 percent chance (or about $1/e$, for those with a passion for calculus) that we will; there is a roughly equal probability that no cases of cancer at all will be found, and some probability that we will discover 2 or more such people among the 1 million people we examine. The observed frequency would match the risk rate better if we examine larger populations, but it is always variable; therefore, knowing risk is not sufficient to exactly predict an outcome. On the other hand, a risk of 1 in 1 million also does *not* mean that it is negligible and no one will develop cancer if we examine just a small population. As highly unlikely as they might be, rare events do happen, and each individual in the population does have a finite risk of developing cancer because of BaP exposure. For the person who develops cancer, the risk would no longer be "negligible." In fact, for a population of just 1 individual, the meaning of probability (and risk) becomes largely a metaphysical question, and the use of risk as defined here is perhaps best avoided.

The second set of reasons a risk equation should not be used as a forecast has to do with the procedure used to estimate risk and the assumptions made along the way. We will discuss these procedures and their potential problems in more detail below.

Finally, the information used to characterize both hazard and probability is a simplified selection of all the present information in the real world in the same way that a city map is different from the city itself. There may be other important factors affecting future outcomes that have not been (or could not be) considered.

The purpose of this clarification is for you to understand that risk estimates are best used in the context of risk management and that the numerical values produced are less meaningful by themselves than when used in comparison with other risk estimates. For example, if you computed the risk of mesothelioma from asbestos exposure using a risk assessment, and then compared it to the results of an epidemiological study of mesothelioma in the general population, you should not expect to find the same numbers.

Components of a Risk Assessment

The process of determining risk quantitatively is called *risk assessment*. There are four components to a risk assessment (Figure 10.1), which we will examine in more detail:

1. **Hazard identification**, finding out (qualitatively) what the hazards might be

2. **Dose-response assessment**, finding out (quantitatively) how potent an agent is

3. **Exposure assessment**, finding out (quantitatively) the amount of contact with an agent

4. **Risk characterization**, combining the information from the above components

Hazard Identification

From early childhood we become familiar with threats to our health that we are likely to encounter, typically echoed in parental recommendations. Identifying

FIGURE 10.1 Components of Risk Assessment Considered in Their Physical and Social Context

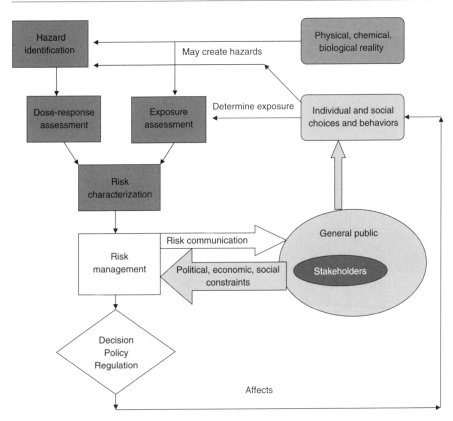

what agents may cause harm is not always simple and straightforward, however. There are tens of thousands of chemicals in current use, for example. Some are innocuous at even very large doses, and some are capable of causing severe toxic effects in minuscule quantities. Furthermore, some hazards are very easily detected and show their effects immediately (think of a hot stove), and others require specialized equipment to be recognized and may take years or decades to show their effects (think of the HIV virus).

A hazard can be an infectious agent (virus, bacteria, protozoa, or parasite), a chemical or physical agent (radiation, noise), or something less neatly classifiable (the prions of Creutzfeldt-Jacob disease). Hazard identification is the first logical step in risk assessment. Its goals are to (1) identify the potential effects to human health and (2) understand under what conditions harm can occur.

The process of identifying the potential hazards and classifying their possible effects may rely on several disciplines, chemistry, epidemiology, microbiology, virology, biochemistry, and qualitative toxicology, depending on the nature of the hazard.

To better understand the effects of a chemical hazard, also called a toxic agent, toxic chemical, or xenobiotic (literally, *foreign to life*), it is useful to examine how an organism reacts when exposure occurs. At the risk of oversimplifying, it can be said that, in general, the organism will try to get rid of the foreign agent, if possible. The most universally effective mechanism of elimination is through urine because the process in the kidneys involves forcing the entire water-soluble component of blood out and then recovering only those molecules that are recognized as useful (a process much akin to that we might use to clean out a refrigerator: taking all the items out and then putting back only those that are still good). The method is highly flexible, thus the body can even rid itself of chemicals it has never encountered before. To facilitate the process, however, some chemicals need to be made more water soluble through metabolic reactions, most of which take place in a dedicated organ, the liver (Figure 10.2). Even though the process is highly effective, there are molecules for which an organism possesses no enzymatic tool to render them more water soluble. These chemicals (such as dioxins, or DDT) will accumulate indefinitely in the fatty tissues, increasing the body burden over time. At other times, metabolism does take place, but it leads to unintended consequences. An essential concept in chemical toxicology is that a chemical agent may not be directly causing an adverse biological effect, but rather the by-products of its biological metabolism are responsible for the adverse effects. An example would be the metabolism of ethanol, which leads to the production of the more toxic acetaldehyde and lipid peroxides[1]. Another example is the metabolism of chloroform (a common contaminant in chlorinated water) to the much more toxic phosgene[2], which is so toxic that it has been used in chemical warfare. Unfortunately, the cascade of biochemical reactions that may take place in the body can be bewilderingly complex, and tools may not exist to effectively predict these developments.

The actual process of identifying a hazard usually involves gathering the preliminary information on the agent, including chemical and physical characteristics and biological testing, and comparing results with epidemiological data, when available.

Biological Testing

The most reliable method of obtaining information on the biological effect of potentially hazardous agents is to produce empirical, experimental data. This

FIGURE 10.2 A Simplified Schematic of the Mechanisms of Urinary Excretion and Oxidative Metabolism of Toxicants

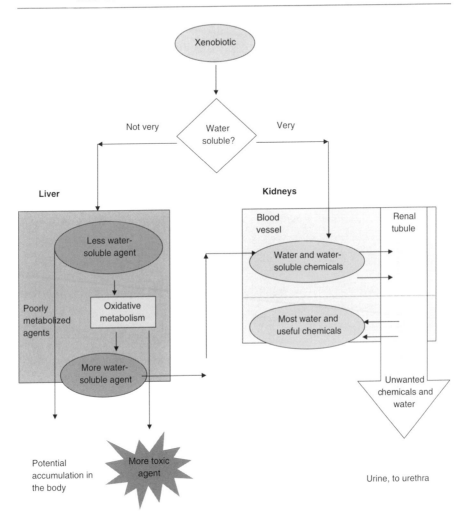

effectively means exposing live organisms to controlled amounts of an agent and observing the effects. Some may find the practice objectionable, but it is the only available approach that can guarantee truly empirical information because our knowledge of the vastly intricate biochemical mechanisms of the human body is not sufficient to allow a satisfactory prediction of all the possible effects based simply on chemical or biological information. To a large extent, we can reasonably predict in which tissues and organs a chemical agent will preferentially accumulate or even how fast it may be excreted using sophisticated mathematical models called physiologically based pharmacokinetic (PBPK) models. But even PBPK models cannot reveal the desired information on the possible effects of toxic agents within tissues and cells.

There are many different types of biological testing, and their use is based on the methods and the kind of information sought. To test for possible mutagenicity (the ability to permanently alter DNA), for example, bacterial or yeast cultures are used. In most other cases, mammals (primarily rodents) are used as surrogates of humans because they are phylogenetically related to us, and at the same time, their use avoids the ethically indefensible approach of exposing humans to agents of unknown hazard. These animals are carefully bred and selected to ensure a measure of genetic uniformity and are typically expensive to purchase and maintain ($100 or more is not uncommon for an adult laboratory rat).

Conditions of exposure are varied in order to understand how they affect toxicity because some effects may not be apparent immediately. A typical battery of tests for chemical hazards will include the following:

1. Acute toxicity: a single high dose administered to determine lethality and immediate effects

2. Chronic toxicity: regular exposures to low doses for the lifetime of the animal

3. Subchronic toxicity: repeated exposures at intermediate doses for medium-term exposures (ninety days in rats)

4. Cancer bioassays: lifetime exposures to establish carcinogenicity (the ability to cause cancer)

5. Reproductive toxicity test: exposure over two or three generations of animals to determine potential interferences with reproductive health

6. Skin/eye tests: to establish if an agent is an irritant

7. Sensitization test: to establish if an agent is an allergen (different from an irritant because it triggers an immunological response)

Additional tests may be performed for effects on a specific organ system, such as neurodevelopmental toxicity, immunotoxicity, or endocrine toxicity tests. In some cases, ecological toxicity tests are also performed to assess the potential for bioaccumulation and biodegradation in the environment that could result in indirect exposures and risks. It is worth pointing out that the same agent can have a variety of different effects simultaneously, including cancer and acute toxicity, although the levels at which each type of toxicity occurs may vary substantially. For example, arsenic is a well-known toxic agent, used since antiquity as a rapid poison (acute toxicity) and the method of choice in many a murder mystery novel. At much lower levels, however, arsenic can also act as a carcinogen and as an irritant.

Epidemiology and Hazard Identification

In many cases, epidemiology can be used as a public health tool to help identify potential hazards. If an association is noted between a particular morbidity and specific exposures or behaviors, a previously unsuspected connection can be made. For example, John Snow linked contaminated water to cholera in a classic and early epidemiological work (see Chapter 1). The process can work the other way around too, with hazard identification supplying plausible agents and mechanisms for epidemiological investigations through which we seek to determine if a plausibly important agent actually does cause measurable deleterious human effects. There are many examples of hazard identification preceding epidemiological evidence, such as polychlorodibenzodioxins (PCDDs), whose toxicity has been well understood even though effects in human population proved comparatively hard to document. There are both advantages and disadvantages to using epidemiology in hazard identification. Some of the advantages include the ability to observe effects in a human (rather than animal) population and the availability of data without expensive toxicological studies. There are inherent drawbacks, however. One of the most important limitations is that exposures in epidemiological studies are not controlled as they can be in a laboratory, there is a much greater uncertainty as to the amount of exposure, and they cannot establish a safe level of exposure (other than none) no matter how many studies are performed.

Dose-Response Assessment

As noted, exposure to the same amount of two different agents may produce drastically different results. Once the nature of the hazard is known, the goals of the dose-response assessment are to find out (1) what levels of exposure lead to what effects and (2) what levels of exposure produce no adverse effects. One of the important results of hazard identification is whether an agent is or is not a carcinogen. The determination of a dose-response relationship changes depending on this difference, based on the concept of threshold. A **threshold** is a level of exposure below which no effects can be detected. It may well be that effects do occur below the threshold, but they are sufficiently subtle that we are unable to distinguish them from those observed in a nonexposed control. Cancer and non-cancer effects differ in this respect: for non-cancer effects we assume a threshold (however small) does exist, and for cancer effects we generally assume that no threshold exists. Consequently, if these assumptions hold, for non-cancer effects there must be a level of exposure that is essentially safe, and for cancer effects any exposure, no matter how small, would increase risk. Although this distinction is somewhat contentious, especially for radiation exposures[3], it is useful in practical applications. It is worth considering the biological reasons for this distinction in more detail.

An agent without carcinogenic potential can exert its effects in a number of different ways, but its effects are counteracted to some extent by the attempts of the organism to eliminate it (as noted above), as well as by other mechanisms used by the body to counteract its effects and maintain homeostasis. The lower the level of exposure, the better able the body is to respond to the agent and neutralize the undesirable effects. At some point, the exposure level is so low that no effects can be detected. A carcinogen, on the other hand, acts by modifying the genetic information of a cell (**initiator**) or by stimulating the growth of a previously mutated cell (**promoter**). Modifications will not always occur, and when they do occur, they may not be at a site in the genome that would lead to cancerous transformation, a cell may be able to repair the damage to its DNA, or the immune system may kill cells that have started replicating out of control. However, both the carcinogenic effect and its countermeasures are hit-or-miss events, rather than events based on the quantity of agents. There is a finite probability (albeit small) that even a single molecule of a carcinogen may initiate the chain of events that lead to a cancer without being intercepted.

Non-Cancer Effects

In a typical dose-response assessment, several genetically similar populations of test animals are exposed to different levels of hazardous agents, and any differences are noted with respect to a nonexposed control population. Each physiological effect is measured separately, and results are plotted on a chart (see Figure 10.3) using levels of exposure as an independent variable (x axis) and the percentage of the exposed population displaying the effect of interest as a dependent variable (y axis). Because the number of available populations of test animals is necessarily limited (recall the cost of each animal), intermediate points are obtained by interpolation. Because exposure levels beyond a certain point produce an effect in 100 percent of the animals, and exposure levels below another point do not produce detectable effects in any animal, data points are typically distributed on an S-shaped curve (Figure 10.3). In some cases, special units (such as probit) are used to allow the points to fall on a straight line, but

FIGURE 10.3 The Typical S-Shaped Curve Produced by Animal Studies for Non-Cancer Effects

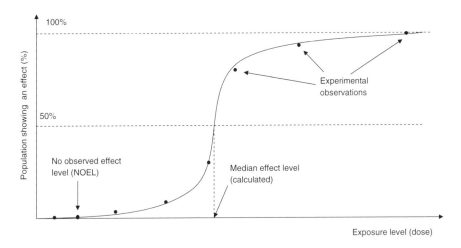

Note that the curve is produced by interpolation of experimental observations, which need not lie exactly on it. The median effect level in acute toxicity studies is the LD_{50}, and it is usually calculated. The no observed effect level (NOEL), on the other hand, must correspond to an experimental data point.

the nature of the relationship does not change. These are representations of the dose-response relationship for each particular effect. In an acute toxicity study, for instance, the effect of interest will be death, whereas in a sensitization test, it will be the appearance of an allergic reaction. Notice that not all the animals, even very genetically homogeneous animals in controlled conditions, will display an effect at the same level of exposure. This variability within a population reflects differences in genetics (still present), social status (where applicable), prior history, and generally everything that makes an individual animal different from another. This is an important characteristic of a dose-response relationship to keep in mind when considering human populations as well.

Several different measures of toxicity can be obtained from the analysis of these dose-response relationships. A common one resulting from acute toxicity studies is the lethal dose for 50 percent of a population (**LD_{50}**), normalized by the weight of the animal, which can be used as a relative indication of acute toxicity. The lower the LD_{50} (in milligrams per kilogram of body weight for chemicals), the more toxic is the agent. For example, in rats, the LD_{50} of sucrose (table sugar) is almost 30,000 mg/kg[4], whereas that of potassium cyanide (another agent favored in murder mysteries) is 5 mg/kg[5], making cyanide almost 6,000 times more toxic than sugar. The example illustrates how any substance or agent can be considered hazardous at high enough doses, a principle identified in toxicology as *the dose makes the poison*. It also shows that the inherent toxicity of different agents can vary over several orders of magnitude.

Other useful measures of non-cancer toxicity are the lowest level at which an effect is observed (**lowest observed effect level**, or LOEL) and even more importantly, the level at which no effect is observed (**no observed effect level**, or NOEL). In some cases, small amounts of an agent may actually produce beneficial effects in the exposed animals, so it is more useful sometimes to identify the **no observed *adverse* effect level** (NOAEL). These measurements are the essential benchmarks of toxicity used to establish risk guidelines.

Extrapolation of Animal Data

One of the downsides of using animals to assess dose response is that toxicity thresholds are not established in humans. As similar as rodents may be to humans, biochemical differences do exist. The use of primates, particularly the great apes, who are virtually indistinguishable from humans from a biochemical standpoint, might provide a better model, in theory. In practice, however, the cost of a full battery of toxicological tests using primates would be prohibitive; these tests in rodents, who are relatively small, prolific, and have short life cycles, can already exceed $1 million[6]. Furthermore, there is greater resistance in both the general public and researchers to using primates rather than rodents as laboratory animals.

Because we cannot know a priori what the differences are in the effects of a particular agent, a solution has been found in the use of multiplicative factors for extrapolation of dose-response studies from rodents to humans. Typically, a multiplicative factor of 1/3 to 1/10 is used to account for possible biochemical differences between humans and rodents, and another factor of 1/10 is used to account for the possibility of greater population variability in humans compared to rodents. These multiplicative factors are known as safety factors, and they are applied to the NOEL or NOAEL observed in the most sensitive animal model (mouse, rat, guinea pig). Thus, the corresponding safe levels in humans are up to 100 times lower than that measured in laboratory animals. This quantity is called the **reference dose** (RfD), and it is deemed the maximum acceptable daily exposure in humans[7]. If studies were unable to produce a NOEL or NOAEL, and only a LOEL is available, or if chronic toxicity studies are unavailable, a further factor of up to 1/10 is applied. The choice of values of 1/10 for these uncertainty factors is regarded as conservative; in cases in which more detailed information is available, larger factors (such as 1/3) might be applied, following research reviews by expert panels.

PUBLIC HEALTH CONNECTIONS 10.1

REFERENCE DOSE (RFD) CALCULATION

1. The most sensitive effect in animal tests for vinyl chloride (an agent used in chemical manufacturing) has been reported in the liver of rats, with a NOAEL of 0.09 mg/kg/day, during chronic exposures[8]. A safety factor of 1/3 is then applied to account for differences between humans and rodents, and another 1/10 for sensitive individuals (i.e., potentially greater variability in humans). The reference dose was then calculated as

$$\text{RfD} = 0.09 \text{ mg/kg/day} \times 1/3 \times 1/10 = 0.003 \text{ mg/kg/day}$$

2. Changes in body weight were reported as the most sensitive effect in rats exposed to nickel for two years (chronic exposure), with a NOAEL of 5 mg/kg/day[9]. A safety factor of 1/10 is then applied for differences between humans and rodents, another 1/10 to protect sensitive individuals, and 1/3 to reflect inadequacy in reproductive toxicity studies, as judged by the U.S. Environmental Protection Agency expert panel. Therefore,

$$\text{RfD} = 5 \text{ mg/kg/day} \times 1/10 \times 1/10 \times 1/3$$
$$= 0.02 \text{ mg/kg/day (with rounding for significant digits)}$$

The use of these safety factors may seem arbitrary, but it is strictly precautionary, with its goal as public health protection rather than exact knowledge. It is worth noting that such safety factors are used in other disciplines where protection from failure is more important than efficiency. Thus buildings and bridges are routinely designed with greater structural specifications (and more materials) than are strictly necessary to stand; military plans usually commit more forces than deemed necessary to achieve an objective; and (responsibly) calibrated bungee jumping cords can withstand greater mechanical stress than expected with a particular participant. This is a concept called *redundancy*, and it is even more important in risk assessment because the magnitude of the variability accounted for by these safety factors is actually unknown.

Cancer Effects

The development of dose-response relationships for cancer effects is similar to that for non-cancer effects in chronic studies, but with the underlying assumption that no threshold exists. This assumption is actually debated, and in several studies[3,10,11] there is evidence that a threshold does exist or even that small levels of exposure may produce beneficial effects, a concept known as **hormesis**. Nevertheless, the assumption of no threshold is generally applied, both for precautionary reasons (since evidence to the contrary is very limited) and for practical reasons. In fact, one of the difficulties of performing dose-response studies for cancer effects with laboratory animals is that the low-probability occurrence of cancers at low exposure levels requires impractically large populations of animals. The assumption of a linear response (see Figure 10.4), on the other hand, allows the extrapolation of risk from exposing animals at several very high levels, far higher than that which humans are likely to encounter. The slope of the dose-response line is taken as a measure of carcinogenic potential, and for toxic chemicals, it is usually given as probability of cancer per unit of

FIGURE 10.4 Typical Results of an Animal Study for Cancer Effects

Experimental observations are possible only at high levels of exposure because observation of effects at low doses would require impractically large populations. A linear dose response is assumed by extrapolating high-dose observations. The actual form of the dose-response relationship at low dose is unknown and could conceivably assume other nonlinear shapes, perhaps with a threshold (patterns A and B). If the dose-response relationship dipped below the background cancer level observed in controls (B), exposure at low levels would actually be beneficial (hormesis).

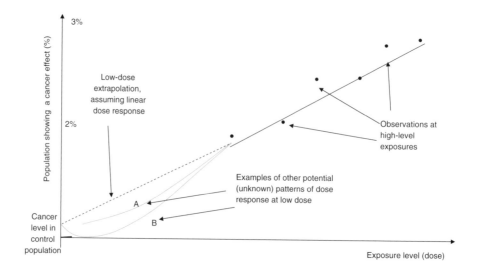

daily dose, in units of (milligrams per kilogram of body weight per day)$^{-1}$. This measure is commonly, and descriptively, called the cancer slope factor (CSF). Greater slope factors imply a greater carcinogenic potential. For example, the CSF for 2,3,7,8-tetrachlorodibenzo-*p*-dioxin (TCDD) has been calculated at 1.5×105 (mg/kg/d)$^{-1}$ [12], whereas that of arsenic is 100,000 smaller at 1.5 (mg/kg/d)$^{-1}$ [13].

Exposure Assessment

The levels of exposure to hazardous agents can be controlled easily among experimental animals in laboratory conditions, but knowing to what levels human individuals and populations are exposed presents challenges of its own. The discipline concerned with understanding the mechanisms of exposure and determining the levels of potentially hazardous exposures to various agents is called **exposure science**, and the process used to achieve that understanding is called **exposure assessment**. The concepts and findings of exposure science are essential to disciplines other than risk assessment, especially environmental epidemiology and occupational health. In the context of an exposure assessment, exposure is defined as the contact between an agent (chemical, physical, or biological) and a target (such as a person) at its boundary over a certain period of time[14]. The concept is most easily understood for chemical agents. For example, a person breathing air that contains carbon monoxide is making contact with that agent both on his or her skin (the boundary) and through inhalation (boundary is the entrance of the airways).

Exposure Routes and Pathways

As for the case of carbon monoxide, there are several ways in which exposure may occur and several mechanisms for an agent to enter the body. There are four distinct mechanisms for entry in the body for a chemical agent, called **routes of exposure**:

1. Inhalation: breathing in

2. Ingestion: eating or consuming

3. Dermal absorption: passing through the skin

4. Puncture: piercing skin and other layers (as in a needle stick)

It is possible for an agent to enter the body through two or more routes simultaneously. For instance, polycyclic aromatic hydrocarbons (PAHs) are produced as combustion by-products by anything from a furnace, to a cigarette, to charred burgers, and they are emitted in the air on fine particles. When those particles deposit on soils, water, or vegetation, PAHs can be taken up by organisms that ingest or absorb them and accumulate them in their tissues. We can then receive an exposure to PAHs both through inhalation, as they are by-products of combustion, and through ingestion, as these chemicals can be taken up and accumulated by organisms that are part of our diet. The sum of all the exposures through different routes is called **total exposure**. In many cases, however, one or two routes dominate the total exposure, whereas others may contribute negligible amounts. To continue the example of PAHs, the general population in the United States has been estimated to receive 1–5 μg/day through ingestion and 0.16 μg/day through inhalation, whereas dermal absorption is deemed negligible[15]. Smoking, however, may change this pattern and contribute as much as 15 μg/day through inhalation.

Knowing the route(s) of exposure is important because the toxicity of an agent can vary with exposure through different routes due to the different ability of the organs to absorb and metabolize toxic agents. For instance, absorption of inorganic mercury through inhalation is about 75 percent, but through ingestion it is less than 15 percent[16]. In addition, different routes of absorption may cause the agent to be routed through different organs (such as the liver) before being distributed through the rest of the body. In general, toxicological benchmark levels like NOAEL can be different for different routes of exposure.

From the standpoint of managing risk, it is also important to know how an agent reached a target from its original source. For instance, how does mercury emitted from coal power plants end up in tuna fish and eventually enter the diet of human populations? The sequence of processes and events that lead from a source to an exposure is called **pathway of exposure**, and it is traditionally the object of environmental science. These exposure pathways can be complex and sometimes lead through unexpected and surprising mechanisms. Children, for example, can receive high exposures to lead, a metal known to cause neurodevelopmental effects including reducing IQ, by ingesting soil and dust contaminated by chipping paint in older houses where lead-based paint was used[17].

Exposure, Contact Rate, and Dose

Intuitively, the greater the concentration of an agent in the medium of contact (air, water, food) and the longer the duration of the contact, the greater the

FIGURE 10.5 Exposure Is Defined as the Product of Concentration and Time at Any Given Instant

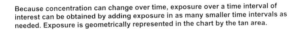

Because concentration can change over time, exposure over a time interval of interest can be obtained by adding exposure in as many smaller time intervals as needed. Exposure is geometrically represented in the chart by the tan area.

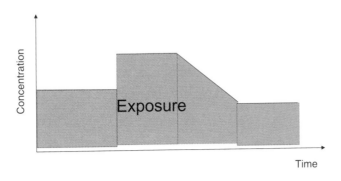

amount of the agent that can be absorbed and the greater the potential for any adverse effects. To account for both of these factors, exposure is mathematically defined as the product of concentration and duration of contact. Because the concentration may vary with time, different exposures may be computed for different time intervals and added to obtain the exposure for the entire duration of interest (see Figure 10.5). Yet, exposure does not convey the amount of an agent that actually crosses the contact boundary and enters the body, a quantity known as **dose**. The two concepts are connected through the **contact rate**, the amount of contact between the body and the medium that contains the agent:

$$Dose = Exposure \times Contact\ rate$$

An example of contact rate is the inhalation rate, the amount of air an individual breathes per unit of time. Other examples are the rate at which one consumes milk or the absorption rate of a chemical through the skin. In most cases, these contact rates vary not only between individuals according to sex, age, ethnicity, and other factors but also by the specific activity that a person is performing. While jogging, for instance, a person's inhalation rate is much higher than while sleeping. In exposure science, the specific activities that people perform in their daily lives, their duration and frequency, are referred to as time-activity patterns, or simply as **activity patterns**.

PUBLIC HEALTH CONNECTIONS 10.2

CALCULATING EXPOSURE AND DOSE

A person breathing air that contains $15\,mg/m^3$ of carbon monoxide (CO) for 2 hours while doing light activity might breathe at the rate of $0.8\,m^3/hr$. The person's exposure will be

$$\text{Exposure} = 15\,mg/m^3 \times 2\ \text{hours} = 30\ mg\ hr/m^3$$

The dose of carbon monoxide that they will receive during those 2 hours is:

$$\text{Dose} = 30\ mg\ hr/m^3 \times 0.8\ m^3/hr = 24\ mg$$

Estimating Exposure

From the definitions of exposure, dose, and contact rate, a rather inconvenient conclusion can be drawn: to estimate the total exposure levels of an individual, which are needed for risk assessment or epidemiology, it is essential to know the concentration of the agent of concern in all the media (air, water, soil, dust, and every food) that the person has come into contact with, as well as what that person was doing and where he or she has been. This information burden is correspondingly expanded when the exposure of a population is sought, and it explains the difficulty and cost of such undertakings. Several different approaches have been developed to make this information more manageable, and these are categorized as direct and indirect methods of exposure assessment. Both types of methods rely on statistical selection of individuals within a population that are representative of its variability in terms of age, sex, socioeconomic status, geographic location, and other parameters[18]: in other words, a representative sample. Although this statistical sampling approach works well, it is wise to remember that some pathways of exposure are so surprising and hard to imagine at the study design stage, and may affect such specific populations, that representativeness is never truly guaranteed.

Direct Methods

The direct approach to measuring exposure consists of following the selected individuals for a period of time (with their consent) and measuring the agent(s) of interest in every medium he or she comes into contact with by taking appropriate samples. Specific methods differ based on the route of exposure.

Inhalation Participants are asked to wear a relatively small portable air sampler, usually consisting of a pump and a collection device, such as a filter or chemical trap. Air is drawn from the breathing zone of the person, and participants must wear it at all times, wherever they go, including their workplace. Because such devices can weigh 1–2 kg and generate a substantial amount of noise and vibration, this method can be a burden, and the duration of the study is necessarily limited. For a few agents, it is possible to use passive samplers that do not rely on a pump and are therefore much lighter and easier.

Ingestion Study participants are asked to set aside a sample of everything they eat or drink (split sample) or to prepare or purchase additional amounts of food (duplicate sample). Samples are then collected and analyzed for the agent of interest. It is important that the food sample undergo the exact preparation as the food the participants actually eat because some contamination may occur during preparation rather than from the original ingredients. Careful compliance by the study participants is essential in this method.

Dermal Participants are asked to wear patches of material that simulate the property of the skin, and the amounts of agents (usually in dust particles) collected on these patches is scaled to the skin size to determine the overall dermal exposure. Many factors can affect the reliability of this method, and the similarity between patches and skin is far from perfect. Alternatively, the skin is washed at regular intervals with an appropriate solvent (such as rubbing alcohol), and the liquid is collected and analyzed. This is especially useful for hands, for example. Even a thorough washing, however, may not completely collect the agent from the skin.

An alternative and still direct approach to these methods is to measure the amount of an agent that is already inside the body by taking samples of bodily fluids, such as blood or urine, or tissues, such as adipose tissue or hair. The agent or any of its by-products measured in these samples is called a **biomarker**. This approach is familiar and commonly used for workplace drug testing or antidoping testing in professional sports. Biomarkers can provide useful information, but they are far from a perfect answer to every exposure question. The primary limitation is that they do not convey information on the route of exposure, only on total exposure. Another important limitation is that, due to the body metabolism and excretion, biomarkers for exposure to certain agents may be available for only a limited time. Cost and difficulty of the analysis are also to be considered, as is the willingness of participants to provide samples (easy for hair or urine, harder for blood or fat tissue samples). Finally, individual differences (genetic or lifestyle) in metabolism may lead to different biomarker concentrations, even with similar exposures[18].

Indirect Methods

In many cases, the cost and burden of direct methods may render them impractical, particularly in large studies. Indirect methods are based on measuring concentration in a few representative locations or rely on existing data for concentrations in environmental media. Indirect methods also use known contact rates and activity patterns to determine exposure. For example, to estimate the ozone exposure among people living in Manhattan, one might use the monitoring network of the state of New York and use the daily ozone concentration collected at sites in the area. Then, making the assumption that people in Manhattan breathe at the same rates as people measured in published studies, one could use daily average inhalation rates to produce an estimate of the dose of ozone in Manhattan. This approach is simple, cheap, and places no burden on the population. The obvious downside is that it does not yield an empirically determined exposure; rather, it is based on a series of assumptions. In particular, it assumes a few monitoring sites represent the entire area of interest. This assumption may at times be correct, but the limited number of monitoring sites within the area limits the ability to capture the true patterns of ozone concentration. Worse, in some areas of interest there may be no monitoring sites available, or the agent of interest may not be monitored at all.

Time-Activity Patterns

Knowledge of time-activity patterns is essential for both direct and indirect methods of exposure assessment, particularly if we want to identify the reasons for certain exposures. For example, if a personal air sampler captures particularly high levels of exposure to suspended particles between 5:00 and 5:30 p.m., it is useful to know where the study participant was and what he or she was doing. To characterize time-activity patterns for an individual or in a population, which is done with a statistically representative sample of people, several methods can be used. One of the simplest and most common approaches is to interview study participants using a questionnaire. The ability to recall times and events, even within a recent time frame, is relatively limited, however, and subject to numerous biases. In particular, people typically remember unusual events and situations better than they recall ordinary ones. In exposure assessment, however, it generally is the ordinary experiences that are of the most interest. To avoid this recall bias, participants may be asked to keep a diary of their activities. These diaries may be a form to be completed at prescribed times or perhaps be an online reporting system[19]. The disadvantage of a diary is that it can prove burdensome for participants, especially if the prescribed time intervals are short. More sophisticated methods include the use of data loggers[19,20], on which participants simply press a button to indicate their activity, and the use of GPS-capable devices to track the location of the study participants[21]. Finally, to avoid reliance on participants' actions, researchers may opt to physically observe and videotape a participant's activities for a certain period. This option is very objective and reliable but takes a lot of observer hours and is intrusive, and participants may act differently when they know they are being observed. Nevertheless, it has been successfully used with young children, who generally ignore the camera once the novelty has worn off[22].

Much information has been collected over the years about a wide array of activities of interest. Data are available for the general population regarding the frequency and duration of activities as diverse as showering, commuting, gardening, eating meats or dairy products, sleeping, and swimming in public pools. The EPA compiled these data in an essential publication for exposure science, the *Exposure Factors Handbook* (see Resources). The need to factor in activity patterns, which strongly depend on social and behavioral characteristics, as well as the individual differences within a population during an exposure assessment, makes the quantification of exposures interesting and challenging and partly explains why exposure assessment is often the weakest aspect of environmental epidemiological studies.

Risk Characterization

The final step in a risk assessment is to integrate the information from hazard identification, dose-response assessment, and exposure assessment to produce an estimate of risk that may be used by risk managers to make decisions and set regulations. At its most basic, a **risk characterization** estimates the risk to a population from a specific level of exposure to a particular agent. A detailed risk characterization, however, needs to take into account the following:

- the nature of the risks involved (such as cancer versus non-cancer)

- the quality of the available evidence

- the size of the affected populations

- the possible presence of especially sensitive, or especially highly exposed subpopulations

- the uncertainty of dose-response and exposure assessments

For non-cancer effects, exposure below the reference dose is not expected to produce any undesirable effect. However, it may be important to assess at a glance how close to the risk threshold an individual or a population may be. The ratio of the chronic (lifetime) daily intake calculated from exposure assessment to the reference dose is called the **hazard index** (HI).

$$\text{Hazard index} = \text{Exposure dose}/\text{reference dose}$$

A hazard index much smaller than 1 indicates that exposures are far from the critical level defined by the RfD so there is an ample margin of safety in public health protection. Conversely, an HI close to 1, or worse, above 1, indicates that steps must be taken to reduce exposures[23].

For cancer effects, no level of exposure is considered safe, and risk characterization produces estimates of risk based on the observed exposure. Traditionally, risk characterization produced point estimates, or single values that expressed the average risk from a hazardous agent given the estimated exposure. This approach is quick and simple but somewhat unsatisfactory, especially in regard to risk in specific subpopulations. In more recent years, the limitations of this approach have led to the production of statistical distributions of risk within a population such that the range of possible risks and the size of the populations involved for each level of risk are properly represented. This may be accomplished through such techniques as Monte Carlo simulations, in which a large number (around 10,000) of individual risk scenarios are created by drawing from the exposure assessment data according to their probability[24]. In addition, as you may have noticed at several points in this chapter, much of the information supplied by exposure and dose-response assessments contains important elements of uncertainty and ambiguity. A risk characterization that does not convey this uncertainty information is unintentionally misleading (at best), or deliberately manipulative (at worst), because the amount of uncertainty alters the confidence that decision makers have in the data and may well affect the outcome of any risk management process.

PUBLIC HEALTH CONNECTIONS 10.3

RISK ASSESSMENT

Consider the simple scenario of a person weighing 70 kg and drinking water that contains arsenic at 10 µg/L at the rate of 2 L/day for a lifetime (80 years), with no other exposure. Arsenic has both cancer and non-cancer effects.

Exposure Assessment

This person has a constant exposure through his life. The dose of arsenic can be calculated as

$$10\ \mu g/L \times 80\ yr \times 365\ days/yr \times 2\ L/day = 584,000\ \mu g$$

If we want to express this as an average daily dose per unit of body weight, we could calculate

$$\text{Lifetime average daily dose} = 584,000\ \mu g/(80\ yr \times 365\ days/yr)/70\ kg$$
$$= 0.286\ \mu g/kg/day$$

Non-cancer Effects

The RfD for arsenic is $0.3\ \mu g$ /kg/day. The hazard index (HI) is then

$$HI = 0.286/0.3 = 0.952$$

Because the HI is less than 1, no harmful effect is expected; however, we are not especially confident in this judgment, given the proximity to 1 and the possible uncertainty in our estimate that we have not factored in.

Cancer Effects

The cancer slope factor for arsenic ingestion is 1.5 $(mg/kg/day)^{-1}$, so we estimate risk as

$$\text{Risk} = \text{Hazard} \times \text{Exposure}$$
$$= 1.5\,(mg/kg/day)^{-1} \times 0.286\ \mu g/kg/day \times 0.001\,mg/\mu g = 4.3\ 10^{-4}$$

In other words, drinking water containing this level of arsenic would increase this person's odds of developing cancer during his or her lifetime by about 4 in 10,000.

Risk Management

Simply knowing what risks are associated with various hazards and what levels of exposure may be safe is not enough. This information must be applied to make policy decisions, set regulations, choose manufacturing options, determine what to do after accidents, and most importantly, limit risk to public health. These decisions require more than scientific knowledge because they have the potential to affect social, economic, and lifestyle aspects of individuals, businesses, and communities and depend on the value preferences and risk tolerance of a society. The people, institutions, and groups that may be affected by a risk management decision are referred to as **stakeholders**. The involvement of stakeholders in the risk management process adds a degree of complexity (see Figure 10.1), and yet this involvement is important to ensure the success of a risk-based decision. Stakeholders are often those whose compliance will be needed for a policy to be implemented after a decision has been made, and although they may seek primarily to protect their own interests, their involvement can help them feel invested in the success of a policy. Just as importantly, stakeholders may have unique perspectives and knowledge to contribute to the risk management process; for example, knowledge of a specific local community or of technological options.

The basic principle of risk management is that the scope of the action is limited to managing exposures. The hazard component of risk is strictly dependent on chemical, physical, and biological realities that are not susceptible to change or regulation. Because risk is a product, however, it can be made arbitrarily small (in principle) by limiting exposure: in the extreme case, with no exposure there is no risk, by definition. Regulatory standards for agents with only non-cancer effects are usually produced by working back from the RfD and the exposure levels to set maximum allowable concentrations that do not cause exposures to exceed the RfD. In the arsenic example (see Public Health Connections 10.3), one might set the maximum allowable concentration at $10\,\mu g/L$, for example. However, exposure levels within a population differ, sometimes by orders of magnitude, and a decision needs to be made on what fraction of the population can realistically be protected. Because setting lower, more protective limits comes at a higher cost, we might ask whether it is fair for a majority to bear higher costs to protect the health of a very small minority whose exposures (or susceptibility) are especially high. The concepts of social justice (see Chapter 1) are called into play here, and the answer will reflect the specific preference of a society as well as the reasons behind these extreme exposures.

When cancer hazards are involved, the situation can be even more complex, and managing risk requires a decision on what risks are acceptable, a definition that has changed over time and in different situations. One might consider zero risk to be the only acceptable option, or perhaps the best technologically achievable level of risk is acceptable. In other situations, a level of risk that does not entail excessive economic burden is agreed upon, or a specific small number is selected, such as 1 in 1 million. It is important to realize that all these definitions may have a proper place. For example, if it is technologically feasible to remove a carcinogen completely from drinking water, then setting the goal of risk from that hazard at zero may be appropriate. If, as is more often the case, exposure cannot be completely eliminated, concepts such as the best available control technology (BACT) or the lowest achievable emission rate (LAER) are invoked by legislation such as the Clean Air Act (which is not based on risk). In other cases, the costs involved in eliminating exposure might have such dire consequences that they would completely outweigh the risks that are being managed. For instance, it is possible to drastically cut the risks of exposure to suspended particles in the air by closing down every fossil-fuel power plant. Without a ready substitute, however, the lack of available energy for heating and other necessities and the ensuing economic upheaval are nearly guaranteed to produce many more casualties than the carcinogenic particles may be producing at present.

These comparisons of risks for different scenarios highlight one of the most important features of risk management, namely the relative nature of risk estimates. Although risk estimates are not necessarily an exact expression of our best knowledge, the fact that they are obtained through a consistent procedure makes them comparable. This is, in fact, the best use of risk assessments: to compare risks rather than focus on the specific magnitudes of estimated risks. In other words, it is far less important to know that the risk from current exposures to agent X in a population is, say, 10^{-4}, than it is to know that that risk is 2,500 times greater than that from present exposures to agent Z. This relative comparison allows us to set priorities in policy and interventions.

The use of specific numbers as a definition of acceptable risk has found consistent application in the environmental regulatory framework of risk management in the United States. The Comprehensive Environmental Response, Compensation, and Liability Act of 1980 (better known as *Superfund*), for example, required that cleanup of toxic waste sites be undertaken if the lifetime cancer risk to the affected populations exceeds 1 in 1 million. This number has achieved a perhaps undeserved popularity, and it is often used in the public discourse as a synonym for *acceptable* risk, despite the fact that no societal feedback has ever been solicited on such a figure and that it is not even clear how it was originally produced[25]. Ranges of numbers for acceptable risks are best used to allow risk managers sufficient flexibility, taking into account that the background lifetime cancer rate in the United States and other developed countries stands at between 1 in 2 and 1 in 3[26,27], thus even additional risks of 1 in 10,000, for instance, cannot be said to appreciably increase that rate.

One of the limitations of risk assessment and risk management is that the risk for each individual agent is estimated and managed on its own, as if it were independent of any other risk. In reality, people are exposed to many different hazardous agents at the same time, and it is possible for some of these agents to interact, either by adding to each other (**additive** effects), enhancing one another (**synergism**), or counteracting (**antagonism**) one another's effects. These interactions are not easily captured by the present mechanisms of risk assessment, even though we are aware of the potential interactions in many cases, such as the synergistic interactions of tobacco smoke with asbestos or radon. Much remains to be done in this area of risk assessment.

Risk Communication

As a part of stakeholders' involvement in risk management, it is important to be able to communicate the technical knowledge derived from risk assessment and its components to larger audiences. In addition, successful behavioral change through public health campaigns requires communication of risk information to the general public to be effective. Technical experts often dislike such risk communications because of the great effort they entail[28]. In turn, this attitude results in mistrust of experts on the part of stakeholders and the general public, who may resort to less reliable and less objective sources of information. Yet, this need not be the case. Considerable research effort has been dedicated to understanding the most effective ways to communicate risk, what barriers may be present, and how they can be avoided.

Actual Versus Perceived Risk

One of the important barriers to risk communication lies at the receivers' end of communication, and it is effectively described by the concept of **cognitive dissonance**. This is the idea that we find it hard to hold conflicting information in our minds and therefore need exceptionally convincing evidence to change our mind on a particular issue and reject a previously held belief. As it turns out, we hold numerous beliefs about the nature and magnitude of the risks we face in our lives. These beliefs affect our risk perceptions and prevent us from accepting new information about the risks we face. In particular, the following are some of the factors that distort our risk perception[29]:

- **Control:** We are inclined to underestimate the magnitude of risks over which we perceive we have some form of control and overestimate those for which we lack control. Thus we may fear airplane crashes much more than automobile accidents, even though the latter is ten times more likely per mile traveled.

- **Voluntary versus involuntary:** We underestimate the risks we choose to take, such as smoking or skydiving, and overestimate those forced upon us, such as catastrophic industrial accidents or residual pesticide exposure.

- **Natural versus manufactured:** We generally prefer and underestimate risks from natural causes over those of anthropogenic nature; thus, we'd rather move to Denver, Colorado, and endure its higher background radiation than move next to a nuclear power plant, a far less risky option.

- **Familiarity:** New or exotic risks such as SARS or terrorism are perceived as being worse than those risks we are acquainted with, including X-rays or eating peanut butter.

- **Scale:** We are more moved by single events that kill a large number of people, such as a tsunami or plane crash, than by many events that kill a small number of people at a time, such as occupational accidents.

- **Proximity:** We are more moved by events affecting people we know than those affecting strangers, especially those living in faraway, unfamiliar places.

- **Dread factor:** Some hazards simply evoke more intense emotional response than do others, such as radiation or hemorrhagic fevers like Ebola versus the less terrifying but more likely diabetes or malaria.

It is important to realize that these perceptions affect our mind naturally, and absent contrary evidence, even risk experts are subject to these distortions. Recognizing that these perceptions are natural, rather than simply a product of ignorance, is a first step in developing a solid, open communication strategy.

Guidelines for Effective Risk Communication

The first step when communicating risk is to accept that the public may not simply be uninformed and governed by prejudice but rather may have different sets of concerns and values. It is also important to understand that resistance to information from sources that are not trusted (such as a spokesperson from an academic or government organization) is quite natural, and risk communicators themselves tend to question such information. Furthermore, it must be clear that the goal of good risk communication is not necessarily persuading the target audience to a particular point of view but rather making sure that the understanding of the issues of concern has increased and that the people involved are informed[28].

In order to convey technical information to the public, it is often effective to convert abstract information to a concrete form that nontechnical audiences may be able to relate to without prior knowledge. An example of this approach is to convert risk given as a probability to risk given in form of years or days of life lost. As a bonus, such a concept incorporates information about the age of people involved, so that the deaths of younger people receive proportionally more weight, reflecting a common societal preference. The World Health Organization use of **disability adjusted life years** (DALYs) is an example of a technical measure of risk that can be readily understood by larger audiences and yet holds great advantages even for the expert's own use. Developing easy and clear communication tools is often hard work and requires a deliberate effort, but these efforts pay off in terms of effectiveness and credibility.

For environmental risks in particular, the EPA has developed a set of cardinal rules to serve as guidelines for effective risk communication to the general public, although they may be useful for all stakeholders and different types of risk (see Resources for additional information):

1. Accept and involve the public as a legitimate partner.

2. Plan carefully and evaluate your efforts.

3. Listen to the public's specific concerns.

4. Be honest, frank, and open.

5. Coordinate and collaborate with other credible sources.

6. Meet the needs of the media.

7. Speak clearly and with compassion.

Following these or similar guidelines, along with an attitude of acceptance for the public's attitude and the use of concrete references, can help improve risk communication and prevent the mistrust/misinformation cycle. It is also worth remembering that risk communication is a field of research in itself and that those selected to communicate risk should deliberately dedicate time and effort to become familiar with its findings and tools rather than improvise the transformation from risk assessor to risk communicator.

Summary

The concepts and methods of risk assessment are used to manage potential threats to public and environmental health. Risk, the probability of an adverse health outcome, can be estimated through a series of steps: hazard identification, dose-response assessment, exposure assessment, and risk characterization. Hazard identification investigates which agents (chemical, physical, or biological) may result in health problems. Dose-response assessment is the process of determining, primarily through testing on animals, at what doses these hazardous agents lead to adverse health effects and at what doses they can be considered safe. There are important differences between agents that may cause cancer and those that do not, most importantly the fact that no doses can be considered entirely safe for carcinogens. There are also important differences between individuals in the levels that each can tolerate without harm. Exposure assessment is the process of determining the actual doses of hazardous agents that specific individuals or populations are likely to receive from their environment and through their activities. This is typically accomplished by observing and measuring contact between people and hazardous agents or by monitoring the levels of these agents in environmental media. Finally, risk characterization combines the information from the dose-response assessment and exposure assessment to produce quantitative estimates of risk from hazardous agents.

Estimates of risk are used to set regulatory limits for toxic agents in air, water, food, and other media at levels that are considered protective of public health. They are also used to issue permits, determine if cleanup interventions are needed, and prioritize resources. Such decisions are complex and require considering competing risks, economical welfare, and societal preferences for and tolerance of different risks. For these reasons, it is important for public health officials involved in risk assessment to adequately communicate risk information to other stakeholders involved in these decisions and to the general public. Risk communication is discipline of its own, requiring considerations about human perceptions of risk and methods to ensure trust between the risk assessors and their intended audiences.

Resources

Health Canada Risk Assessment website: A compact review of risk assessment, including a more detailed look at risk from physical agents (radiation) than addressed in this chapter. www.hc-sc.gc.ca/ewh-semt/pubs/radiation/98ehd-dhm216/assessment-evaluation-eng.php.

Exposure Factors Handbook: The definitive compilation of contact rate and time-activity studies, for exposure research. http://cfpub.epa.gov/ncea/cfm/recordisplay.cfm?deid=12464.

Sigma-Aldrich, material safety data sheets: Information on physical, chemical, and toxicological characteristics of a variety of chemical agents is best obtained from the manufacturers. This site is especially comprehensive. www.sigmaaldrich.com/site-level/msds.html.

ATSDR, toxicological profiles: Detailed studies on toxicological characteristics, pathways of exposure and risk estimates for a variety of chemical agents. www.atsdr.cdc.gov/toxpro2.html.

U.S. EPA cardinal rules of risk communication: Fundamental rules for risk communication explained. www.epa.gov/CARE/library/7_cardinal_rules.pdf.

Key Terms

activity pattern, 247

additive, 256

antagonism, 256

biomarker, 249

cognitive dissonance, 256

contact rate, 247

disability adjusted life year, 258

dose, 247

dose-response assessment, 234

exposure, 233

exposure assessment, 234, 245

exposure science, 245

hazard, 233

hazard identification, 234

hazard index, 252

hormesis, 244

initiator, 240

LD_{50}, 241

lowest observed effect level, 242

no observed *adverse* effect level, 242

no observed effect level, 242

pathway of exposure, 246

precautionary principle, 232

promoter, 240

reference dose, 242

risk, 233

risk assessment, 232

risk characterization, 234, 251

routes of exposure, 245

stakeholders, 254

synergism, 256

threshold, 239

total exposure, 246

Review Questions

1. Researchers in the agricultural division of a chemical company have developed a new, exceptionally effective pesticide to protect wine grapes from mold. Explain what specific steps they should now take to establish limits for its safe use.

2. Imagine that chocolate ice cream had been subjected to toxicological tests such as those used for hazardous agents and that its LD_{50} had been set at 50 g/kg and its NOAEL at 10 g/kg. How much chocolate ice cream could you consume, in total? If potato chips had an LD_{50} of 60 g/kg and a NOAEL

of 5 g/kg, which would you say is more toxic, chocolate ice cream or chips? Explain.

3. Using the resources suggested in the chapter, find the toxicological information for benzidine, a chemical that was used in the production of dyes. What are the *reference dose*, *cancer slope factor*(s), and *LOAEL* (or *NOAEL*)? What is the combined value of the safety factors used to derive a reference dose? Explain.

4. Do you think it is possible for two people living in the same place, breathing the same air, eating the same food, drinking the same water, and performing the same activities to be exposed to different doses of a chemical agent in their environment? Why or why not?

5. Why is collecting data about the concentration of hazardous agents in environmental media (air, soil, food, water, etc.) not sufficient to characterize the exposure and risk from that agent? What else must be known?

6. How would you measure your own exposure to polycyclic aromatic hydrocarbons (PAHs) present in air, food, soil, and dust, if you had access to adequate equipment? Explain your procedures.

7. Why is the hazard index calculated without taking into account carcinogenic potential?

8. Calculate the hazard index and the lifetime cancer risk from exposure to the pesticide chlordane for a person weighing 55 kg (121 lb.) who is ingesting 0.01 mg/day as a residual on food for a lifetime of 80 years. The reference dose of chlordane is 5×10^{-4} mg/kg/day, and the cancer slope factor is 0.35 $(\text{mg/kg/day})^{-1}$. Would you be more concerned about acute, short-term effects, or the risk of cancer from chronic exposures? Justify your interpretation.

9. Why is the relative magnitude of risks from different hazards generally more important than the absolute value of risk estimates?

10. Find information on the Web about a specific Superfund site (check the U.S. EPA Web site), including the details of the contamination and the toxicology of the agent. Then imagine you are the public health official in charge of communicating risk information about this site to local citizens. Write a one-page executive summary for the city authorities and a list of talking points for the person presenting the results at a town hall meeting.

References

1. Lieber CS. Role of oxidative stress and antioxidant therapy in alcoholic and nonalcoholic liver diseases. *Adv Phrmacol.* 1997;38:601–628.

2. Gemma S, Vitozzi L, Testai E. Metabolism of chloroform in the human liver and identification of the competent P450s. *Drug Metab Dispos.* 2003;31(3):266–274.

3. Royal HD. Effects of low level radiation–what's new? *Semin Nucl Med.* 2008;38(5): 392–402.

4. Sucrose [material safety data sheet]. Fisher Scientific. Available at: http://fscimage. fishersci.com/msds/22174.htm. Accessed March 25, 2009.

5. Potassium cyanide [material safety data sheet]. Fisher Scientific. Available at: http:// fscimage.fishersci.com/msds/19350.htm. Accessed March 25, 2009.

6. Amdur M, Doull J, Klaassen CD. *Casarett & Doull's Toxicology.* 4th ed. New York: McGraw-Hill; 1993.

7. U.S. Environmental Protection Agency. Reference Dose (RfD): Description and Use in Health Risk Assessments. Background Document 1A, March 15 1993. Available at: www.epa.gov/iris/rfd.htm. Accessed March 25, 2009.

8. Agency for Toxic Substances and Disease Registry (ATSDR). Toxicological profile for vinyl chloride, 2006. www.atsdr.cdc.gov/toxpro2.html.

9. Agency for Toxic Substances and Disease Registry (ATSDR). Toxicological profile for nickel, 2005. www.atsdr.cdc.gov/toxpro2.html.

10. Jamall IS, Willhite CC. Is benzene exposure from gasoline carcinogenic? *J Environ Monit.* 2008;10(2):176–87.

11. Cohen SM, Ohnishi T, Arnold LL, Le XC. Arsenic-induced bladder cancer in an animal model. *Toxicol Appl Pharmacol.* 2007; 222(3):258–263.

12. U.S. Environmental Protection Agency. *Health Assessment Document for Polychlorinated Dibenzo-p-Dioxin.* Cincinnati, Ohio: Environmental Criteria and Assessment Office, Office of Health and Environmental Assessment, Office of Research and Development; 1985. EPA 600/8–84–014F.

13. Tseng WP, Chu HM, How SW, Fong JM, Lin CS, Yeh S. Prevalence of skin cancer in an endemic area of chronic arsenism in Taiwan. *J Natl Cancer Inst.* 1968:40: 453–463.

14. Zartarian V, Bahadori T, Mckone T. Adoption of an official ISEA glossary. *J Expos Anal Environ Epidemiol.* 2005;15:1–5.

15. Menzie CA, Potocki B, Santodonato J. Exposure to carcinogenic PAHs in the environment. *Environ Sci Technol.* 1992; 26(7):1278–1284.

16. Hrudey S, Chen W, Rousseaux CG. *Bioavailability in Environmental Risk Assessment.* Boca Raton, Fla.: CRC Press, Inc.; 1995.

17. Linakis JG. Childhood lead poisoning. *R I Med.* 1995;78(1):22–26.

18. Ott W, Stinemann AC, Wallace L. *Exposure Analysis.* Boca Raton, Fl.: CRC Taylor & Francis; 2007.

19. Lu C, Pearson M, Renker S, Myerburg S, Farino C. A novel system for collecting longitudinal self-reported dietary consumption information: The internet data logger (iDL). *J Expo Sci Environ Epidemiol.* 2006;16:427–433.

20. Waldman JM, Bilder SM, Freeman NCG, Friedman M. A portable datalogger to evaluate recall-based time-use measures. *J Expos Anal Environ Epidemiol.* 1989;3: 39–48.

21. Elgethun K, Yost M, Fitzpatrick CTE, Nyerges T, Fenske RA. Comparison of global positioning system (GPS) tracking and parent-report diaries to characterize children's time–location patterns. *J Expo Anal Environ Epidemiol.* 2007;17:196–206.

22. Freeman NCG, Hore P, Black K, et al. Contributions of children's activities to pesticide hand loadings following residential pesticide application. *J Expos Anal Enviro Epidemiol.* 2005;15:81–88.

23. National Research Council (NRC). *Science and Judgment in Risk Assessment, 1994.* Washington, D.C.: National Academies Press; 1994.

24. Biesiadia M. Simulations in health risk assessment. *Int J Occup Med Environ Health.* 2001;14(4):397–402.

25. Kelly KE. The myth of 10^(-6) as a definition of acceptable risk. Presented at: The 84th Annual Meeting of the Air & Waste Management Association; June 16–21, 1991; Vancouver, B.C., Canada.

26. Bender AP, Punyko J, Williams AN, Bushhouse SA. A standard person-years approach to estimating lifetime cancer risk. *Cancer Causes Control.* 1992;3(1):69–75.

27. Kamo K, Katanoda K, Matsuda T, Marugame T, Ajiki W, Sobue T. Lifetime and age-conditional probabilities of developing or dying of cancer in Japan. *Jpn J Clin Oncol.* 2008;38(8)571–576.

28. National Research Council (NRC). *Improving Risk Communication.* Washington, D.C.: National Academies Press; 1989.

29. Maxwell NI. *Understanding Environmental Health.* Sudbury, Mass.: Jones & Bartlett Publishers; 2009.

BEHAVIOR AND HEALTH

CHAPTER 11

SOCIAL AND BEHAVIORAL SCIENCES IN PUBLIC HEALTH

Ellen D. S. López, MPH, PhD
Barbara A. Curbow, PhD

LEARNING OBJECTIVES

- Express the purpose and goals of social and behavioral science in public health.
- Discuss the roots of social and behavioral science.
- Understand the importance of taking a social-ecological approach to research and practice.
- Describe several social and behavioral science theories and frameworks at different levels of the social-ecological framework.
- Explain the importance of community participation throughout the research and intervention process.

In this chapter, we will introduce the public health area of social and behavioral sciences and describe how this discipline strives to improve the health and health behavior of individuals, groups, and populations. Because our health issues and health behaviors are often extremely complex, we will discuss them within the context of the social-ecological framework. This public health framework is also described in the context of public health systems in Chapter 2. The social-ecological framework assists public health professionals in identifying and organizing the important factors that pertain to us as individuals (such as knowledge, attitudes, beliefs, and skills), as well as those factors found in our relational, community, and societal environments that either do or do not support health and healthy behaviors (such as friendships, community resources, organizational policies). We will then devote a majority of this chapter to the social and behavioral science theories and models that are commonly used at each ecological level for the purpose of understanding health behavior and developing and evaluating health-promoting interventions. We will end the chapter with a discussion about the importance and principles of community participation in social and behavioral science research and practice.

Setting the Stage: Hookah Smoking as a Public Health Issue

Meet Anna and Janie. Both are juniors at State University. They are discussing their Friday night plans.

Anna: Hey Janie, Sam said that everyone is meeting at the Happy Hookah Cafe on Friday night. We should join them!

Janie: I'm not sure. I've never even smoked a cigarette. Do you think it's safe?

Anna: Definitely! That's the beauty of hookah! It's totally safe because you smoke out of a water pipe that filters out all the bad stuff. I tried it last week. It's really fun because everyone shares the same pipe, and the tobacco comes in great flavors like apple and mint. Plus, it must be safe. Why else would it be legal to smoke hookah when there's a ban on indoor tobacco smoking within city limits?

Janie: Well, my mom read an article that said that smoking hookah can be as bad or worse for you than smoking cigarettes. She would kill me if she knew I was going to the Hookah Cafe. I'm just not sure that I want to try it.

Anna: What your mom doesn't know won't hurt her. Anyway, it's not like you're going to become *addicted* to hookah smoking!

PUBLIC HEALTH CONNECTIONS 11.1

THE TRUTH ABOUT HOOKAH SMOKING

Myth: Many people think that smoking hookah is harmless fun and safer than cigarettes.

Truth: According to the Centers for Disease Control and Prevention (CDC), hookah smoking is far from safe, and it poses a major public health threat.

- Hookah tobacco and its smoke are dangerous to both the smoker and any others who are exposed.

- Even after it passes through the water pipe, hookah smoke contains the same harmful and addictive drugs and toxins found in cigarette smoke.

- Because a hookah session lasts forty to sixty minutes, smokers take in as much as one hundred times the volume of smoke inhaled from a single cigarette.

- Even the charcoal and wood cinders used to heat the hookah tobacco emit harmful toxins.

- Sharing hookah mouthpieces can increase chances of transmitting communicable diseases (e.g., herpes, tuberculosis, and hepatitis).

- Hookah is most popular with eighteen to twenty-four year olds, even those who would never consider smoking a cigarette.

- In many cities and states hookah cafes are exempt from laws that enforce clean air laws and smoking bans.

Source: Adapted from reference 1

Social and Behavioral Science in Public Health

In our Happy Hookah Cafe scenario, Janie and Anna were uninformed about the potentially adverse health consequences associated with smoking hookah. Personal knowledge and attitudes toward a behavior can be strong determinants of health-related decision making. But even if Anna and Janie did know that smoking hookah can be as or more dangerous than smoking cigarettes, do you think that they might still join their friends at the Happy Hookah Cafe? As we all know, there are many considerations besides health that influence our health behaviors. For Anna and Janie, those other factors might include whether there are fun alternatives to smoking on a Friday night or if they feel pressured to go along with what their friends are doing. Another factor for Janie might be how much she cares about pleasing her mom, who does not want her to smoke anything. Think about it: Have you ever made a health-related decision because you wanted to fit in or please another person?

Nearly half of all deaths in the United States can be linked to risky health behaviors such as smoking tobacco, using drugs and alcohol, eating an unhealthy diet, not getting enough physical activity, or practicing unprotected sex[2–4]. The primary aims of **social and behavioral science** in public health are to understand, predict, and influence health behaviors of individuals, groups, and entire populations. The main goals are to prevent **morbidity** (disease and health problems) and premature mortality, especially as they are caused by unhealthy behaviors. Our decisions and health behaviors are inextricably linked to the environments in which we live, work, and play. As such, social and behavioral science is concerned with understanding and addressing how our health behavior decisions influence and are influenced by the world around us[3].

Roots of Social and Behavioral Science in Public Health

Social and behavioral science in public health is steeped in the rich influence and traditions of a variety of disciplines, such as psychology, health communication, sociology, anthropology, political science, and economics[5]. Although each discipline offers its own area of study, perspectives, and methodological approaches, each is predominately centered in the study of humans and their relationship to society. When focused on health, each discipline explores how health issues are influenced by human nature, behavior, and the surrounding environment[5]. For example, although psychologists often focus on the individual's behavioral and mental processes, specific subfields of psychology, such as health, community, and social psychology, are also interested in the broader social and cultural forces that impact human behavior[6,7]. One such force is how health information is offered and received. Health communication is the study of how different communication strategies inform and influence individual, community, and population health decisions[8]. Anthropologists study humans from a social, biological, and cultural perspective. Their use of ethnography or field research to describe different cultures is often used in public health to better understand and address the inequalities experienced by underserved populations. These inequalities (such as poor access to health care) often pertain to poverty, which is one of the strongest risk factors associated with poor health across the globe[9,10]. Economic and political science theories focused on wealth, power, poverty, trade, and industry often inform public health efforts aimed at addressing poor health outcomes that result from economic disparities[10].

In summary, social and behavioral science in public health draws from a wide array of disciplines and traditions and focuses on the interplay between and among individuals and their environments. With the aim of reducing preventable illness and premature death, public health as a whole has achieved great success in health promotion and disease prevention efforts related to AIDS/HIV, cancer, asthma, diabetes, injury, reproductive health, environmental health, employment, housing, access to care, and countless other health issues[5].

Using a Social-Ecological Framework to Understand Health Factors

Public health problems are complex and influenced by many variables that interact with each other. Even issues that on the surface might appear to be relatively easy to grasp, such as deciding whether to smoke hookah on a Friday night, can pose a great dilemma. A **social-ecological framework** (recall Figure 2.2) can help us consider the complicated relationships that exist between individuals and the world around them. With this consideration, we can better understand and actually target our efforts to reduce or eliminate public health problems[11].

The social-ecological framework forms the conceptual basis of social and behavioral science research and practice. The framework organizes the numerous factors that influence health and health behaviors into several defined categories or levels. For the most part, these categories include the factors that are associated with us as at the *individual* level (such as knowledge, attitudes, beliefs, experiences), *relationship* level (such as influence or support from friends, family, professors), *organizational* and *community* level (such as norms and regulations), and *societal* level (such as policies and mass media) (see Figure 2.2)[12,13]. By organizing our efforts around multiple levels of influence, as opposed to solely focusing on either the individual or an aspect of the environment, public health professionals can positively and comprehensively address the underlying causes of health problems.

As described in Table 11.1, each ecological level has a target, focus of change, and strategies for change. Let us think about the social-ecological framework as it might apply to Janie and whether she will decide to start smoking hookah. At the **individual level**, Janie is the target, especially in terms of increasing her knowledge about hookah smoking and her attitude toward pleasing her disapproving mom. At the **relationship level**, interpersonal influences such as Anna's and Janie's families might be targets of a university-based campaign that provides tips to parents regarding successfully talking with their college-aged children about avoiding all forms of smoking, including hookah. At the **organization and community level**, the target of change is the social environments in which Anna and Janie live, work, study, or socialize, primarily their university campus and the surrounding area. A public health **intervention** (a program or initiative developed with the goal of producing behavior changes or improved health status)[14] might involve creating a university policy that requires all students and faculty to attend a seminar about the dangers of hookah smoking to the smokers and those around them. The hope is that hookah

Table 11.1 Social-Ecological Levels and Their Targets of Change, Focus of Change, and Strategies

Level	Target of Change	Focus of Change	Strategies to Address Hookah/Water Pipe Use
Individual	Individual person	Characteristics of person: knowledge, attitudes, beliefs	Educational programs Incentives
Relationship	Social influences: family, coworkers, roommates	Nature of social relationships: social norms, access to support	Support groups Peer mentoring Social modeling
Community	Social environment	Community norms, values, attitudes, and power structures	Education/awareness campaigns Community organizing Leaders speak out against hookah Smoke-free areas and events
Societal	Local, state, and national laws and policies	Government regulations and other regulatory processes, procedures, or laws to protect health	Taxation and pricing Restrictions and bans Enforcement and litigation Voter awareness campaigns Education for policy and decision makers Mass media campaigns

Source: Adapted from reference 12.

smoking will be regarded as unattractive, unhealthy, and plain foolish. Finally, at the **societal level**, the targets of change are local, state, and national laws and policies. Interventions at this level might include regulations that require all hookah bars to display information (on their tables and in their menus) about the adverse effects of hookah smoking.

It is important to understand that although any of these levels might be helpful in changing health behavior, intervening at multiple levels with numerous strategies that discourage hookah smoking would increase chances that Anna and Janie will abstain because they are supported by the environment in which they live.

Using Social and Behavioral Theories to Inform Public Health Research and Practice

Given the tiny bit of information you know about Anna and Janie, what do you think is the likelihood that they will join their friends at the Hookah Cafe? What theories can you develop to make this educated guess? We all develop our own commonsense theories about day-to-day experiences. These personal theories represent a system of beliefs that can assist us in making sense of how things work and why things happen[15]. Often, our personal theories are based on the things we observe and experience in our everyday lives. An example of a personal theory might be, "If I bite into that piping hot slice of pizza, I am going to burn my tongue!" For social and behavioral researchers and practitioners, similar types of **theories** (although usually a bit more complex than avoiding scalding cheese burns) can be used to systematically organize the numerous factors that influence health and health behavior into manageable groupings, or **constructs**. Relationships among these constructs can then be hypothesized and tested with the goal of predicting behavior. If we can understand not only which factors impact health and health behavior but also how these factors work in relation to others, we can then develop and evaluate interventions focused on modifying these key behavioral influences[15,16].

Several tested and validated theories exist and are used in social and behavioral science research and practice. Many theories originate as commonsense ideas that are based on observations and experiences of what is going on in the environment. For example, it is not too difficult to hypothesize that if Anna and Janie do not know the dangers of smoking hookah, they will probably see no reason to avoid it. For this commonsense theory to be validated, it must be tested to make sure it holds true when used in different situations and with different populations[15,16]. As described in Public Health Connections 11.2, theories are composed of concepts, constructs, variables, and linkages. It is important to remember that a theory is more than just the sum of its parts. As a whole, a theory represents relationships among several factors that may influence health and health behavior[17].

Let us take a look at a selection of commonly used social and behavioral science theories and models. There are many theories from which to choose. Here we provide an introduction to a few theories and frameworks that can be applied to health and health behaviors from different levels of the social-ecological framework. Of course, we will be sure to apply these theories to Anna and Janie's hookah dilemma!

PUBLIC HEALTH CONNECTIONS 11.2

THEORIES COMPRISE THESE ELEMENTS

- **Concepts** are the primary structures or building blocks of theory. For example, a concept of interest might be whether or not a person feels *at risk* for developing a health problem.

- **Constructs** are key concepts that are named and defined for use in a particular theory. For example, in the health belief model (discussed later in this section), feeling at risk is called *perceived susceptibility*.

- **Variables** are ways to measure constructs to evaluate their importance. For example, to see if perceived susceptibility to cancer is associated with a person's decision to quit smoking, survey questions could focus on assessing the person's fear about getting cancer.

- **Linkages** show how constructs are related to each other. What leads to what? For example, according to the health belief model, if individuals perceive that they are susceptible to a disease, they might change their health behavior.

- **Models and frameworks** draw on several theories or theoretical constructs to understand a health issue.

Source: Reference 17.

Individual-Level Theories

Although the goal of public health is to improve health for the entire population, it is important to recognize that individual people make up our populations, communities, and groups. At the individual level of the social-ecological framework, the focus of behavior change is the individual's knowledge, attitudes, beliefs, motivations, intentions, history, experiences, and skills[17]. There are several theories and models that strive to predict individuals' health behaviors. Here we discuss three that are commonly used in public health research and practice: the health belief model, the theory of planned behavior, and stages of change.

Health Belief Model

The **health belief model** (HBM) is one of the most widely used public health theories for explaining health behavior (Figure 11.1). It was developed in the

FIGURE 11.1 The Health Belief Model

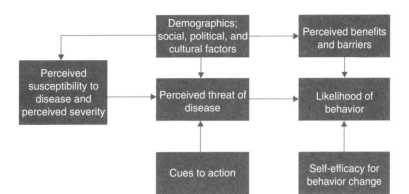

1950s by Godfrey Hochbaum, a social psychologist working for the U.S. Public Health Service who wondered why relatively few people decided to take part in a free and conveniently located chest X-ray screening for tuberculosis (TB). To gain a better understanding about people's motivations, Hochbaum and others studied probability samples of over 1,200 adults to understand the factors that influenced their decisions to obtain a TB X-ray. They found that people were more likely to be screened if they believed they were at risk for TB and if they believed that the screening would be beneficial[18]. Over time, the HBM has evolved to include six main constructs that together have been shown to statistically explain individuals' likelihood of performing one-time behaviors, such as TB screening, and long-term health behaviors, such as yearly cancer screening, medication adherence, condom use, smoking cessation, and emergency preparedness[19].

The HBM stipulates that the likelihood of a new behavior (such as being screened for TB) or a behavior change (such as quitting smoking) is an outcome of six components. Let's look at smoking cessation in the context of Figure 11.1. Individuals believe[19]:

1. that smoking will put them at risk of developing cancer (**perceived susceptibility**);

2. that having cancer would be serious (**perceived severity**);

3. that quitting smoking would reduce their risk of developing cancer and its severity (**perceived benefits**);

4. that quitting smoking will be difficult or uncomfortable (**perceived barriers**);

5. that they are exposed to internal or external prompts, reminders, or cues to quit smoking (**cues to action**); and

6. that they feel confident that they can successfully quit smoking (**self-efficacy**).

Let's consider our friend Janie, who is not sure that she wants to smoke hookah. According to the HBM, Janie's decision to smoke or abstain will be contingent on the perceived threat she feels for developing a tobacco-related disease such as cancer. **Perceived threat** is the combination of how *susceptible* Janie feels to developing cancer (does she think that she is too young to get cancer?) and how *severely* she feels that cancer would impact her life. Her decision is also contingent on whether she feels that the benefits of not smoking hookah (avoiding cancer, saving money) will outweigh the barriers (pressure from friends, missing a fun evening). In addition, Janie's decision will depend on the prompts or cues she receives that either encourage her to smoke or not smoke (for example, receiving an article from her mom about the evils of hookah smoking, learning about a cousin who was recently diagnosed with cancer). Finally, Janie will assess her level of confidence or self-efficacy to avoid smoking hookah, even though all of her friends are doing it. Think about this: Would Janie's decision-making process be different if, instead of focusing on cancer, she focused on something more near term, such as being exposed to an infectious disease from sharing the mouthpiece of the hookah? Do you think college students would be more influenced by long-term consequences such as cancer or short-term consequences such as infectious disease? This would be an important topic to explore, particularly if you wanted to develop a public health education campaign targeted toward young adults. The HBM can be used to inform health promotion programs and campaigns that increase perceptions about disease threat while enhancing the perceived benefits and self-efficacy for taking positive health action. One feature that is unique to HBM is the emphasis on having cues to action (a feature of the environment) as part of a campaign.

Theory of Planned Behavior

Another commonly used individual level theory is the **theory of reasoned action** (TRA), which was developed in 1967 by Fishbein and later updated by Azjen and colleagues to become the **theory of planned behavior** (TPB) (Figure 11.2). In this theory, performing a health behavior is determined by the individual's readiness or intention to perform that behavior. Originally, this behavioral intention was thought to be dependent on two concepts: the individual's attitude toward the behavior and the importance the individual places

FIGURE 11.2 The Theory of Planned Behavior

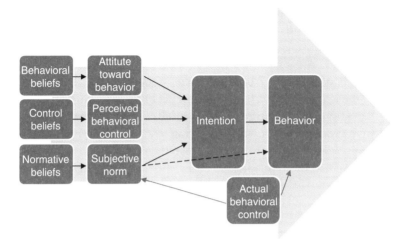

Source: Adapted from reference 21.

on what others think he or she should do (**subjective norm**). The TPB extended the original model to take into account circumstances in which an individual's behavior is influenced by factors that are out of his or her control. As such, TPB includes **perceived control**, in which behavioral intention also depends on how confident the person is that he or she has control over performing the behavior[20].

Suppose Anna and Janie's friend, Sam, has been smoking hookah for a long time. He just heard about a guy in his dorm that had to undergo surgery for a cancerous spot on his lip. Worried about his own health, Sam is now considering stopping all tobacco use, including hookah. According to the TPB, Sam's intention to stop smoking will be determined by his belief that quitting would decrease his own chances of developing cancer, which he perceives to be a good thing (attitude toward the behavior). His intentions to quit would also depend on whether he believes that the people who are important to him (his friends, parents, roommates) want him to quit and how motivated he is to please these different people (subjective norms). For example, does Sam want to please his dad, who wants him to quit, or does he want to please his smoking buddies? Finally, Sam will be more likely to quit if he feels he has control over his ability to quit in different situations, such as when he is with his friends who will pressure him to smoke with them or when he is stressed about his final exams (perceived behavioral control).

The TPB provides a thoughtful blueprint for understanding the reasons individuals do or do not perform health behaviors. Using this model, interventions can be designed to target and change beliefs about behaviors, social norms, and control with the goal of increasing the likelihood these healthy behaviors will be performed.

Stages of Change (Transtheoretical Model)

In the late 1970s, psychology researchers Prochaska and DiClemente developed the **stages of change** or **transtheoretical model** (Figure 11.3)[22]. They were trying to find a way to integrate concepts from more than three hundred psychological and behavioral change theories.

Across these theories (hence, the name *transtheoretical*), Prochaska and DiClemente identified ten common strategies that are used to change behavior (Table 11.2).

DiClemente and Prochaska conducted studies to assess how individuals used these ten processes as they attempted to quit smoking. What became evident to

FIGURE 11.3 The Stages of Change Model

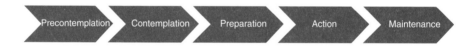

Table 11.2 Ten Strategies Used to Change Behavior

• **Consciousness raising**	Learning new facts that support behavior change
• **Dramatic relief**	Feeling negative emotions (fear, anxiety) associated with unhealthy behavior
• **Self-reevaluation**	Seeing behavior change as important to one's self-identify
• **Environmental reevaluation**	Seeing negative impact of unhealthy behavior on important others
• **Self-liberation**	Making commitment to change
• **Helping relationships**	Seeking social support for behavior change
• **Counterconditioning**	Finding healthier alternative behaviors for unhealthy behaviors
• **Reinforcement management**	Increasing rewards for healthy behavior and decreasing rewards for unhealthy behavior
• **Stimulus control**	Increasing cues for healthy behavior and decreasing cues for unhealthy behaviors
• **Social liberation**	Seeing society as changing to better support healthy behaviors

Source: Reference 21.

Table 11.3 The Stages of Change: Definitions and Strategies

Stage	Definition	Process of Change Strategies
Precontemplation "Never!"	No intention to change behavior within next six months	Provide personalized information about risks and benefits of change (*consciousness raising, dramatic relief, environmental reevalution*)
Contemplation "Someday"	Intends to change behavior in next six months	Reinforce person's self-identify as a healthy person (*self-reevaluation*)
Preparation "Soon"	Intends to make change in next month and has taken some steps to do so	Help develop behavior change plans (*self-liberation*)
Action "Now"	Has changed behavior for less than six months	Provide feedback, social support, and reinforcement (*reinforcement management, social liberation*)
Maintenance "Forever?"	Has changed behavior for more than six months	Provide helpful cues, alternatives to unhealthy behavior (*stimulus control, counterconditioning*)

Source: Adapted from reference 21.

the researchers is that smoking cessation is not a one-time event but rather is a process that involves movement through five stages of change: precontemplation, contemplation, preparation, action, and maintenance. They found that people differed in their *readiness* to stop smoking. That is, some people were at the very beginning of the change process (precontemplation), and others were farther along. They also found that as people progressed through the stages they made use of the ten different change strategies[22].

Each stage is described in Table 11.3. Let's apply the stages of change theory to our friend, Anna, who started smoking hookah several times a week and now even enjoys cigarettes ... a lot! In the **precontemplation stage**, Anna is not even considering changing her behavior. She just has not thought about it. To move her to contemplation, Anna might require basic education about the risks associated with smoking, possibly from a person who has experienced tobacco-related cancer or some other health effect. In the **contemplation stage**, Anna is now considering refraining from all smoking activities, but she has no concrete plans to do so. To move her to preparation, Anna might be encouraged to think how nice her life could be without smoking (whiter teeth, clean-smelling clothes, extra spending money). In the **preparation stage**, Anna is not only considering quitting smoking, but she has actually bought a supply of nicotine patches and breath mints. To progress Anna to action, she might be supported in setting a specific quit date and even announce it to others who will support her efforts. In the **action stage**, Anna has quit smoking for less than six months. To progress her to maintenance, Anna might be encouraged to call a supportive friend (such as Janie) when she feels the urge to smoke. She might also use the money she is saving to buy herself a reward for not giving into temptation. In the **maintenance stage**, Anna has quit smoking for more than six months. To refrain from relapse, she might be convinced to get rid of all of her lighters and to start spending time with friends who also chose to abstain from smoking.

Since its inception, the stages of change model has been applied to a variety of behaviors. Although the five stages of change are progressive in nature, the model is not meant to be linear and one directional because the potential for relapse to an earlier stage is expected. That is, although some individuals progress from one stage to the next, others might cycle forward and backward. Individuals vary in their readiness or stage of change. As public health professionals, it is important to identify where the individual is in his or her readiness to change and work from there. Once the stage of readiness is determined, the ten processes of change can be used as guides for developing stage appropriate intervention strategies.

Relationship/Interpersonal Level Theories

People have evolving and reciprocal relationships with their social environments; this idea forms the central premise of social and behavioral theory at the relationship or interpersonal level of the social ecological framework. Our **social environment** comprises the individuals and groups with whom we interact or that we encounter, such as our family members, friends, coworkers, roommates, doctors, and even our store clerks and fellow bus riders. Whether we like it or not, during our interactions with others we receive advice, opinions, pressures, and support. We also gain education by observing how others behave. Consciously and unconsciously, we are influenced by these interactions, as they help to form our own decisions. Because our social interactions influence our behaviors, our social environment is viewed as an important determinant of health. Numerous theories and frameworks focus on factors at the relationship/interpersonal level. In this section we discuss the social cognitive theory and social support/social networks.

Social Cognitive Theory

The **social cognitive theory** (SCT) (formerly known as social learning theory), developed in the 1960s by Albert Bandura, is one of the most frequently used interpersonal health behavior theories. During the 1960s, most psychological theories took a behavioral approach to personality and essentially proposed that individuals learn and adopt behaviors solely through direct, personal experiences. However, during his famous Bobo doll experiment (Public Health Connections 11.3), Bandura actually found that behavior was also influenced by **vicarious experience**, or observing the behaviors of others and the outcome of their behaviors[23]. Think about it. Have you ever imitated someone else's behavior because you saw that person rewarded for his or her actions? For Anna and Janie, a scenario might go like this: Friday finally arrives, and Janie decides to join Anna and her other friends at the Happy Hookah Cafe. Still, she makes it clear that she is only going along for the ride and does not want to smoke … anything! During the evening, Janie sees how much fun Anna is having as she shares the hookah experience with her friends. Janie starts to feel left out and wants the same reinforcement she sees Anna receiving. So, before the night is over, Janie is also smoking hookah. In a different scenario, let's say that Janie refrains from smoking hookah, but finds that she still has a great time with everyone! Anna sees through Janie's actions that she does not have to smoke to have fun with her friends. As a result, Anna also decides to forego smoking the rest of the night.

Underlying this ability to process vicarious experience is SCT's premise that learning and behavior change involve an interdependent relationship between the person, his or her behavior, and the environment. This interdependence, called **reciprocal determinism**, stresses the mutual impact these three components have on each other. As such, change in a person's behavior is inherently dependent on the way he or she thinks about and processes what is going on in the social environment, and this will most likely produce changes to the environment[24]. Just think: If Anna decides to model Janie's behavior by not smoking hookah, she might also influence the behavior of her friends. Ultimately, the group might find alternative places to go on a Friday night.

Respected peers, celebrities, and other influential people are often used in health promotion efforts to endorse a wide variety of healthy behaviors. By modeling health behaviors and the rewards or punishments they produce, others can develop a repertoire of responses to different situations and circumstances.

Social Networks and Social Support

What if you took a blank sheet of paper and drew a circle to represent yourself? Then, you drew small circles for each of the people you consider to be close to

PUBLIC HEALTH CONNECTIONS 11.3

BANDURA'S BOBO DOLL EXPERIMENT

In Bandura's research, nursery school-aged children watched (on a TV monitor) an adult male modeling aggressive behavior by hitting, punching, and yelling at a life-size plastic Bobo doll. The children then saw the adult receive rewards, a scolding, or no reinforcement for his aggressive behavior. Bandura found that when the children were placed in the same room with the Bobo doll, those who saw the adult receive either positive or no reinforcement were more likely to reenact the similar aggressive behaviors on the doll.

Source: Reference 22.

FIGURE 11.4 Social Networks Are a Web of Social Relationships

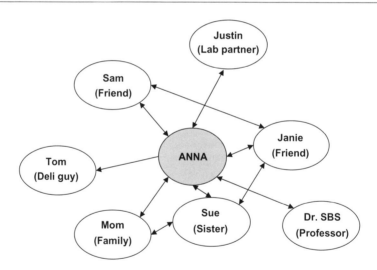

you and then circles for all of the other people you know, but with whom you do not feel such a strong connection. Finally, what if you drew lines between people who know each other? Like Figure 11.4, your paper might start to look pretty messy, possibly resembling an elaborately spun spider web. This web of social relationships represents your **social networks**. Your social networks can serve several functions, such as providing you with employment opportunities, services, connections to others, and grief and social support[25].

Networks are often described in terms of their **size** (how many members are in the network?), **homogeneity** (how similar are the members?), **geographic dispersion** (how far apart do members live or work?), **density** (how well do members know each other and interact?), **reciprocity** (is support both given and received?), **intensity** (how emotionally close are members?), and **complexity** (do relationships serve a variety of functions?)[26].

What do you think would be the pros and cons of having a large network that is not well connected? A benefit of such a network is that you would have access to a diverse array of people who can offer different skills and resources, but a con is that you might find yourself feeling alone in a crowd. On the other hand, if your network is small, dense, and well-connected, you would have intimate relationships with people to whom you could turn for support, but these few people could become overburdened and need support themselves.

Social support is one of many important functions of our social networks; it is intentional aid and assistance that is received through our social interactions. Four different but overlapping types of social support have been proposed: **emotional** (expressions of empathy, love, and caring), **instrumental** (tangible aid and services that provide assistance to meet your needs), **informational** (advice, suggestions, and information to solve problems), and **appraisal** (constructive and useful feedback and affirmations for self-evaluation). Different types of support are often provided simultaneously[25, p. 186].

Research suggests that social support can work as a protective factor to decrease one's vulnerability to the negative effects of stress on health. In fact, studies have found that social support might even influence whether or not a person develops or survives a major illness or disease.[27] Social interactions with others can provide reinforcement and help in times of need and influence our health behavior choices. Just think of how Anna and Janie might be influenced by their friends who want them to smoke hookah. For support to be considered supportive, the giver must provide it within a context of caring, trust, and respect. The recipient must also perceive it as positive support. This perception is important because individuals are affected by how they interpret the world and not necessarily how the world might actually be. For example, to help nudge Janie into smoking hookah, Anna might offer to pay for the first bowl of tobacco (tangible support). Janie could see this as positive (because she really does want to try hookah) or negative (because she is using expense as an excuse not to try it). Janie might find it more helpful if Anna publicly supported her decision not to use hookah (emotional support). In public health, the goal is to enhance skills and perceptions of support for positive behaviors in terms of how it is provided and received.

Community-Level Models

Social and behavioral science in public health, in essence, strives to develop interventions and programs that promote health and prevent disease and illness for communities and populations, especially those that experience health disparities that can lead to poorer health and well-being. In this section, we will explore how communities (such as Janie and Anna's university community) can address health-related issues through community-organizing strategies and participation. To work with a community, public health professionals must understand the community as a unit of identity. Only then can they move forward to learn about the factors that influence the community's current health situation, such as its demographic makeup, historical and political culture, and norms.

When you hear the word *community*, what comes to your mind? We often think about communities in terms of their geographical location, such as neighborhoods, towns, or reservations. Yet, beyond geography, the concept of **community** can convey a variety of meanings. Communities can be defined by their shared interests (baseball fans, art lovers, hookah aficionados) or by their shared identities (Hispanic community, Lutheran community, campus Greek fraternities or sororities)[28, p. 33]. Communities can also be defined by their ability to harness collective power and influence (gangs, political parties, and membership organizations such as Doctors Without Borders [doctorswithoutborders.org] or Mothers Against Drunk Driving [www.madd.org][29]). Given these definitions, to what community (or communities) do you belong? Possibly, you belong to several communities at the same time, and it might be that these communities influence your health and health behaviors in different directions.

Community Organizing

After listening to Janie hem and haw for days about whether or not she should go to the hookah cafe, Anna finally proposes the following challenge: "If you think going to the Happy Hookah will be so bad for us, find something better for us to do on Friday night." Janie takes on this challenge and seeks out other options that will allow them to socialize with their friends, but in a healthful environment. To Janie's surprise, she finds that there are actually few available options. In her attempt to find something (anything!) to do on a Friday night near State University, Janie has actually conducted a small-scale community assessment. In her assessment, she identified a specific community need. **Community needs** are the reality of how things *are* versus how they *should be* for individuals, groups, and communities. These needs might be concrete, such as the need for nutritious food and clean water, or abstract, such as the need for communities to be able to come together to solve important problems. For State University students, a community need is for fun activities that are not health compromising. **Community assets**, on the other hand, are the strengths and resources available, such as schools, parks, arts, churches, businesses, leaders, and other residents[30]. Community organizing is based on the assumption that the people most affected by local concerns can do something about them. This strengths perspective highlights people's assets and abilities, not their deficits and limitations.

What if Janie and Anna decided to engage other students and local organizations and businesses in an effort to create new and fun social opportunities that can rival those that are not so healthful? They would be taking on the role of community organizers! **Community organizers** are individuals who believe that regular folks can make a difference. Organizers might be paid or unpaid, trained or untrained, and they require a keen sense and understanding of the community and the underlying issues that influence the health of its members. Community organizers strive to challenge people to act on behalf of their common interests. In part, organizers meet this challenge by linking people and networks together so that they can pool their assets and resources and by creating opportunities for people to come together to critically assess their circumstances with the goal of discovering new possibilities for taking action.

Community organizing is the "process by which community groups are helped to identify common problems or goals, mobilize resources, and in other ways develop and implement strategies for reaching the goals they collectively have set."[28, p. 30] Essentially, community organizing involves people (even college students who are looking for better ways to spend their Friday nights) working together to improve their lives. Embodied in this definition are the concepts of empowerment, competence, critical consciousness, and participation. **Empowerment** is a process through which community members develop the belief in their ability to make a difference in their own lives and the lives of others[31]. **Community competence** is a community's ability to engage in problem solving by collectively identifying common needs; by establishing agreed-upon goals, priorities, and strategies for meeting these needs; and by undertaking necessary action[28]. **Critical consciousness** is the community's awareness of the underlying or root causes of the way things are, often with the goal of taking action to change the status quo[32]. Finally, **participation** is the engagement of community members, leaders, and structures (such as local programs, centers, organizations, churches, schools) in all organizing efforts, including problem identification, priority setting, intervention development, and evaluation[33]. In community organizing, the main premise is that power is an infinitely expanding commodity that doesn't require one person lose power for another person to gain it. Through participation, caring, sharing, and the emphasis on social responsibility to others, communities can create and maintain positive social change.

Community Organizing Strategies

Janie and Anna decide to get started making positive changes in their community. Community organizing involves a diverse array of strategies, including those associated with locality development, social planning, social action, and coalition building[28,34].

Locality development (also called community development) is based on the concept of helping people help themselves. The focus is on individuals working together to improve how things are done. Locality development is a process approach and involves achieving group consensus about common concerns and collaborating in problem solving. Community competence is enhanced through leadership development, training in facilitation, and critical thinking with the goal of building harmonious relationships among people from different groups and classes. Initiatives based on locality development include Peace Corps, VISTA, and Habitat for Humanity, where individuals or groups of volunteers join communities in determining their needs and assets and in achieving their goals.

Social planning (also called policy change) is based on the assumption that there are deficiencies in the manner in which services and resources are offered and distributed. It involves solving social problems through coordination of social services and program development and planning so that there is adequate resource allocation. Health and welfare councils, city planners, urban renewal authorities, and large public bureaucracies often use social planning. It is task oriented and focused on building agreement about goals and means to achieve winnable and tangible outcomes. Social planning relies on information and analysis from research and systems analysis. For example, as organizers, Anna and Janie might point out to the university administration that over 50 percent of State University students report that they drink and smoke because they are bored. The desired outcome might be that increased resources are allocated to create non-alcohol- and non-smoking-related student events! Because it is driven primarily by statistics and other types of data, social planning may be seen as being more scientific than locality development. Examples include war on poverty programs, Head Start, and other community action agencies.

Social action (also called systems advocacy) is what most people think about when they think of community organizing. It is more publicly demonstrative than the other types of organizing because of the "in your face" and some-times adversarial methods (strikes, boycotts, protests, sit-ins, marches) that are used to bring attention to issues. The focus of social action is on **social justice** (the demand for equitable allocation of goods, resources, and opportunities)[35], especially in situations that involve conflicting interests and an imbalance of power between the haves and have-nots. Social action strategies are primarily used by groups and organizations that seek to alter institutional policies or to make changes in the distribution of power. The idea is to stir things up and shift power by creating conflict with power holders. In social action, participation is highly valued and necessary. Social action strategies are typically used when conventional negotiations are not working. Examples of groups and activities that have used social action strategies include unions, Black Panthers, civil rights demonstrations, AIDS activists conducting "die-ins" in front of the White House in the 1980s, and other social movements. Think about this. What if Anna and Janie were able to convince the entire student body to boycott all establishments that served only alcohol and tobacco products? Do you think these places could survive without offering more healthful options?

Community coalitions can be an effective way to organize the community around issues with the purpose of bringing about social change. Coalitions are broad groups that bring together people and organizations throughout the community, including many groups that may not normally work together. For example, a campus-based coalition working to increase AIDS awareness through-out a university might bring together officials from student services, representatives from faith-based groups, student leaders, on-campus business owners, and members of GLBT (gay, lesbian, bisexual, and transgendered) groups. Although these individuals and groups typically might not see eye to eye on many issues, they often are able to find a common ground for building a coalition around this particular public health problem. In the process, they might develop better relationships that will enable them to support each other on other important issues (such as demanding entertainment options that are less detrimental to one's health). The value of coalitions resides not only in their strength in numbers but also the momentum and power they generate when diverse people and organizations (and the resources they each offer) come together to achieve a desired change that could not be attained by each entity acting alone[34].

These four strategies of community organizing are not completely distinguishable because there is a lot of overlap between them. Anna and Janie's group might rely on the information and analysis involved with social planning while also using some of the more strident tactics of social action to achieve desired results. Once established, coalitions will choose to use any or all of the three other strategies at some point in their life span.

Community-Based Participatory Research

Community participation is clearly important to successful community organizing, but wouldn't it be important to all social and behavioral science research that strives to result in programs and interventions that benefit people? This poses both philosophical and methodological questions about the nature of research and the relationship that should exist between researchers and those who are supposed to benefit from their work.

Historically, communities that have taken part in research studies have rarely directly benefited from the research process or findings. At times, these communities have even been harmed, especially when the research results have been published in ways that make the community look unfavorable. Imagine how Anna, Janie, and their friends would feel if they completed a survey about life as a college student, and one day they read in the newspaper that a "recent study has found that students attending State University are less intelligent and lazier than students at other universities." Equally regrettable is research that leads to interventions and programs that are culturally inappropriate or inattentive to community needs. Again, imagine how Anna and Janie would feel if their university built a new student recreation facility but did not involve any students in the planning. Did the students really need a new facility? Is it conveniently located? Does it offer all of the equipment, classes, and resources that the students desire? Often, when we take action to address complex issues without involving the expertise of community leaders and members, we wind up developing programs that fail because they do not meet the community's needs or expectations. As a result of these and other issues, many individuals and communities have lost trust in researchers and the usefulness of their studies and programs.

Community-based participatory research (CBPR) is an approach to conducting research that emphasizes the engagement of community partners in all phases of the research process to ensure that the priorities of the communities are addressed in a manner that is culturally appropriate and sensitive[36]. CBPR has its underpinnings in several of the theories, models, and concepts we have already discussed in this chapter. Particularly relevant are those located at the interpersonal and community levels, including social ecological framework, social support, models of community organizing, concepts of empowerment, community competence, and of course, participation. Ultimately, this approach may produce more meaningful and sustainable public health activities.

Although there are many ways to conduct participatory research, the main goal is to bring together researchers and communities to examine and address community-identified needs and public health problems. Often, when CBPR partnerships are initiated, they will develop a set of guiding principles that reflect their collective vision and structure for making important decisions (Public Health Connections 11.4). These principles are intended to help ensure that all partnership efforts are conducted within a context of trust and shared ownership of the research process. Furthermore, they are meant to foster co-learning among members (where each person offers his or her own unique expertise, skills, and knowledge); the ability to recognize and draw from existing community strengths and resources (as opposed to a focus on deficits); and enhanced community competence to work toward sustainable change[37].

Working within a CBPR framework can be challenging due to the time it demands of all partners in terms of partnership development, mutual education, and appropriate decision-making processes[36,38]. Nevertheless, the benefits of

PUBLIC HEALTH CONNECTIONS 11.4
GUIDING PRINCIPLES OF CBPR

Community-based participatory research

1. acknowledges community as a unit of identity;

2. builds on the strengths and resources within the community;

3. facilitates a collaborative, equitable partnership in all phases of research, involving an empowering and power-sharing process that attends to social inequities;

4. fosters co-learning and capacity building among all partners;

5. integrates and achieves a balance between knowledge generation and intervention for the mutual benefit of all partners;

6. focuses on the local relevance of public health problems and on ecological perspectives that attend to the multiple determinants of health;

7. involves systems development using a cyclical and iterative process;

8. disseminates results to all partners and involves them in the wider dissemination of results; and

9. involves a long-term process and commitment to sustainability.

Source: References 36, 37.

CBPR include appropriate study design and implementation procedures, increased quality and validity of research findings, and the potential for research findings to be used to develop culturally sensitive and useful interventions[36].

Societal Level Strategies

At the social level, social and behavioral science researchers often focus on the role of the mass media, such as radio and Web blogs, in how individuals and populations develop healthy and unhealthy behaviors. For example, when we look at unhealthy behaviors, researchers often focus on product placement or the use of specific products within mass media (such as television or movies). Have you ever noticed the brand of soda that the judges on the show *American Idol* drink? It is quite evident and could influence consumer behaviors. This is a perfect example of product placement.

Researchers are often concerned about unhealthy behaviors that are portrayed in the media, such as television or movie personalities who are shown engaging in unprotected sex or smoking cigarettes. You would think that smoking in movies would be a thing of the past, yet a 2004 study by Glanz and his colleagues found the opposite. Their study looked at movies that were released over a fifty-year period and how many times per hour these movies depicted people smoking. They found that the rate of smoking scenes in the 1950s was 10.7 per hour. It then decreased to 4.9 scenes per hour between the years 1980 and 1982. But in 2002, the rate of smoking scenes actually increased to 10.9 scenes per hour[39]. How do you think this might influence smoking behaviors, especially among teenagers? If you think that young adults are impacted by watching people smoke in movies, you are absolutely right! This influence on smoking behavior has prompted suggestions for smoke-free movies, incorporating anti-smoking advertisements into movies, and better parental control of the movies seen by children[40]. Many times social and behavioral scientists choose to use the mass media to change negative health behaviors or to promote healthy ones. Often, their method of choice is to develop health communications campaigns. A **health communications campaign** is a strategy that uses different types of media (such as newspapers, movies, radio, television, Internet, magazines) to get one or more health-promoting messages out to a defined audience[41]. You might remember the truth® Campaign that conveyed edgy antitobacco advertisements using magazines, the Internet, and television to counteract the untrue claims about smoking that were coming from the tobacco industry. The campaign was found to be a success. In a study to evaluate its effectiveness, it was found that youth who saw truth Campaign advertisements were more likely to have negative attitudes about smoking and less likely to have intentions to smoke[42].

Edberg and Abroms[41] describe four stages used when developing, implementing, and evaluating communications campaigns (Table 11.4). Let us say that Janie and Anna made the decision to not smoke hookah. Furthermore, after learning more about its potential adverse health effects, they actually started working with their social and behavioral science professor to develop a health communications campaign that targeted other State University students. Table 11.4 shows the process they used to develop, implement, and evaluate their campaign.

Managing Multiple Theories

Social and behavioral science in public health strives to improve health by understanding and addressing factors of influence across social-ecological levels (individual, relational, community, and societal). Theories, models, and frameworks are tools that can help us understand, predict, and explain why people behave the way they do[15]. This information can guide our selection of targets and strategies for successful interventions. Nevertheless, because there are so many theories from which to choose, it is sometimes difficult to find the theory that best fits our work[16]. Unfortunately, often our response to this challenge is to avoid using theory altogether. As a result, we might miss the mark when developing interventions for health issues. For example, based on our intuitions, we might put all of our resources into educating college students about the evils of hookah smoking. Yet, when theoretically informed, we might discover that our efforts should also be devoted to increasing students' self-efficacy and control over their abilities to resist peer pressure to smoke.

To help manage the daunting challenge of understanding each and every theory, Jackson[43] identified a set of principles about health and health behavior that cross numerous social and behavioral science theories. Although these principles were developed over a decade ago, they still hold true. They also provide a nice summary of the issues we must consider in social and behavioral science research and practice. Let us apply them (for the last time, we promise!) to Anna and Janie and their decision about the Happy Hookah Cafe.

- **We are influenced by (and influence) the world around us.** By taking a social-ecological approach, we can help ensure that Anna and Janie's decision to avoid smoking is supported by their environment.

Table 11.4 Stages of Communications Campaign Development, Implementation, and Evaluation

Communications Campaign Stages	Anna and Janie's Decisions
Stage 1 Planning and strategy development: Who is the intended audience? How will you find out about the audience? What type of communications activities will you use?	Anna and Janie decide to focus on students at State University. To find out about their hookah-related attitudes, knowledge, and behaviors, they decide to conduct a baseline survey of all enrolled students. From this survey they find that most students do not know about the dangers of smoking hookah. Anna and Janie decide to develop a brief video that can be posted on YouTube and shown during student orientations and Parents' Weekend.
Stage 2 Developing and pretesting concepts, messages, and materials: What is your health message? How will you test it to make sure it works?	Anna and Janie's health message is: *"You are smart enough to get into State University. Don't be dumb enough to smoke hookah."* Anna and Janie plan out the images, dialogue, and music for their video, and present their ideas to other students for feedback. They also recruit other students to be featured in the video.
Stage 3 Implementing the program: How will you get started? How will you know that people are getting your message?	Anna and Janie ask the Registrar's Office to send an e-mail to all students announcing the video's debut on YouTube. They also show the video during student orientation and Parent's Weekend. They monitor exposure to the video by tracking orientation and Parents' Weekend attendance, and the number of "hits" the video receives and comments viewers make about it.
Stage 4 Assessing effectiveness and making refinements: How will you know if it is working or not? What changes might be needed?	Six months after the video's debut, Anna and Janie send the same survey to all students to see if their attitudes, knowledge, and behaviors about hookah have changed. They also invite comments from students about how their video might be improved.

Source: Adapted from reference 40.

- **We differ in our readiness to change and the rate at which we change our behaviors.** We must know at what stage of change Anna is before we can choose appropriate strategies to help her quit smoking. We must expect that quitting smoking will be a gradual process and not a one-time event.

- **Our beliefs, attitudes, and values influence how we behave.** To help Janie make the decision to not start smoking hookah, we may need to help her focus on her own antismoking beliefs and attitudes. To do this we can point out how not smoking is consistent with the importance she places on staying healthy.

- **How we behave is influenced by others.** Consciously and unconsciously, social support, social norms, and vicarious learning experiences will influence Janie. These influences should be considered when developing interventions.

- **Participation is important.** Janie and Anna want to be in control of their decision about smoking hookah rather than feeling forced or coerced. Engaging individuals and communities as partners in the research and practice process will help ensure that the root determinants of health are addressed in a culturally appropriate and sensitive way.

Summary

Social and behavioral science in public health strives to improve health by understanding and addressing factors of influence across social-ecological levels (individual, relational, community, and societal)[12,13]. The goal is to facilitate the adoption and maintenance of healthy behaviors within a supportive and helpful environment. Drawing from the rich traditions of an array of social and behavioral science disciplines, the field of public health has achieved success in understanding and addressing many complex public health issues.

Key Terms

action stage, 280

appraisal support, 283

community, 284

community assets, 285

community coalitions, 287

community competence, 285

community needs, 284

community organizer, 285

community organizing, 285

community-based participatory research, 288

Review Questions

1. List several ways that social and behavioral theories can be helpful tools in our work as public health researchers and practitioners.

2. Explain why it is important to consider the multiple levels of the social-ecological framework (individual, relationship, community, and societal) when addressing public health problems and concerns.

3. Imagine that you have been hired by a county commission to recommend strategies they might undertake to address the growing childhood obesity problem. On your own or in a small group, identify at least two factors that are associated with childhood obesity at each level of the social-ecological framework (individual, relationship, community, and societal). Next, based on these factors, recommend programs and interventions that might be developed. You might complete your work using a grid, such as the one found below.

	Factors	Intervention Strategy
Individual		
Relationship		
Community		
Societal		

4. Look up a journal article that uses the health belief model. Briefly define the public health issue that is the focus of the article. In one or two paragraphs, describe how the authors used the health belief model in their work. Be sure to cite the article you use.

5. According to the stages of change (transtheoretical model), individuals progress through five stages when attempting to make a significant behavioral change. List and define these five stages of change, and describe a case in which a person might not progress through the stages in a linear manner.

6. Describe and give an example of each of the four types of social support that a person can receive or provide.

7. Choose two people with whom you can conduct a brief interview. Ask each person to describe the different groups, organizations, or communities to which he or she belongs. For each group, organization, or community mentioned, you might also ask about the type of social support (if any) they might receive or provide (for example, does one group provide emotional support and another provide instrumental support)? In one to two pages, summarize the answers you received during these interviews and explain how the communities to which each person belongs are similar or different.

8. In community organizing, what are some of the strategies that a community might use to try to address a priority health problem (such as neighborhood violence, teen smoking, or childhood obesity)?

9. Community-based participatory research (CBPR) is a type of research that involves community partners in all phases of the research process. Explain why you think it is important to include community leaders and members in planning and implementing public health programs, as opposed to developing these programs without community involvement.

10. Describe the four stages involved with developing, implementing, and evaluating a public health communications campaign. Apply these stages to develop a communications campaign about a public health issue that interests you.

References

1. Centers for Disease Control and Prevention (CDC). Factsheet: hookah. Updated April 2007. www.cdc.gov/tobacco/data_statistics/fact_sheets/tobacco_industry/hookahs/index.htm. May 2009.

2. VanDevanter N, Shinn M, Niang KT, Bleakley A, Perl S, Cohen N. The role of social and behavioral science in public health practice: A study of the New York Department of Health. *J Urban Health*. 2003;80(4):625–634.

3. Cohen, NL, Perl S. Integrating behavioral and social science into a public health agency: A case study of New York City. *J Urban Health*. 2003;80(4):608–615.

4. McGinnis JM, Foege WH. Actual causes of death in the United States. *JAMA*. 1993;270(18):2207–2212.

5. Holzman D, Neumann M, Sumartojo E, Lansky A. Behavioral and social sciences and public health at CDC. *MMWR*. 2006;55(Suppl):14–16.

6. Myers DG. *Psychology*. 8th ed. New York: Worth Publishers; 2007.

7. Edberg M. Social/behavioral theory and its roots. In: Edberg M, ed. *Essentials of Health Behavior: Social and Behavioral Theory in Public Health*. Sudbury, Mass.: Jones and Bartlette Publishers; 2007.

8. Schiavo R. What is health communication? In: Schiavo R, ed. *Health Communication: From Theory to Practice*. San Francisco, Calif.: Jossey-Bass; 2007.

9. World Health Organization. The World Health Report 2008. *Primary Health Care: Now More than Ever*. Geneva: World Health Organization; 2008.

10. Coreil J, Bryant CA, Henderson JN. *Social and Behavioral Foundations of Public Health*. Thousand Oaks, Calif.: Sage Publications; 2001.

11. Reifsnider E, Gallagher M, Forgione B. Using ecological models in research on health disparities. *J Prof Nurs*. 2005;21(4):216–222.

12. CDC. Violence Prevention. The Social Ecological Model: A Framework for Prevention. Updated August 2007. www.cdc.gov/ncipc/dvp/Social-Ecological-Model_DVP.htm. Accessed May 30, 2010.

13. McLeroy KR, Bibeau D, Steckler A, Glanz K. An ecological perspective on health promotion programs. *Health Edu Q*. 1988;15(4):351–377.

14. Modeste N, Tamayose T, eds. *Dictionary of Public Health Promotion and Education*. 2nd ed. San Francisco, Calif.: Jossey-Bass, 2004: p. 78.

15. van Ryn M, Heaney CA. What's the use of theory? *Health Educ Q.* 1992;19(3): 315–330.

16. Hochbaum GM, Sorenson JR, Lorig K. Theory in health education practice. *Health Edu Q.* 1992;19(3):295–313.

17. Glanz K, Rimer BK, Lewis FM. Theory, research, and practice in health behavior and health education. In: Glanz K, Rimer BK, Lewis FM, eds. *Health Behavior and Health Education: Theory, Research, and Practice*. 3rd ed. San Francisco, Calif.: Jossey-Bass; 2002.

18. Hochbaum GM. Psychosocial aspects of smoking with special reference to cessation. *Am J Public Health*, 1965;55(5):692–697.

19. Janz NK, Champion VL, Strecher VJ. The health belief model. In: Glanz K, Rimer BK, Lewis FM, eds. *Health Behavior and Health Education: Theory, Research, and Practice*. 3rd ed. San Francisco, Calif: Jossey-Bass; 2002.

20. Montano DE, Kasprzyk D. The theory of reasoned action and the theory of planned behavior. In: Glanz K, Rimer BK, Lewis FM, eds. *Health Behavior and Health Education: Theory, Research, and Practice*. 3rd ed. San Francisco, CA: Jossey-Bass, 2002.

21. Ajzen, Icek. Home page. www.people.umass.edu/aizen/index.html. Accessed May 30, 2010.

22. Prochaska JO, Redding CA, Evers KE. *The Transtheoretical Model and Stages of Change. Health Behavior and Health Education: Theory, Research, and Practice*. 3rd ed. San Francisco, Calif.: Jossey-Bass; 2002.

23. Bandura A. Influence of models' reinforcement contingencies on the acquisition of imitative responses. *J Pers Soc Psychol.* 1965;1(6):589–595.

24. Baronowski T, Perry CL, Parcel GS. How individuals, environments, and health behavior interact: Social cognitive theory. In: Glanz K, Rimer BK, Lewis FM, eds. *Health Behavior and Health Education: Theory, Research, and Practice*. 3rd ed. San Francisco, Calif.: Jossey-Bass; 2002.

25. Heaney CA, Israel BA. Social networks and social support. In: Glanz K, Rimer BK, Lewis FM, eds. *Health Behavior and Health Education: Theory, Research, and Practice*. 3rd ed. San Francisco, Calif.: Jossey-Bass; 2002.

26. House JS, Umberson D, Landis KR. Structures and processes of social support. *Annu Rev Sociol.* 1988;14:293–318.

27. Berkman LF, Glass T. Social integration, social networks, social support, and health. In: Berkman LF, Kawachi I, eds. *Social Epidemiology*. New York: Oxford University Press; 2000.

28. Minkler M, Wallerstein N. Improving health through community organization and community building: A health education perspective. In: Minkler M, ed. *Community Organizing and Community Building for Health*. New Brunswick: Rutgers University Press; 1997.

29. Eng E, Parker EA. Measuring community competence in the Mississippi Delta: The interface between program evaluation and empowerment. *Health Edu Q* 1994;21(2): 199–220.

30. Kretzmann JP, McKnight JL. *Building Communities from the Inside Out: A Path Toward Finding and Mobilizing a Community's Assets.* Chicago, Ill.: ACTA Publications; 1993.

31. Rappaport J. Research methods and the empowerment social agenda. In: Tolan P, Keys C, Chertok F, Jason L, eds. *Researching Community Psychology: Issues of Theory and Methods.* Washington, D.C.: American Psychological Association; 1992:51–63.

32. Freire P. *Pedagogy of the Oppressed.* 30th anniversary ed. New York: Continuum; 2003.

33. U.S. Department of Health and Human Services. National Institutes of Health. *Theory at a Glance: A Guide for Health Promotion Practice.* Part 2. 2005. Available at: www.cancer.gov/cancerinformation/theory-at-a-glance. Accessed May 10, 2010.

34. Butterfoss FD, Kegler MD. Toward a comprehensive understanding of community coalitions: Moving from practice to theory. In: DiClemente RJ, Corsby RA, Kegler MC, eds. *Emerging Theories in Health Promotion Practice and Research: Strategies for Improving Public Health.* San Francisco, Calif.: Jossey-Bass; 2002:557–193.

35. Hofrichter R. The politics of health inequality. In: Hofrichter R, ed. *Health and Social Justice: Politics, Ideology, and Inequity in the Distribution of Disease: A Public Health Reader.* San Francisco, Calif: Jossey-Bass; 2003.

36. Israel BA, Schulz AJ, Parker EA, Becker AB. Review of community-based research: Assessing partnership approaches to improve public health. *Annu Rev Public Health.* 1998;19:173–202.

37. Israel BA, Eng E, Schulz AJ, Parker EA. Introduction to methods in community-based participatory research for health methods. In: Israel BA, Eng E, Shulz AJ, Parker EA, eds. *Methods in Community-Based Participatory Research for Health.* San Francisco, Calif: Jossey-Bass; 2005.

38. López EDS, Parker E, Edgren K, Brakefield-Caldwell W. Planning and conducting community forums to disseminate research findings using a CBPR approach: A case study from community action against asthma. *Metro Universities Journal.* 2005;16: 57–76.

39. Glanz SA, Kacirk KW, McCulloch C. Back to the future: Smoking in movies in 2002 compared with 1950 levels. *Am J Public Health.* 2004;94(2):261–263.

40. Sargent JD. Smoking in movies: Impact on adolescent smoking. *Adolesc Med.* 2005;16:345–370.

41. Edberg M, Abroms L. Application of theory: Communications campaigns. In: Edberg M, ed. *Essentials of Health Behavior: Social and Behavioral Theory in Public Health.* Sudbury, Mass.: Jones and Bartlett Publishers; 2007.

42. Farrelly MC, Davis KC, Jennifer D, Messeri P. Sustaining "truth": Changes in youth tobacco attitudes and smoking intentions after three years of a national antismoking campaign. *Health Educ Res.* 2009;24(1):42–48.

43. Jackson C. Behavioral science theory and principles for practice in health education. *Health Educ Res.* 1997;12(1):143–150.

CHAPTER 12

QUALITATIVE DATA AND RESEARCH METHODS IN PUBLIC HEALTH

Sharleen Simpson, PhD, ARNP
Mary Ellen Young, PhD, CRC/R

LEARNING OBJECTIVES

- Define and describe qualitative research.
- Explain how qualitative research differs from the more well-known quantitative research.
- Understand why qualitative research is used in public health.
- Identify qualitative data.
- List the qualitative traditions most appropriate for public health use.
- Describe how to evaluate and use qualitative research.

In this chapter, we define qualitative research and describe two specific approaches that are particularly relevant for public health: ethnography and grounded theory. We briefly discuss the differences between qualitative and quantitative research and the rationale for using either a qualitative approach or a combination of qualitative and quantitative data collection methods, also known as mixed methods. We describe the philosophical underpinnings of ethnography and grounded theory. We also talk about how to design qualitative research projects using either of these approaches, and we describe sampling, data collection, and data analysis, including use of newer techniques such as computer-assisted data analysis systems.

What Is Qualitative Research?

Qualitative research (also known as interpretive research) is a holistic approach to answering questions. It derives from recognition that human lives are complex and that in-depth understanding is not described by numbers. The focus of this research is on the human experience: the context of human behavior, or in other words, what people do and how and why they do it. Research strategies generally feature sustained contact with people in settings in which they normally spend their time, such as the community, their homes, or where they work. Usually, the researcher is very involved with the participants, using in-depth unstructured interviews, observations, documents, and field notes to collect information that becomes the data that are analyzed. Because of the nature of these data, the researcher becomes the instrument used to collect the data. What is produced is a description or **narrative** of people living through events in various situations.

Albert Einstein once said "not everything that can be counted counts, and not everything that counts can be counted."[1, p. 12] Even the foremost mathematician of the twentieth century recognized the limits of math, of counting, in our understanding of the world.

PUBLIC HEALTH CONNECTIONS 12.1
QUALITATIVE AND QUANTITATIVE RESEARCH

The way we now approach the study of things that cannot or should not be counted is called *qualitative research*. That term is often used in contrast to *quantitative research*, implying that there are two types of research, quantitative and qualitative, and that you should know about both of them. Chapter 5 describes common epidemiological study designs and methods that are typically quantitative in nature. Quantitative research has become the dominant paradigm in health care research. In this chapter, we will provide you with a little background to help you understand the differences between quantitative and qualitative research and why qualitative research is as important to understanding the provision of health care services and public health as the quantitative studies that abound.

Qualitative Versus Quantitative Research

In the philosophy of science, students are taught that there are two types of reasoning: inductive and deductive. Simply put, **inductive reasoning** is the thinking process by which theories are developed, and **deductive reasoning** is the thinking process by which those theories are tested. Qualitative research fits nicely into the long-standing research tradition of inductive reasoning[2]. For example, as discussed in Chapter 8, in the late eighteenth century Edward Jenner noted that milkmaids who had contracted cowpox (an occupational hazard) seemed to be immune to the more virulent, deadly, and disfiguring smallpox. Based on this observation, he developed the theory that someone could be vaccinated with one disease-causing organism in order to prevent another, more serious, disease. His theory is based in the natural world and his experience of that world: the *qualitative* experience that leads him to his explanation of that world. His laboratory work came *after* his observational work.

That distinction leads us to the second characteristic that distinguishes qualitative from quantitative research in public health: it is naturalistic[3]. **Naturalistic research** is not conducted in a laboratory but is conducted in the real world. In public health, that real world consists of the lives and experiences of the people, patients, clients, or populations with whom we work. A third characteristic of qualitative research is that it is **phenomenological**[1]. By this we mean that we seek to capture the lived experience of the individuals or groups about whom we have questions. We do not abstract that experience into things that can be counted (as in questions that score people's symptoms of depression), rather we focus on the entirety of the experience and the meaning of that experience to our research participants.

PUBLIC HEALTH CONNECTIONS 12.2
QUALITATIVE THINKING

Innovators are told to think outside the box.

Qualitative scholars tell their students, Study the box. Observe it. Inside. Outside. From inside to outside, and outside to inside. Where is it? How did it get there? What's around it? Who says it's a box? What do they mean? Why does it matter? Or does it? What is *not* box? Ask the box questions. Question others about the box. What's the perspective from inside? From outside? Study diagrams of the box. Find documents related to the box. What does *thinking* have to do with the box anyway? Understand *this* box. Study another box. And another. Understand *box*. Understand. Then you can think inside *and* outside the box. Perhaps. For awhile. Until it changes. Until you change. Until outside becomes inside again. Then start over. Study the box[1, p. 2].

Qualitative Research in Public Health

The method used for a research project depends on the purpose of the research and the questions you are asking. Qualitative research is usually conducted to explore problems about which relatively little is known[4]. Quantitative research requires enough prior data and research to be able to put together surveys and questionnaires that can gather appropriate information that is countable or that has specific categorical responses (such as yes and no or a finite list of experiences that can be checked off). If not enough is known about a particular topic to be sure what questions should be asked, then that topic is a good candidate for a qualitative study that might generate a theory for testing or at least suggest the appropriate questions for inclusion in a survey or questionnaire. The term **mixed methods** is sometimes used to describe research in which qualitative methods, data, and analysis are followed explicitly by quantitative surveys or for which qualitative methods are used to further interpret quantitative surveys[2]. Qualitative research can also be used to explain data that do not fit within the parameters of a quantitative study. For example, **outliers**, or answers that are not typical, in a quantitative study are frequently excluded; however, these same outliers may provide clues for understanding the behavior or motivations of certain population groups, a problem that is familiar to public health professionals. One way to use qualitative research is to do follow-up interviews with the participants who are the outliers and do not fit the typical patterns or hypothesized model. Another way is to conduct open-ended interviews first, in whatever group, institution, or community is the focus of the study, to determine the best way to frame the questions or create a survey. **Open-ended interviews** may have several forms: they may be informal conversations, they may use an interview guide of general topics to be covered, or they may be statements requiring the participants to fill in the blanks[1]. Quantitative interviews may use questionnaires that have been developed based on previous work for which the possible responses are already presented. The participant merely chooses the answer that he or she thinks is correct.

What Are Qualitative Data?

Collecting qualitative data is an ongoing, collaborative process between the participants and the researcher[5]. Open-ended questions and interviewer probes yield in-depth responses about people's experiences, opinions, perceptions, feelings, and knowledge. Because the questions and responses are not fixed, we do not always know exactly where the interview will take us in terms of the topics.

These interviews may be audio recorded and then transcribed. Activities, behaviors, and conversations observed during the interviews or in the particular setting where the people being studied spend their time are also described in rich detail in written **field notes**. These observations describe the context of the activities. Written materials, particularly reports, official publications, personal diaries, letters, Web materials (such as blogs), artistic works, and photographs may also be used to describe these experiences, opinions, and feelings. In short, qualitative data consist of words, both those of the participant and those of the researcher. They may also include visual images such as photos or videotape. The following is an excerpt from field notes compiled in a methods course research project about the barriers persons with mobility disabilities face when they try to participate in community activities. The excerpt adds context and sets the stage to illustrate the researcher's uncertainty about the interview process:

So before the interview she said she was going to introduce me to her partner, so again I am not sure if the person will be in a wheelchair. She had a very nice long wheelchair ramp up to her house. So I meet L ... who is a man and now I am really confused and L.T. refers to "him." Well now I cannot figure the situation out because I got her name through a lesbian group and all her friends are lesbians and her partner is a man. So I am trying to figure the situation out, but do not want to ask and decide to proceed with the interview and see if anything comes up. But I am now very curious.

So I meet her two dogs and we begin. Most of the people she mentions I know or know of, and all the events and things I am familiar with, so I know she is a lesbian.... I keep trying to place the partner in the situation and decide that perhaps the partner was a woman and transitioned to a man.... I am thinking this is kind of interesting, and I am thinking I want to interview her about that. I mean here you are a lesbian and you are hanging out with a fairly radical crowd who has "no male" events and now your partner is a man ... so now what? But I keep on with the interview and decide to try to confirm the situation later. But it was a distraction.

AC, 2006

Below is an excerpt from a focus group conducted as part of the same study on barriers faced by persons with mobility disabilities in trying to move about the community.

P2: They just, that's not just (this city), like you know I've traveled all over the country and I found it everywhere, its everywhere.

Int: ... I'm sorry, are there other places in town that are particularly difficult for you to go out to?

P1: Well, number 1 talking, you see this fresh tear in my chair, that's because ah, a ___ store, that's what it's called ... where you mail packages?

Int: Right, uh huh.

P1: The door is so heavy, that I hardly had the strength in my arms to open it and then, anyway, trying to get out of it is just as bad and my wheelchair got caught on the handle ... and it just tore my chair. You get these doors that are so heavy and there is no way to get in unless you get some help and someone comes along and holds it for you.

P2: The merchants put merchandise in the stores and they don't think about people ... that have mobility problems, cause they jam as much merchandise as they can. There is a major store in the mall which I won't mention here, and I actually had to write letters to the regional manager to get them to take some of the merchandise out so that I can get through.

As these excerpts demonstrate, individual and focus group interviews and field notes let us see the way both the researchers and the participants are thinking and how they are interacting.

Qualitative Traditions in Public Health

Although there is no one best approach for doing qualitative research, good research has a purpose and good methods have a good fit or **congruence** among scientific question, method, data, and strategies for analysis[5]. In other words, the method used will depend on the question being asked, the feasibility of the project, and the time frame available to complete it. In this chapter, we will be focusing mainly on ethnography and grounded theory, recognizing that photovoice and narrative analysis may be techniques used in the context of either an ethnographic or a grounded theory study.

Ethnography and Public Health

Ethnography has been the primary method of anthropology and was the earliest distinct tradition of qualitative inquiry[1, p. 81]. Ethnography is a means of exploring cultural groups. Traditionally, the ethnographer presented a background of the history of a group, community, or institution; the social geography; the conflicts between various factions within the community; and an explanation of some of the core meanings of the culture. Although there are many definitions of culture, most include the idea that it consists of "beliefs, behaviors, norms, attitudes, social arrangements, and forms of expression that form describable patterns in the lives of members of a community or institution."[6, p. 21] Because these assumptions are embedded within cultural groups, they may not be evident to insiders or group members. Some believe that ethnography is best conducted by outsiders because they may more easily see these patterns.

In recent years, ethnography has moved from a **community focus** to a **problem focus**. Communities are no longer isolated exotic groups, but rather they may be groups or institutions such as businesses, health departments, schools, or professional people. Some have questioned if this is still *real* ethnography. One of the foremost voices in ethnography, Michael Agar, in the preface of the second edition of his classic introduction to ethnography, *The Professional Stranger*, speaks of the differences between the ethnography of the original volume published in 1980 and the "new ethnography" of today, calling it both current and out-of-date[7]. The ethnography outlined in the original book viewed the group being studied as isolated, whereas the new ethnography considers "the political and personal circumstance of the research, [and] views the local group as a diverse crowd in a world of blurred edges" that is also influenced by historical forces[7, p. 6]. He also notes, however, that on the ground and in the trenches, where the new ethnography is done, "one still makes contacts, finds a trail into a new research site, hangs around and asks questions, struggles to figure out how to analyze uncontrolled material, and worries about the generalizability of the results"[7, p. 7]. In other words, although the information gathered may be different now, the way it is gathered is still much the same.

In his book, *Health Culture and Community*, anthropologist Benjamin Paul was one of the first to point out the ways that culture and social organization affect the health of communities[8,9]. The concept of individuals and their community group, in context, also resonates with the public health social-ecological model (see Chapters 2 and 11). However, even though there has been a growing recognition of the impact of social factors on health, systematic use of this knowledge to translate public health knowledge to actual practice is not very common[9].

How Do You Do Ethnography?

In ethnography, you learn what is going on by paying attention to behavior, whether it is movement, or sound, or smell or taste, or anything else that is happening[7]. You then ask questions about what the things you observed mean and why they are happening at this particular time (context), because ethnography translates events from one point of view to another. Using ethnographic research to fully understand problems and how to effectively communicate with communities and understand their needs is a way to begin the process of translating knowledge to practice.

Ethnographic data collection includes interviews, observation, and use of documents such as reports, scrapbooks, diaries, photo albums, and audio taping and videotaping. Multiple sources of information are collected and used because no single source of information can be trusted to provide a complete picture of the problem or community being studied. In ethnography, data collection may be referred to as **fieldwork**, which means that the researcher is on-site wherever the action is happening, observing, talking with people, looking at documents, and just generally hanging around.

In the early years, these data-collecting activities required writing voluminous notes every night after the day's activities. At present, voluminous notes are still recorded, but they may be dictated using battery-operated digital recorders. These recordings can be directly downloaded from either interviews or field notes onto a computer that has a software program that facilitates transcription of the spoken word.

One of the ways that qualitative methods differ from quantitative methods is that quantitative researchers are on the lookout for *variables*, or things that can be measured; ethnographers are on the lookout for *patterns*[7, p. 17]. Ethnography can use both quantitative and qualitative information. For example, you may conduct observations and open-ended interviews, but you may also wish to do a community survey. Ethnographers were among the first to use what we now call *mixed methods* or *mixed data*, combining open-ended interviews and observations with survey data.

How Do We Design Ethnographic Studies?

A **research design** is a plan or proposal to conduct research and should involve a philosophical point of view, strategies of inquiry, and specific methods[2]. For example, the **social constructivist** worldview is a philosophical point of view compatible with ethnography. One of the basic assumptions of this viewpoint is that meanings are constructed by human beings as they engage with the world they are interpreting[2,10]. Another assumption is that humans engage with their world and make sense of it based on their historical and social perspectives: we are all born into a world of meaning bestowed upon us by our culture. And finally, the social constructivist view assumes that the basic generation of meaning is always social, arising in and out of interaction with a human community[2, pp. 8–9].

Strategies of inquiry focus on data collection, analysis, and writing, but they originate out of disciplines and flow throughout the process of research[2]. These strategies result directly from the nature of the problem to be investigated and the research questions to be answered. An example of this is illustrated by a community-based mosquito net intervention in Tanzania, described by Winch[11]. Three research questions were addressed, each using different strategies: Why did many villagers not view malaria as a high priority? How could year-round net use be promoted? How could the project create a demand for regular retreatment (adding more insecticide) of the nets?[11, p. 45] These questions could not be answered without understanding the local culture, thus an ethnographic approach was well suited for this project.

Using pile sorting (organizing items or events into groups based on similarity) and unstructured interviews, the project researchers discovered that there were many definitions of malaria and many kinds of fever, making it difficult to focus on malaria using definitions derived from Western medicine. Use of local healers in the campaign improved the ability of project organizers to communicate with villagers about malaria[11, p. 49]. To understand why nets were not used all year, interviews were done to define the seasons, and a survey was completed to document use[11, p. 54]. To determine why there were low rates of retreatment of the nets, additional interviews were done. Results indicated that a series of factors influenced whether nets would be retreated, including access to facilities where retreatment could be done and the cost of retreatment. The results showed that the major problems in maintaining this intervention were administrative and political, including poor communication and lack of a public system to make the nets and retreatment easily available[11, p. 60]. None of these questions could have been answered with survey data alone.

Sampling, or choosing research participants, depends on the unit of analysis, that is, whether the focus is on the individual, families, groups, gender, ethnicity, or some other unit. The kinds of sampling frequently used in ethnographic research are purposive or judgment sampling, snowball or referral sampling, and convenience sampling. According to Bernard "in [**purposive** or] **judgment sampling** you decide the purpose you want informants (or communities) to serve, and you go out to find some."[12, p. 176] Purposive sampling can be applied to any units of analysis, such as families, communities, or individuals engaged in certain activities or having certain characteristics. An example of purposive sampling is illustrated by Erickson's study on people who spent time in Montana radon health mines as an alternative treatment for some chronic diseases such as arthritis[13]. Participants in this study were recruited from the ranks of the health mine users. In this study, Erickson herself spent time in the radon mines and interviewed other people using the mines while she was there.

Snowball sampling (or **referral sampling**) involves locating some key individuals to interview and then asking them to recommend others who might be willing to participate[12]. This kind of sampling is especially useful for obtaining participants from a difficult-to-reach population. An example of snowball sampling is illustrated in a recent study on becoming a male sex worker in India[14]. Researchers recruited leaders among the population of men who have sex with men (MSM) to train to do the interviews. These MSM workers then used a form of referral sampling to recruit other MSM sex workers for interviews. Finally, **convenience sampling**, or simply talking to whoever will agree to answer your questions is a commonly used technique[15].

How Do We Analyze Ethnographic Data?

As mentioned earlier, ethnographic data may consist of transcriptions of individual interviews, focus group interviews, field notes, existing text data in reports, or other documents. Data analysis often begins while the data are being collected. In fact, field notes and memos written while transcribing and reading interviews are usually the first phase of data analysis. According to Ryan and Bernard, analyzing textual data involves discovering themes and subthemes, narrowing them to a manageable number, deciding which are the most important, conceptualizing how they fit together, and linking these themes to theoretical models[16, p. 85]. This involves reading and rereading the text and analyzing it line by line. Thematic analysis is the basis of much social science research. "Without thematic categories, investigators have nothing to describe, nothing to compare, and nothing to explain."[16, p. 3] An example of thematic categories as they relate to cultural explanatory models can be drawn from the study of the Montana health mines cited above. Some of these themes, which also illustrate how participants were able to justify use of the mines, are as follows: (1) Radon in the mines is different from the radon you might find in a run-down basement; (2) radon is natural, therefore it is good; (3) radon is mild, not strong radiation; (4) radon is dangerous but controllable[13, pp. 8–11]. These ideas or themes emerged from analysis of participant interviews and provide insights about the reasons people used the mines. They constitute an *explanatory model*, which Kleinman[15] defines as the way people develop their own specific ideas about the cause and treatment of certain illnesses. Finding out about these models allows practitioners to understand the patient's perspective and develop effective strategies of care.

Most qualitative researchers accept that there are several forms of ethnography that may be used depending on the problem to be investigated[5, p. 57–59].

Traditional ethnography is usually done in a single setting, such as a village or a community that is unfamiliar to the researcher. This research has a broad focus and describes the group as completely as possible, including such attributes as language and kinship systems, and it requires a long residence and time in the field (usually at least a year). An example of this type of ethnography is a recent ethnographic study examining the response to a community-based participatory project reform in behavioral health care in New Mexico[17]. This study collected data using participant observation, formal interviews, critical readings of newspapers and official documents in the local community, and it considered the behavioral health system by focusing upward on those with power. The themes generated from this study fell into two broad categories: (1) structure and function and (2) participation and collaboration. The first category had to do with such issues as concerns about the greater input of providers compared to consumers, lack of resources, administrative demands by the state, and lack of state response to local efforts. The second category had to do with information flow problems, transportation, and how stigma affected the program[17, p. 283]. The researchers concluded that attempts at change and participation-based reform can only succeed in an open process of mutual learning and discovery where all voices can be heard, regardless of ethnicity, class, and cultural and geographic differences[17, p. 293]. When the voices of the people and the community need to be heard, ethnography is a good method to use.

Focused ethnography is used to evaluate or to obtain information on a special topic or shared experience. The topic is specific and may be identified before the researcher begins the study. An example is a recent dissertation on becoming a man in Black culture, a study that focused on Black adolescents growing up in the inner city and the obstacles they faced in this process[18].

Critical collaborative ethnography is one of the newer approaches[19, p. 303]. This perspective has grown out of critical social theory and reflects a growing discontent with the positivist notion of an objective social science that produces value-free ethnographies. It critiques modern society and its institutions as they affect race, gender, class, sexuality, and disability[19, p. 305]. Critical collaborative ethnography includes participatory, action-based, indigenous, and collaborative ethnographic practices that focus on resistance, social change, and political action[19, p. 314]. The work of many feminist ethnographers has illustrated how gender has influenced the ways that cultural practices are perceived. For example, prior to the emergence of the feminist perspective, ethnographic reports available about the women of certain cultures were minimal and usually reported by the men of that culture as told to male anthropologists. Because the health of a group is often linked more strongly to the work of women's roles, this perspective is extremely important. The work of Margaret Mead in *Coming of Age* *in Samoa*[20] and later in *Sex and Temperament*[21] is an early example of feminist efforts to separate sex (biological) and gender (culturally defined). Robbie Davis Floyd, who wrote *Birth as an American Rite of Passage*[22], a critique of the impersonal, technological approach to childbirth currently used by hospitals and providers in the United States, is a current feminist anthropologist. Emily Martin[23], who has written about the subordination of women's bodies in health care, is another example.

An example of the work of critical medical anthropologists is that of Nancy Scheper-Hughes, who criticized the idea of innate maternal/infant bonding in her book on mother love and child death in northeastern Brazil, *Death Without Weeping*[24], and who has also studied the organ-trafficking underworld[25].

At present, the goal of critical ethnography is to find ways to bring multiple voices into any research study and break down the dominant structures and practices. Early proponents of this approach include Merrill Singer and Hans Baer, who have written numerous works on critical medical anthropology[26,27], which has largely the same focus.

Participatory action research (PAR) is an example of critical collaborative ethnography in which researchers conduct field research, but community participants are collaborators in the process. This means that community members have a say in what the research questions are and what data should be collected. Community participants may help collect the data rather than just being the subjects of the study. Proponents of this method believe that cooperative inquiry is less likely to undermine the self-determination of the participants[5,28]. An example of this method is a recent report on preventing teen pregnancy done by Cornerstone Consulting in conjunction with community members, teachers, counselors, and health care providers of Palm Beach County, Florida[29]. Several key questions were addressed, including which teenagers were getting pregnant, where in the county they lived, what were common characteristics of the communities most affected by the problem, whether appropriate resources were available to these teens, and what could be done to change the situation. This is very similar to community-based participatory research (CBPR, described in Chapter 11). PAR had its origin in international development projects, whereas CBPR seems to have developed in the context of public health.

Grounded Theory and Public Health

Another major tradition in qualitative research is called **grounded theory**. We use grounded theory to develop explanations for or theories about the phenomena we observe or the narratives our participants provide for us. In grounded theory, we work up from the data to develop theory; thus our explanations are *grounded* in the data.

Barney Glaser and Anselm Strauss were pioneers of the grounded theory method. In *The Discovery of Grounded Theory*, they describe the methods that they used to study how people who are given a terminal prognosis (expectation that a disease will be fatal) are treated by health care professionals in a hospital setting[30]. In their seminal work, Glaser and Strauss describe their fieldwork at a number of hospitals in the San Francisco Bay area[31,32]. Their focus was the experience of health care workers caring for dying patients. Through extensive interviews and observations, Glaser and Strauss documented a key theoretical construct, the "awareness of dying," which is the knowledge of an individual, his or her loved ones, and the medical staff that the condition is terminal. Four "awareness contexts" are described: closed awareness, suspected awareness, mutual pretense awareness, and open awareness[31]. In situations of closed awareness, doctors and health care workers know that a patient is most likely terminal but do not disclose this to the patient or family. In suspicion awareness, the patient is seeking out clues to his or her condition, and the health care worker is trying to hide them. In mutual pretense awareness, all parties pretend that dying is not imminent, and in open awareness all parties are aware and act upon that awareness[31]. It is important to note that this theory did not exist prior to the authors spending an extensive amount of time in the field, observing and documenting what they saw and what was said to them in the hospitals, followed by extensive analysis of the data.

Characteristics of Grounded Theory

Grounded theory is by nature inductive rather than deductive. The research does not start out to test or verify a hypothesis but to develop an explanation for or generate a theory about what is observed. This theory is constructed from and invariably linked to the data[32].

PUBLIC HEALTH CONNECTIONS 12.3
FOOD FOR THOUGHT

Fundamentally, grounded theory allows for a subjective or interpretivist approach to data analysis[33]. Contrast that with the objective stance of most quantitative researchers, who seek to minimize what they term *threats to validity*. Qualitative researchers know that they develop their research questions based on their own beliefs, values, and experiences. However, they are challenged to articulate those beliefs, values, and experiences so that the reader can understand the lens through which the data are interpreted.

Grounded theory research is best used when very little is known about a phenomenon. For example, in Nosek and coworkers' study of the sexuality of women with disabilities, researchers (including women with disabilities themselves) initially felt that very little was known about the topic[34]. In order to prepare a national survey, in-depth interviews about their sexuality were conducted with thirty-one adult women with physical disabilities. Six major domains emerged from the data analysis: sense of self (how a woman feels about herself as a sexual being); sexuality information (what she was told about sex in general or in relation to her condition); relationships (a history of family, friendship, and intimate relationships); sexual functioning; abuse; and health maintenance (general as well as specific to reproductive health care). These six areas composed a theoretical model for the development of the final national survey and provided the context and, in some cases, the wording of the survey items.

Data Collection

Rather than state hypotheses to be tested, grounded theory researchers pose research questions. The questions are open-ended and usually address the who, what, where, when, how, and why questions rather than how many or how much questions[1]. Random sampling is not expected in grounded theory research because individuals or cases are selected based on their characteristics, either theoretical (selected on the basis of the emerging theory)[32] or purposive (selected to get representation from participants with differing characteristics such as sex, ethnicity, or socioeconomic status)[1]. The research questions typically are answered by interviewing participants (not called subjects in qualitative research), conducting observations of them, or reviewing other relevant material, such as archival material or reports. Glaser and Strauss spent approximately three years observing and interviewing in their hospital settings. Extensive time in the field and in-depth questioning of the individuals who are involved leads to a rich dataset consisting of interview transcripts, field notes describing what was observed, and memos documenting the insights and ideas of the researcher.

Data Analysis

Data analysis in grounded theory consists of preparing and verifying narrative data, coding data, constructing theory, analyzing more data, and constantly comparing new data with emerging theory until an interpretive framework is established[32]. For example, in Nosek and coworkers' study, the thirty-one women identified were each interviewed in their homes, with each interview lasting approximately one hour[34]. Interviews were conducted using an **interview guide**, a series of suggested questions in a suggested order in which the wording and order of the questions were changed based on the language and direction of the participant[1]. Interviews were transcribed verbatim and then checked for accuracy by the interviewer. Coding was conducted by an interdisciplinary team of researchers, including women with disabilities themselves. **Coding** refers to reading the data and identifying major themes, and then assigning labels to and defining categories that emerge. Strauss defines two levels of coding: **open coding**, referring to an approach to data with no preconceived ideas about what will be found, and **axial coding**, referring to reviewing data for the purpose of more richly coding on a particular theme[35]. A grounded theory researcher goes back and forth between the data and the emerging analytic framework, employing *constant comparison* of new data with already coded data and new categories with previously analyzed text[32]. The result of this iterative process is an explanatory model or theory for the phenomenon being studied. The model contains major categories and well-defined properties of those categories, all linked to or grounded in the data, especially the words of the participants. These words are powerful in conveying the meaning of the model. For

> I always felt like a neutral sex. It's like I'm not a woman, nor a man. I don't know what I am because I was never approached like a woman and I guess that as I grow older and mature more, I have begun to proclaim that identity as a woman and thinking even if no man approached me, I am still a woman. I am still attractive.[34, p. 5]

example, this excerpt from Nosek and coworkers' study illustrates one of the major findings with a power that cannot be captured in research language.

The goal of grounded theory research is the development of what Glaser and Strauss called substantive theory, an explanatory model of a discrete phenomenon[32]. Enough work in substantive theory might lead to the development of formal theory about a larger phenomenon.

Computer-Assisted Data Analysis Systems

Traditionally, qualitative research involved pieces of paper, note cards, colored pencils, thumb tacks, and cork boards to capture the emerging analysis. Fortunately, we now have computer programs to assist us with the organization, coding, and retrieval of our data. Examples of available software include NVivo[36] and Atlas.ti.[37]. These programs give us the capability to handle larger datasets and approach the data in ways that are complex and sophisticated. We must realize, however, that these programs do not do the analytical or thinking work for us.

For example, in her study of stroke survivors and their caregivers, Lutz[38] used NVivo v. 7 to manage the data analysis. Interviews with stroke patients and caregivers were transcribed and then imported into NVivo. Coding was done directly in the software by highlighting passages of text and labeling those passages with words representing the themes emerging from the analysis. Each passage was then easily retrievable when the code was used to search the data. Coding could be arranged in a hierarchical structure, searched by attributes of the participants (such as male or female), or displayed in models much more readily using the software than conducting the analysis by hand. Interpretive writing was done within the software itself in the form of memos, capturing the thoughts, feelings, reactions, and emerging analysis of the research team. These memos are retained as a way of creating an **audit trail** for the analysis, which enhances data credibility.

Mixed Methods and When to Use Them

Mixed methods research is considered an emerging, innovative research strategy that is moving across disciplines. It is an approach in which the different methods inform one another to provide a more layered, multipronged approach to research[39]. Mixed methods research seeks to combine quantitative and qualitative methods using a variety of approaches or designs. Tashakkori and Teddlie published the first comprehensive overview of this research strategy[40]. At present, there are several journals that emphasize this type of research[2], including the *Journal of Mixed Methods Research, Quality and Quantity,* and *Field Methods.* According to Creswell, this research strategy has evolved because of the complexity of the questions addressed by public health and social science researchers[2]. This means that neither quantitative nor qualitative approaches by themselves are sufficient to adequately answer these questions. There may also be questions that can only be answered by comparing, contrasting, and combining findings from both strategies[2,41]. However, it should be noted here that, as mentioned earlier, ethnography has long incorporated both quantitative and qualitative methods of data collection.

Visual Research Methods as Emerging Qualitative Research Strategies

Holm notes that three major kinds of visual images are used in visual research[42, p. 327]. First, there are **subject-produced images**, such as autophotography[43,44]. In this method, the researcher asks the participants to either photograph or videotape aspects of their world to allow the researchers an insider view[42, p. 327]. Subject-produced images can generate more authentic data because researchers view the world of the participants through their own eyes[44]. The second type of visual image is rooted in the use of documentary photography in anthropology and consists of **researcher-produced images**. The third type of image is the **preexisting image**, including family pictures, newspaper photographs, photographs of rituals, archival materials, and more recently, photoblogs[42, p. 328].

Recently, a technique called **photovoice** was introduced as a part of participatory action research[42,45]. The main goals of photovoice are (1) to empower and enable people to reflect on their personal and community concerns; (2) to encourage a dialogue and transfer knowledge through discussions about photographs among participants and with the researcher/audience; and (3) to access the perception of those not in control of various problem issues (for example, people with disabilities or from minority backgrounds who traditionally have not been asked about their experiences) and share it with those who make policy, programmatic, or individual treatment decisions[42, p. 329].

Photos may be analyzed using content analysis and a predetermined code, or they may be used as a prompt to elicit interviews. Visual methods are becoming more common in evaluation research and in public health research. Some of the issues associated with these new techniques include confidentiality, consent, and power relations[42, p. 339].

Evaluating Qualitative Research

Traditional methods for evaluating quantitative research, such as validity, reliability, and generalizability, just do not apply to qualitative research. Efforts to make the quantitative criteria fit the qualitative designs usually result in the number of participants being deemed too small, the analysis being characterized as too subjective, and the process criticized as lacking rigor. Qualitative researchers might counter with arguments that there is trade off between sample size and depth of understanding, that subjectivity is embraced as enhancing meaning, and that the process of data collection and analysis is just as rigorous (if not more so) as in traditional quantitative research. To counter the arguments about validity and reliability, qualitative researchers stress that their studies must be trustworthy and credible[46]. Techniques such as maintaining audit trails and **peer debriefing** enhance the credibility of the data. An example of an audit trail would be a series of memos organized by date to document how and when analytical decisions were made. Peer debriefing is a process by which other researchers provide feedback on the data collection and analysis. Researchers establish trustworthiness by presenting enough details of how the data were collected and analyzed so that the reader has confidence in the conclusions reached.

Summary

In this chapter we have described what qualitative research is and how it differs from quantitative research. We have focused on two primary approaches to qualitative data collection that are useful for public health, ethnography and grounded theory, including where and with what type problems they may be used. We have discussed research design, data collection, and data analysis for each of these approaches, including computer-assisted data analysis. We have also looked at some newer strategies for data collection, such as using mixed methods (combining quantitative and qualitative methods or data), using visual images instead of words as data with such strategies as autophotography and photovoice. Finally we have addressed issues related to evaluation of qualitative research such as reliability (trustworthiness) and validity (credibility) of qualitative research.

Key Terms

audit trail, 314

axial coding, 313

coding, 313

community focus, 305

congruence, 304

convenience sampling, 308

critical collaborative ethnography, 309

deductive reasoning, 301

ethnographic data collection, 306

ethnography, 305

field notes, 303

fieldwork, 306

focused ethnography, 309

grounded theory, 310

inductive reasoning, 300

interview guide, 312

judgment sampling, 307

mixed methods, 302

narrative, 300

naturalistic research, 301

open coding, 313

open-ended interviews, 302

outliers, 302

participatory action research, 310

peer debriefing, 315

phenomenological, 301

photovoice, 315

preexisting image, 315

problem focus, 305

purposive sampling, 307

qualitative research, 300

referral sampling, 308

research design, 306

researcher-produced images, 315

sampling, 307

snowball sampling, 308

social constructivist, 306

subject-produced images, 314

traditional ethnography, 309

Review Questions

1. Write three questions that cannot be answered by counting something.
2. Pick a research topic that you think might need both quantitative and qualitative data. Why do you think the topic you chose needs both types of data? Write one qualitative question and one quantitative question that might provide data to answer questions about this topic.
3. How would you go about purposive sampling for your qualitative question? Give some examples.
4. What would your sources of data be and what form would your data take?
5. Would your question be best answered by ethnography or grounded theory, or another design? Defend your answer.
6. What techniques might you use to analyze your data?
7. How might you establish credibility and trustworthiness in your qualitative study?

References

1. Patton MQ. *Qualitative Research & Evaluation Methods*. 3rd ed. Thousand Oaks, Calif.: Sage Publications; 2000.
2. Creswell JW. *Research Design: Qualitative, Quantitative and Mixed Methods Approaches*. Thousand Oaks, Calif.: Sage Publications; 2009.
3. Lincoln Y, Guba EG. (1985). *Naturalistic Inquiry*. Belmont, Calif.: Wadsworth.
4. Morse JM, Field PA. *Qualitative Research Methods for Health Professionals*. 2nd ed. Thousand Oaks, Calif.: Sage Publications; 1995.
5. Richards L, Morse JM. *Readme First for a User's Guide to Qualitative Methods*. 2nd ed. Thousand Oaks, Calif.: Sage Publications; 2007.
6. LeCompte MD, Schensul JJ. *Designing and Conducting Ethnographic Research. The Ethnographer's Toolkit*. Vol. 1.Walnut Creek, Calif.: Altamira Press; 1999.
7. Agar MH. *The Professional Stranger*. 2nd ed. San Diego, Calif.: Academic Press; 1996.
8. Paul BD, ed. *Health, Culture and Community: Case Studies of Public Reactions to Health Programs*. New York: Russell Sage Foundation; 1955.
9. Hahn RA, ed. *Anthropology in Public Health: Bridging Differences in Culture and Society*. New York: Oxford University Press; 1999.
10. Crotty M. *The Foundations of Social Research: Meaning and Perspective in the Research Process*. Thousand Oaks, Calif.: Sage Publications; 1998.
11. Winch PJ. The role of anthropological methods in a community-based mosquito net intervention in Bagamoyo District, Tanzania. In: Hahn RA, ed. *Anthropology in Public Health: Bridging Differences in Culture and Society*. New York: Oxford University Press; 1999:44–62.

12. Bernard HR. *Social Research Methods: Qualitative and Quantitative Approaches*. Thousand Oaks, Calif.: Sage Publications; 2000.

13. Erickson BE. Toxin or medicine? Explanatory models of radon in Montana health mines. *Med Anthropol Q.* 2009;21(1):1–21.

14. Lorway R, Reza-Paul S, Pasha A. On becoming a male sex worker in Mysore: Sexual subjectivity, "empowerment," and community-based HIV prevention research. *Med Anthropol Q.* 2009;23(2):142–160.

15. Kleinman A. *The Illness Narratives: Suffering, Healing and the Human Condition*. New York: Basic Books 1988.

16. Ryan GW, Bernard HR. Techniques to identify themes. *Field Methods*, 2003;15(1): 85–109.

17. Kano M, Willging CE, Rylko-Bauer B. Community participation in New Mexico's behavioral health care reform. *Med Anthropol Q.* 2009;23(3):277–297.

18. Thomas RLM. *The Impact of Black Masculinity on Identity Development and Sexual Attitudes of Inner-City Black Adolescents: An Ethnographic Analysis [dissertation]*. Gainesville, Fla.: University of Florida; 2006.

19. Bhattacharya H. (2008). New critical collaborative ethnography. In: Hesse-Biber SN, Leavy P, eds. *Handbook of Emergent Methods*. New York: The Guilford Press; 2008: 363–387.

20. Mead M. *Coming of Age in Samoa*. New York: Harper Collins; 1928.

21. Mead M. *Sex and Temperament in Three Primitive Societies*. New York: Harper Collins; 1950.

22. Davis Floyd R. *Birth as an American Rite of Passage*. Berkeley, Calif.: University of California Press; 2004.

23. Martin E. *The Woman in the Body*. Boston: Beacon Press; 1987.

24. Scheper-Hughes N. *Death Without Weeping: The Violence of Everyday Life in Brazil*. Berkeley, Calif.: University of California Press; 1993.

25. Scheper-Hughes N. Parts unknown: Undercover ethnography of the organs-trafficking underworld. *Ethnography*. 2004;5(1):29–73.

26. Singer M, Baer H. *Critical Medical Anthropology*. Amityville, N.Y.: Baywood Publishing Company; 1995.

27. Baer HA, Singer M, Susser I. (1997). *Medical Anthropology and the World System: A Critical Perspective*. Westport, Conn.: Bergin & Garvey.

28. Reason P. *Human Inquiry in Action: Developments in New Paradigm Research*. London: Sage Publishing; 1988.

29. Cornerstone Consulting Group, Inc. (2001). A report for The Palm Beach County Health Department and Governor's Council for Community Health Partnerships, Inc. Available at: www.pbchd.com/pdfs/2003/PBC_Final_Report%20.pdf. Accessed February 12, 2009.

30. Glaser BG, Strauss AL. *The Discovery of Grounded Theory*. Chicago, Ill.: Aldine; 1967.

31. Glaser BG, Strauss AL. *Awareness of Dying*. Chicago, Ill.: Aldine; 1965.

32. Glaser BG, Strauss AL. *Time for Dying*. Chicago, Ill.: Aldine; 1968.

33. Glesne C. *Becoming Qualitative Researchers: An Introduction*. 2nd ed. New York: Longman; 1990.

34. Nosek MA, Howland C, Rintala DH, Young ME, Chanpong GF. National study of women with physical disabilities: Final report. *Sex Disabil.* 2001;19:5–39.

35. Strauss A. *Qualitative Analysis for Social Scientists.* New York: Cambridge University Press; 1987.

36. QSR International. NVivo 8 Web page. Available at: www.qsrinternational.com. Accessed May 15, 2010.

37. Atlas.ti. Atlas.ti v6 Web page. Available at: www.atlasti.com/index.html. Accessed May 15, 2010.

38. Lutz BJ, Young ME. Rethinking intervention strategies in stroke family caregiving. *Rehabil Nurs* 2010; 35(4):152–160.

39. Hess-Biber SN. Innovation in research methods design and analysis. In: Hesse-Biber SN, Leavy P, eds. *Handbook of Emergent Methods.* New York: The Guilford Press; 2008:359–362

40. Tashakkori A, Teddlie C., eds. *Handbook of Mixed Methods in Social and Behavioral Research.* Thousand Oaks, Calif.: Sage Publications; 2003.

41. Plano Clark VL, Creswell JW, Green DO, Shope RJ. Mixing quantitative and qualitative approaches: An introduction to emergent mixed methods research. In: Hesse-Biber SN, Leavy P, eds. *Handbook of Emergent Methods.* New York: The Guilford Press; 2008:363–387.

42. Holm G. Visual research methods. In: Hesse-Biber S, Leavy P, eds. *Handbook of Emergent Methods.* New York: The Guilford Press; 2008.

43. Ziller RC. *Photographing the Self: Methods for Personal Orientation.* Newbury Park, Calif.: Sage Publications; 1990.

44. Noland CM. Auto-photography as research practice: Identity and self-esteem research. *Journal of Research Practice.* 2006; 2(1):1–19.

45. Wang CC, Pies CA. Family, maternal, and child health through photovoice. *Matern Child Health J.* 2004;8(2):95–102.

46. Miles MB, Huberman AM. *Qualitative Data Analysis: An Expanded Sourcebook.* 2nd ed. Thousand Oaks, Calif.: Sage Publications; 1994.

CHAPTER 13

TUBERCULOSIS

Michael Lauzardo, MD, MSc
Joanne Julien, MD
David Ashkin, MD

LEARNING OBJECTIVES

- Distinguish between latent tuberculosis infection and active tuberculosis disease.
- Identify major risk factors for tuberculosis infection and disease.
- Describe the epidemiology of tuberculosis globally.
- Explain the relationship between HIV and tuberculosis.
- Describe directly observed therapy and its role in tuberculosis control.
- List current research and development efforts in tuberculosis prevention, diagnosis, and treatment.

Tuberculosis (TB) is arguably the most important infectious disease in the history of humankind. About one-third of the world's population carries the organism in a dormant state known as latency, and another 8 to 10 million people around the world develop the active form of the disease each year. Between 1.5 and 2 million people die from tuberculosis each year[1]. To put that into perspective, imagine a commercial jetliner with just over two hundred passengers crashing every hour on the hour, twenty-four hours a day, 365 days a year, with no survivors. That is how many people die from TB each year, a disease for which there has been an effective cure and prevention for over half a century. Distributing the medicines that cure and prevent the disease is hampered by a variety of social, political, and economic barriers that have led many to consider TB as a social disease with a medical aspect.

TB is caused by the organism *Mycobacterium tuberculosis*. Mycobacterium is a type of bacteria with a characteristic cell wall that has a propensity to affect the lungs. Because the biology and life cycle of this organism is quite different from other bacteria, treatment with antibiotics is effective but requires much longer treatment, and the organism can develop resistance; that is, the antibiotics don't work against the germ after a period of time, with much more serious consequences than occurs with some other bacteria. Today, drug-resistant TB is one of the biggest challenges faced by public health authorities and policy makers around the globe.

Infection with the human immunodeficiency virus (HIV) poses another challenge to the control of TB. HIV weakens the immune system mostly by affecting what is known as cell-mediated immunity, the precise arm of the immune system that is required to prevent the progression from latent TB infection to active disease. Persons who are infected with HIV will develop active TB disease more rapidly and at higher rates than those not infected with HIV. Also, they will develop disseminated forms of TB more frequently, making diagnosis more difficult and increasing the mortality from TB. Worldwide, TB is the number one cause of death among persons with HIV infection[2].

So how did we here? How can a disease with a known cure since the middle of the twentieth century grow to such enormous proportions that in 1993 the World Health Organization declared TB a global emergency? The reasons for this are as complex as the disease itself, but they stem from the fact that when TB therapy was developed and gained widespread use in industrialized countries, there was a widespread belief that disease would soon be relegated to the annals of history. Gradually, public health commitment to TB control eroded, as did the infrastructure to provide care. Research dollars and innovative strategies vanished along with advocacy for a disease that had lost its voice. In the meantime, a new player emerged on the scene, HIV, and the TB epidemic would never be the same. Developing countries, where the TB epidemic never abated, continued an unprecedented process of urbanization and crowding that further fueled the TB epidemic. These and other factors conspired to ensure TB's membership in an exclusive club of pandemic diseases that has shaped human history and will continue to do so for the foreseeable future.

Microbiology, Disease Types, Diagnosis, and Treatment

Mycobacterium tuberculosis is a member of the bacterial family *Mycobacteriaceae*. The organisms in this family are rod-shaped bacilli and are known for their thick, lipid-filled cell walls. It is the lipid-filled wall that gives mycobacteria their classic microbiological characteristic, acid fastness. An organism is said to be **acid fast** when, after staining and subsequent rinsing with acid, the stain remains in the organism's cell wall and can be seen in clinical specimens using a microscope. When an acid-fast organism is seen microscopically in a clinical specimen, it is most frequently a mycobacterial species, and the specimen will then be termed AFB smear positive, indicating that organisms were actually seen on a smear of the specimen microscopically.

M. tuberculosis is one of several organisms in what is known as the **MTB complex**, a group of very closely related organisms that cause similar disease in humans. The two most important members of the family *Mycobacteriaceae* are *M. tuberculosis* and *Mycobacterium leprae*, the organism that causes leprosy. For the better part of a century, these were the only organisms thought to be important in terms of human disease. However, with the advent of newer molecular diagnostic techniques looking for differences in bacterial DNA, literally dozens of new mycobacteria have been identified. An increasing number of them have been identified as important in terms of human disease, and still others are important in animals. However, the majority of these organisms are found in soil and water, and these organisms are important in breaking down organic matter. Of the non-tuberculous mycobacteria, *Mycobacterium avium complex*, *Mycobacterium abscessus*, and *Mycobacterium kansasii* are the most important in relation to human disease. Other species of mycobacteria may be more important depending on geographical region and individual susceptibilities that are not well understood.

Latent Tuberculosis Infection

Tuberculosis is spread through the air when a person who is sick with the active, pulmonary form of the disease coughs, spits, speaks, or sneezes. The bacilli can stay in the air for several hours and can eventually be inhaled by individuals in close contact with the infectious patient. The immune cells of the lung engulf the bacilli and work to contain the infection by preventing the bacillus from multiplying and spreading. It is important to note that the vast majority of individuals (approximately 90 percent) will never become sick, and this form of tuberculosis is referred to as **latent tuberculosis infection**.

Unfortunately, the body does not have an effective way of eliminating the TB bacteria; therefore, the bacilli continue to reside in the body in a state of dormancy, forever retaining the potential to reactivate, multiply, and cause symptomatic and contagious disease. In those who develop disease, more than half the time this reactivation occurs within two years after the initial infection. However, reactivation can occur at any time and is more likely when the person's immune system is weakened by age, HIV infection, or diabetes. In the immunocompetent adult, there is a 10 percent lifetime chance that latent TB infection will go on to become TB disease. In contrast, individuals with HIV infection may develop active TB at a rate as high as 10 percent per year[3].

People with latent tuberculosis infection are not considered contagious and cannot transmit the disease to others. Despite this, the treatment of affected individuals has significant public health implications. Studies in molecular epidemiology have shown that these patients represent an enormous reservoir of potential cases because the majority of active cases result from reactivation of latent infection.

Diagnosis of Latent Tuberculosis Infection

One of the oldest tests still used in clinical medicine is the **tuberculin skin test** (TST), used in the detection of latent TB infection. The test was first developed by Robert Koch and is accomplished by injecting filtered, heat-sterilized cultures of *M. tuberculosis* intradermally into a subject. The immune cells of individuals who are infected with tuberculosis will recognize the antigens in the injection and produce a local reaction (redness and swelling) at the injection site within two to three days. Unfortunately, the test is imperfect and associated with both false-negative and false-positive results. The protein derivative in the test contains antigens that are shared with other mycobacteria and therefore may elicit a positive result in subjects who have received the TB vaccine known as **BCG vaccine** or been exposed to non-tuberculous mycobacteria. False-negative results occur frequently in immunosuppressed people (for example, people with HIV or older adults) and therefore cannot mount the local immune response to the injection. Consequently, the Centers for Disease Control and Prevention (CDC) recommends that the tuberculin skin test be reserved for patients who are at increased risk for the development of tuberculosis, such as close contacts of active cases or people who are at risk of reactivating after prior infections. It should be underscored that a positive test indicates infection but does not in itself distinguish active disease from latent tuberculosis infection.

More recently, two blood tests, the QuantiFERON® (manufactured by Cellestis in Victoria, Australia) and the T-SPOT.TB® (manufactured by Oxford Immunotec in Oxford, United Kingdom) have been developed to detect latent TB infection. In these tests, the patient's blood is mixed with synthetic proteins that are identical to those produced by tuberculosis. If the individual has been infected with TB, their white blood cells will recognize the proteins and release molecules called interferons, which can then be measured in the blood. The main advantages of these tests are that they are not affected by prior BCG vaccination or prior exposure to non-tuberculous mycobacteria.

Tuberculosis Disease

The progression of tuberculosis from latent infection to active disease can take different forms. Unlike most infectious diseases, tuberculosis rarely makes people sick within the first few weeks of exposure. The exception is young children or people with HIV, in whom progression to active disease can be very rapid. TB can affect virtually any tissue or organ in the body, but the majority of cases are limited to the lung, a form referred to as pulmonary TB. The two other major classifications of TB are extrapulmonary and miliary tuberculosis.

In **pulmonary tuberculosis**, coughing is the most common symptom. Other symptoms include recurrent fevers, night sweats, weight loss, and decreased energy. Because the infection progresses slowly, patients may wait for weeks and often months before seeking medical care. As a result of this delay, it is estimated that the average pulmonary tuberculosis patient will infect ten to fifteen other people before being diagnosed and treated for the disease.

It is estimated that about 25 percent of active tuberculosis cases will present with **extrapulmonary disease**, or disease outside the lung. The kidneys and lymph nodes are the most common sites for extrapulmonary tuberculosis. Other locations include the bones, joints, brain, abdominal cavity, pericardium (the membrane around the heart), and reproductive organs. The risk of extrapulmonary disease increases with the degree of immunosuppression, and HIV is an important risk factor. Some studies have shown that more than 50 percent of patients with concurrent HIV and tuberculosis have extrapulmonary involvement[4]. Most extrapulmonary disease is not considered infectious.

When the TB bacilli gain entry to the bloodstream, they can spread through the body and set up many foci of infection. This form of tuberculosis is called **miliary tuberculosis** because the tiny foci that form in the lungs are the size of millets, the small round seeds in bird food. Infants and the elderly are most at risk of this form of tuberculosis, and it is associated with a 20 percent fatality rate, even with intensive treatment.

Diagnosis of Active Tuberculosis Infection

The diagnosis of active tuberculosis infection is based on risk factors for the disease, the clinical history of symptoms, an abnormal chest X-ray, a positive skin test, and the presence of bacilli in the sputum. Microscopic examination of the sputum is used with special acid-fast staining techniques to detect the bacilli. This technique can yield a result within hours. Unfortunately, the test lacks sensitivity and may fail to detect up to 50 percent of cases. Therefore, the specimens are also sent for culture, which is more sensitive but may take several weeks. Mycobacteria grow very slowly compared to other bacteria; the generation time is approximately twenty hours compared to other bacteria with generation times as short as fifteen minutes[5]. For this reason, patients frequently are started on treatment before the diagnosis can be confirmed by the laboratory. In a minority of patients, a laboratory diagnosis is never established and a presumptive diagnosis is made based on the clinical presentation and response to therapy.

PUBLIC HEALTH CONNECTIONS 13.1

DIAGNOSING TUBERCULOSIS

Mario is a twenty-seven-year-old man from Central America who came to the United States two years ago to find work. His family remains in his home country, and he sends back a portion of his earnings every month. Three months before going to the emergency room, Mario noted that he was more tired than usual, and he noticed his clothes were fitting more loosely. He noted a cough that began mostly in the morning now persisted throughout the day. Over the last three weeks, he noticed a small amount of blood in his sputum. In the last two weeks, he has had fevers and night sweats.

Mario decided to go to the emergency room when he became too weak to work. The nurses and doctors in the emergency room quickly suspected tuberculosis, put him in isolation, obtained a chest X-ray, and contacted the health department. Mario's sputum under the microscope showed organisms typical of tuberculosis, called AFB, on staining of the sputum. A rapid test that checks for TB DNA in the sputum came back positive for TB. He was started on four TB medications (isoniazid, rifampin, pyrazinamide, and ethambutol) and sent home after the health department made arrangements for his care as an outpatient. Two weeks later the cultures came back and confirmed the DNA tests on the sputum. Two weeks after that, his susceptibilities, the test that determines if the germ is going to be susceptible to the medications being used, came back showing his germ was susceptible to all TB medications. He responded well to treatment and went back to work after two weeks. After nine months of therapy he was cured.

This case is a typical example of an uncomplicated case of pulmonary TB. Most patients are ill for a period of several months prior to being diagnosed; Mario's symptoms are common among patients with TB. His X-ray shows the typical **infiltrates**, portions of the lung involved in the infection visible by X-ray (Figure 13.1). TB is a disease that is treated and cured mostly without the need for hospitalization, and many times individuals who, like Mario, are young and otherwise healthy, can return to work after a couple of weeks. About 85 percent of TB cases involve the lung. It is these pulmonary cases that are potentially infectious. People with extensive lung involvement, as evidenced by a positive smear and visible bacilli in stained sputum, are potentially very infectious. In these cases, an investigation into the patient's social, work, and home contacts is necessary to identify anyone who may have been infected. People found to be infected will be offered preventive treatment.

Figure 13.1 Chest X-Ray Showing Tuberculosis Infection

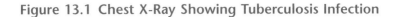

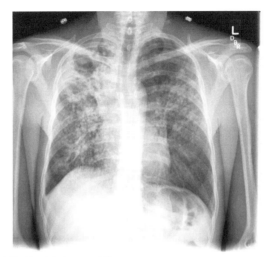

Source: CDC Public Health Image Library.

Treatment Principles

As described, *M. tuberculosis* are very slow-growing bacteria; therefore, the anti-biotics used in TB treatment regimens must be taken for long periods of time, usually six months or longer. When treatment is discontinued too early, the disease tends to recur. In addition, multiple drugs are required to prevent the development of drug resistance, and a standard regimen for patients with pan-susceptible tuberculosis disease would include the four drugs isoniazid, rifampin, pyrazinamide, and ethambutol. Compliant patients who complete therapy can be cured in over 95 percent of cases. When left untreated, the risk of death approaches 50 percent. The most commonly used regimen to treat latent tuberculosis infection is isoniazid for nine months. Under ideal conditions, this treatment can reduce one's chance of progressing to active tuberculosis disease by up to 90 percent[6]. Unfortunately, many patients miss doses or dis-continue the treatment; consequently, the overall efficacy of this treatment is only about 60 percent.

Patients with TB may face barriers such as substance abuse, mental health disease, fear or disbelief about the diagnosis, impoverished social conditions, and drug side effects that prevent them from successfully completing therapy. In some cases, patients choose to stop the treatment early because their symptoms improve and they no longer perceive a useful gain from continuing the drugs.

Because of these factors, the standard of care for the treatment of tuberculosis includes **directly observed therapy** (DOT) in which a health care worker supervises the administration of every dose until the regimen is considered complete. This is one of the most effective tools in achieving a cure and reducing the risk for the development of resistant TB in the community.

Hospitalized patients should be isolated in airborne-isolation rooms, and health care workers and visitors must wear an N95 disposable mask during contact with the patient. Not all patients with active tuberculosis disease require hospitalization, and in fact, many can be treated as outpatients. In such instances, the patient should be instructed to remain at home, without visitors and away from other family members until he or she is no longer considered infectious. Tuberculosis is a reportable disease in the United States, and all persons with confirmed or suspected tuberculosis must be reported to a state or local public health authority. This will instigate a **contact investigation**, an effort to identify close contacts who may have been exposed to TB, which may lead to additional case finding and prevent further spread of the infection in the community.

History

Few things have affected the history of civilization more than human illness. Among illnesses, tuberculosis ranks among the highest in terms of its overall impact on humanity. From ancient societies to the globalized world of the information age, humankind has been shaped by the Captain of Death for centuries. From the earliest recorded plagues to the current HIV pandemic, tuberculosis has exacted its toll on humanity.

The earliest evidence of tuberculosis infecting people comes from ancient Egypt, where the archeological evidence for tuberculosis is strong. Two mummies, one a little girl most likely of humble origin and the other a high-ranking priest of Ramses,

The Lord will strike you with wasting disease, and with fever, inflammation, and fiery heat ... and they shall pursue you until you perish.

Deuteronomy 28:22[7]

I cannot so properly say that he died of one disease, for there were many that had consented, and laid their heads together to bring him to his end. He was dropsical, he was consumptive, he was surfeited, was gouty, and as some say, he had a tang of the foul distemper in his

Nesperehan, had hunchback deformities[9]. Although there are several causes of a hunchback, the most common is known as a tuberculous **gibbous deformity**. This occurs when the tubercle bacillus infects the vertebra and destroys it. As it collapses, the remaining vertebrae protrude outward, leading to not only the deformity but also stunted growth, weakness, and neurological compromise, including paralysis. In the case of the young girl, tubercle bacilli were identified microscopically three thousand years after her death.

bowels. Yet the captain of all these men of death was the consumption, for it was that that brought him down to the grave.

The Life and Death of
Mr. Badman
John Bunyan[8]

Around 3000 BC, people with the gibbous deformity begin to be portrayed quite commonly in Egyptian art[10]. Whether because the deformity was common or because it was an oddity that carried special significance to the artists is unclear, but the fact remains that tuberculosis likely impacted ancient Egyptian culture. Ancient Egypt was not the only society plagued by tuberculosis. There is also strong evidence that precolonial populations in North and South America had contended with tuberculosis. Similar archeological evidence was discovered in parts of North and South America, and perhaps not surprisingly, artistic depictions of gibbous deformities are found in pre-Columbian art not too dissimilar to that found in ancient Egypt. As something of a foreshadowing of the stigma attached to tuberculosis in ages to come, there is evidence among the writings of Spanish conquistadores that indicate the Aztecs preferentially selected people with hunchback deformities for human sacrifice[11].

During the classical period and the time of Hippocrates, the father of modern medicine, tuberculosis was very common in Greece, judging by the amount of writings dedicated to it. Hippocrates accurately described the age groups most afflicted by tuberculosis and many of the clinical presentations of disease. However, Greek physicians working in Alexandria and the outer reaches of the Roman Empire wrote very little of tuberculosis, suggesting, at the least, that other diagnoses seemed more important causes of illness and death.

Very little is known about tuberculosis between the fall of Rome and the Renaissance, but the one form of tuberculosis about which a fair amount was written was tuberculosis of the lymph nodes of the neck. Tuberculosis can infect virtually any organ of the body, and when it affects the lymph glands of the neck it is referred to as **scrofula**. These lymph glands enlarge and eventually ulcerate, leading to very unsightly open wounds on the infected person's neck that can extend to the face and chest. Scrofula became known as the King's Evil in medieval Europe because it was believed that, due to the divine right of kings, a monarch could touch those afflicted and miraculously heal them. Thousands would line up for the royal touch, and most certainly the waxing and waning of the disease's natural course convinced many of the afflicted of the divinity of their rulers[12]. Eventually, during the Renaissance, a vigorous debate arose as to the cause of tuberculosis. Was it hereditary? Was it caused by the environment? Was it infectious and spread from person to person? It was a debate that lasted centuries and engaged the brightest and some of the most famous minds in medicine. It was eventually solved in 1882 when **Robert Koch** reported that he had isolated the organism responsible for tuberculosis.

It would be over fifty years between Koch's discovery and the development of effective therapy for tuberculosis, but during this time science dealt seriously with the causes and potential solutions to the problem of TB. In 1900, French microbiologists **Albert Calmette** and **Camille Guerin**, inspired by the new science of microbiology pioneered by their fellow countryman Louis Pasteur, began to work on tuberculosis with the idea of developing a vaccine. During their work, they observed that when ox bile was added to the liquid media containing tubercle bacilli, the bacilli became less virulent; that is, they became **attenuated**. After more than twenty years of work, personal tragedy, and the disruption of their work by World War I, Calmette and Guerin were ready to try out their vaccine in humans after very encouraging results in cattle. Although Bacille Calmette Guerin, now known as BCG, never proved to be effective against adult forms of pulmonary tuberculosis, its impact on infantile forms of the disease were dramatic, resulting in huge drops in infant mortality in France.

PUBLIC HEALTH CONNECTIONS 13.2
LESSONS FROM HISTORY

Tuberculosis is frequently associated with the poor and marginalized segments of society, and with good reason: the vast majority of tuberculosis cases today occur among the poor. But when you look at history and who has contracted the disease, you quickly realize that TB can strike anyone. In fact, over the course of the recent centuries, some of the most famous and influential artists, writers, and politicians have been counted among the victims of the White Plague. Albert Camus wrote what is his most well-known work, *The Plague*, while dealing with the effects of untreated tuberculosis. The famous Bronte sisters all succumbed to the disease, all at an early age. George Orwell finished *1984* the year he was dying from tuberculosis. Orwell was among the first recipients of streptomycin, the first effective antibiotic for TB. His side effects were so bad that he was unable to continue its use and died from advanced tuberculosis. More recently, Eleanor Roosevelt, former first lady of the United States, died in 1961 from undiagnosed disseminated tuberculosis commonly referred to as miliary TB, despite the fact that she had access to the best medical care available. Tuberculosis can be a challenging and dangerous disease regardless of a person's social standing. Nelson Mandela, the anti-apartheid leader of South Africa, contracted TB while an inmate at Pollsmoor Prison in Cape Town, South Africa. Fortunately, Mr. Mandela was cured and has since become a powerful advocate for TB patients everywhere.

The era of effective medications for tuberculosis was ushered in by Selman Waksman and his colleagues as the world was embroiled in World War II. In 1943, a new compound was identified by Waksman from a soil organism known as *actinomycetes*. This compound killed or impaired the growth of other bacteria and was eventually tested on tuberculosis. After promising results in guinea pigs, the first people received the drug streptomycin with remarkable results. However, it became clear that the medications were hard to tolerate and that the drug did not always kill all of the organisms, resulting in persistent if not fatal disease. Streptomycin resistance developed in as little as a few months, and physicians realized that using multiple drugs at the same time was more effective. And so was born the era of effective medications, the so-called chemotherapy era of tuberculosis.

With a new and expanding regimen of medicines available to treat tuberculosis, the focus in the early 1950s shifted away from procedures and practices of questionable benefit such as **collapse therapy**, the practice of collapsing infected lungs by injecting air or other substances into the chest cavity, to evidence-based treatment with medicines of proven value. **Sanitaria**, large institutions where thousands of tuberculosis patients from across the country went to convalesce and undergo various unproven treatments, became hospitals focused on not only the isolation of patients with tuberculosis but also as places where patients could expect to be cured. The decline of tuberculosis in the United States and Western Europe continued through the early 1980s, and the disease became mostly an outpatient disease treated in the community.

In the early 1980s, public health's focus was moving increasingly away from infectious disease. In fact, most people thought that tuberculosis was soon to become a disease of the past. Programs were gradually eroded, and other public health infrastructure related to TB was dismantled. But the specter of the human immunodeficiency virus (HIV) epidemic was rising, and its impact would be devastating. HIV case rates soared in many cities, and along with them TB began to climb. The more than thirty-year trend of declining tuberculosis rates was reversing. Fortunately, after the development of effective therapy for HIV and an increase in funding for the public health infrastructure, TB case rates began to decline once again by the early 1990s. This ten-year resurgence gives us some very valuable lessons in public health preparedness and the role of public health in controlling tuberculosis and other diseases.

Epidemiology

In the United States, we frequently speak of the resurgence of tuberculosis that occurred in the 1980s, but in much of the developing world tuberculosis has never had a sustained period of decline. The developing world experienced an uninterrupted explosion in the number of TB cases over the latter half of the twentieth century and into the twenty-first century. There are many reasons for this, and there are important risk factors for developing tuberculosis, such as HIV infection and poverty (discussed in more detail below), which are more common in developing countries. It is interesting to point out, however, that the impact of effective medications to treat tuberculosis has had a modest impact on the overall course of the tuberculosis epidemic. Rates of tuberculosis were declining in the United States and Britain decades before the advent of effective therapy[13]. These trends have led many to believe that improving the economic conditions of populations is the most important intervention to reduce the impact of tuberculosis.

The scale of the tuberculosis epidemic is enormous. One-third of the world, or 2 billion people, harbor inactive or dormant tuberculosis (latent TB infection), making tuberculosis the most common infection in humans. Between 8 and 9 million new cases of active tuberculosis develop each year, and between 1.5 and 2 million people die of the disease annually[14]. Among people with HIV, tuberculosis is the single most important cause of death in developing countries. *M. tuberculosis* is the second most deadly microorganism behind the human immunodeficiency virus.

There is a significant difference in how tuberculosis is distributed around the world. As Figure 13.2 shows, Asia, Africa, and Latin America have the highest **incidence rates** (the number of new cases each year divided by the total population at risk) of the disease. To put things in perspective, the incidence of TB in North America is about 0.5 percent to 1 percent the incidence in the countries of sub-Saharan Africa most affected by tuberculosis. In 2008, fewer

Figure 13.2 Estimated Incidence of Tuberculosis by Country, 2007

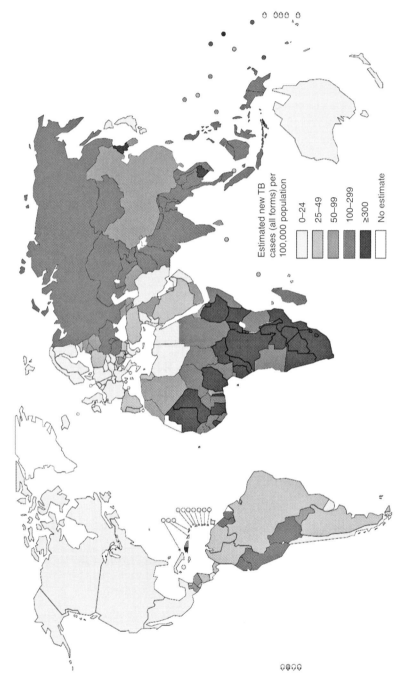

Estimated new TB
cases (all forms) per
100,000 population

- 0–24
- 25–49
- 50–99
- 100–299
- ≥300
- No estimate

Source: Reference 14. Used by permission of the World Health Organization.

than 13,000 of the estimated 9 million cases in the world occurred in the United States; 59 percent of these cases were diagnosed in people born outside of the United States[15]. In fact, 90 percent of cases and 95 percent of deaths from tuberculosis occur in the developing world.

Remember, infection with tuberculosis is different from disease from tuberculosis. When someone is infected with tuberculosis, it means that the germ is in the person's body. When there is evidence of tuberculosis infection, either by a blood test or by a positive skin test, and the person does not have any symptoms, no abnormalities on physical exam, and a clear chest X-ray, that person is said to have a latent tuberculosis infection. A primary risk factor for TB infection is being in contact with people with tuberculosis. This may occur in countries where the rates of tuberculosis are high; settings with a concentrated number of people from high-incidence countries; congregate care facilities such as prisons, refugee camps, or nursing homes; and health care facilities housing patients with tuberculosis or HIV. Although anyone may become infected with tuberculosis and subsequently develop active disease, there are a number of recognized risk factors for developing tuberculosis. Risk factors for developing tuberculosis are conditions or characteristics that reduce the body's ability to kill the organism or to contain the organism in a dormant or latent state.

PUBLIC HEALTH CONNECTIONS 13.3

RISK FACTORS FOR DEVELOPING TUBERCULOSIS DISEASE

Persons at high risk for developing TB disease fall into two categories:

1. People who have been recently infected
   - Close contact with person with infectious TB
   - Skin test converters (within past two years)
   - Recent immigrants from TB-endemic regions of the world (within five years of arrival to the United States)
   - Children five years or younger with a positive tuberculin skin test
   - Residents and employees of high-risk congregate settings (correctional facilities, homeless shelters, health care facilities)

2. People with clinical conditions that increase their risk of progressing from latent tuberculosis infection to TB disease
   - People with HIV infection
   - People with a history of untreated TB or fibrotic lesions on chest radiograph

- People who are underweight or malnourished
- People who use injection drugs
- People receiving TNF-α antagonists for rheumatoid arthritis or Crohn's disease
- People with certain medical conditions such as silicosis, diabetes mellitus, chronic renal failure, or head or neck cancer
- People who have had a solid organ transplant (such as heart or kidney)
- People who have had a gastrectomy or jejunoileal bypass

Source: Reference 16.

Of all the risk factors listed, the greatest impact comes from HIV. In all of history, nothing has changed the face of the tuberculosis epidemic like the arrival of HIV in the 1980s. HIV weakens the immune system by affecting cell-based immunity, the precise way that allows tuberculosis to progress from latent infection to full-blown active disease. HIV also changes the clinical presentation of tuberculosis, delaying the diagnosis and prolonging the time during which patients are infecting others.

There are a number of other factors that likely contribute to the development of tuberculosis that are not listed in Public Health Connections 13.3. Genetics no doubt play some role, but this has been difficult to characterize. Interesting studies in twins point to a genetic contribution to susceptibility to tuberculosis as do population studies that show tuberculosis rates varying between different populations around the world[17]. Stress is another factor that is difficult to characterize but likely plays a role. In a study looking at marriage status, married men had lower rates of tuberculosis, suggesting that increased social support decreases risk of the disease, other things being equal[18]. Poverty is perhaps the factor that historically has been the most closely associated with tuberculosis. However, poverty encompasses many known risk factors, such as poor nutrition, overcrowding, and overall lower health status, that all contribute to developing tuberculosis.

Prevention and Control

Hermann Biggs, a well-known leader in public health who was health commissioner for New York in the early twentieth century, once said, "Public health is purchasable. Within a few natural and important limitations, any community can determine its own health."[19] In Biggs's words, improved rates of tuberculosis were purchased when the resurgence of tuberculosis that occurred in the United States during the 1980s and early 1990s was reversed by an unprecedented infusion of funding. In the ten years from 1993 to 2003, tuberculosis rates in the United States dropped 44 percent, and in 2008 tuberculosis hit a historic low with 12,898 cases recorded[15].

There are four basic strategies to control tuberculosis in the United States. In order of priority they are as follows:

1. Prompt identification of cases and beginning effective therapy on active cases quickly

2. Protection of close contacts of active cases by screening for active disease and beginning preventive therapy as soon as possible

3. Treating latent tuberculosis infection first in those with highest risk for progressing to active disease and then in others who may be infected and represent potential future cases of tuberculosis

4. Implementing effective infection control practices to prevent the spread of tuberculosis in facilities such as hospitals, clinics, prisons, and anywhere else people at risk for tuberculosis may congregate

Perhaps the single most important step to prevent and control tuberculosis is directly observed therapy (DOT). As described earlier in this chapter, DOT occurs when a health care worker such as a nurse, outreach worker, or other non-family member working with public health authorities observes all the doses of tuberculosis medications prescribed to the patient. A well-functioning DOT program provides a number of benefits to the patients and tuberculosis control programs. DOT ensures that patients complete their prescribed regimens and become noninfectious rapidly, ensures that patients are cured in the shortest time possible, prevents drug resistance, and improves adherence to other aspects of care related to tuberculosis. DOT is the standard of care for tuberculosis the world over. A DOT program implies more than just observed therapy; the five elements of the DOT short-course strategy for tuberculosis control are as follows:

- Sustained government commitment to tuberculosis control

- Diagnosis based on quality-assured sputum-smear microscopy, mainly among symptomatic patients presenting to health services

- Standardized short-course chemotherapy for all cases of tuberculosis under proper case-management conditions, including direct observation of treatment

- Uninterrupted supply of quality-assured drugs

- Standardized recording and reporting system enabling program monitoring by systematic assessment of treatment outcomes of all patients registered

A DOT strategy that employs observed therapy as one element can be very effective in reaching the majority of infectious cases.

The World Health Organization (WHO) recommends a similar course of action for countries around the world. The biggest difference is the amount of resources available. Tuberculosis-control programs exist in every corner of the globe and use these same basic principles, but for the most part they are limited to identifying cases of tuberculosis and beginning effective therapy. Resources for protecting close contacts, treating those with latent infection, and conducting infection control in facilities with people at risk for tuberculosis are not available in many parts of the world where tuberculosis is common. In fact, even the first priority of promptly identifying cases is limited by the way that tuberculosis is diagnosed in most low-resource countries. In most programs around the world, the more sensitive and specific method of diagnosing tuberculosis by culture and susceptibility testing is not available, and programs must rely on smear micros-copy only, the technique in which the sputum is stained and reviewed under the microscope for the presence of organisms. Considering the limitations faced by many countries, a well-functioning program employing the DOT strategy can be effective, especially in areas with a low incidence of HIV infection. The WHO DOT strategy has a goal of detecting 70 percent of smear-positive cases (con-sidered the most infectious) and curing 85 percent of those cases[20]. The assump-tion is that this will control tuberculosis and reduce the incidence of drug resistance. In fact, there is some evidence of this. However, only about 40 percent of cases of active tuberculosis are detected by using the smear alone, and in areas of high HIV prevalence, DOT does not adequately reduce the incidence of tuberculosis[21]. In short, DOT alone is inadequate to control tuberculosis, but it is the best strategy available in most parts of the world.

In 2000, the Institute of Medicine (IOM) critically evaluated the prospects for the elimination of tuberculosis from the United States in its report, *Ending Neglect*, and concluded that until tuberculosis is controlled around the world, tuberculosis will remain a problem in the United States[22]. The report outlined the steps necessary to move toward eliminating tuberculosis in the United States. Among its most significant recommendations was the call for increased U.S. involvement in global efforts to control tuberculosis. This involvement has come in several forms, including direct assistance to countries with a high burden of tuberculosis and increased support for research efforts. The goal of the research is to develop new tools to fight tuberculosis, including faster and more effective diagnostic tools, new medicines that can shorten treatment regimens and treat drug-resistant disease, and finally, a vaccine that is more effective than BCG.

Current Public Health Challenges to Control Tuberculosis

A recent slogan for the WHO's efforts to raise global awareness of tuberculosis was "Until tuberculosis is controlled everywhere it is not controlled anywhere." This statement is more than just a slogan because it captures the truly global nature of this disease. As mentioned throughout this chapter, there is a great difference in tuberculosis rates around the world, but with our increasingly globalized society, public health challenges in the most remote corners of the world concern us all.

There are many challenges to control tuberculosis globally, and virtually all of them have significance, to one degree or another, in both high-incidence and low-incidence countries. Adequately training and maintaining capable public health and medical personnel, improving laboratory capabilities, especially in high-incidence countries, and maintaining political support are all specific challenges faced by control programs everywhere. But the two most important challenges that threaten TB control efforts, which have effects that go beyond the control of tuberculosis, are drug-resistant disease and infection with the human immunodeficiency virus.

Drug-Resistant Tuberculosis

Bacteria such as *M. tuberculosis* are said to be **resistant** when medications (antibiotics) used to kill the organism are not effective as expected. The germs can thrive in the presence of medications that would under normal circumstances kill or stop the bacteria from growing. Bacteria develop resistance in many ways, but *M. tuberculosis* develops resistance exclusively by specific mutations in certain genes. These mutations occur randomly and occur rarely, but predictably, under normal conditions in the laboratory or in individuals. The problem of resistance occurs when there is **selective pressure** and the very few organisms with the mutations that create resistance are selected. This selective pressure comes from either inappropriately administered medications or nonadherence to the prescribed treatment regimen.

So how does this work? Think about a patient with tuberculosis, and for argument's sake, let's say that he has a million organisms in his lungs that are making him sick. A random mutation in the gene responsible for resistance to isoniazid, one of the most important medications used to treat tuberculosis, occurs in one of those million organisms. If that patient is given isoniazid alone or decides to take only the isoniazid part of the treatment, all of the organisms that do not have the mutation will die, leaving only the one organism with the resistance mutation to survive. That single organism will then divide and grow and eventually replenish the already damaged lung with other organisms just like it, that is, resistant to isoniazid. This example is an oversimplification, but it serves to illustrate why and how resistance develops. The chances of random mutations occurring in the same organism giving resistance to different medications is highly unlikely and thus serves as the basis of multiple-drug therapy and DOT therapy. These random events are so uncommon naturally that without selective pressure, as described above, drug resistance as we know it would be unheard of. In short, drug-resistant tuberculosis is a completely human-caused phenomenon that would be virtually impossible without poorly administered therapy.

Although there are not as many effective medications to treat tuberculosis as there are for other infections, there are a number of drugs that are available to use in combination. These combinations are used to both shorten the regimen and to avoid developing resistance. In fact, most people with tuberculosis are treated without knowledge of whether or not there is drug resistance. Tests to determine if there is resistance, known as susceptibility or sensitivity tests, take time and are usually not available until after as much as two months after therapy is started. More importantly, however, is the fact that the majority of cases around the world are treated without access to a laboratory capable of doing susceptibility testing.

Resistance to tuberculosis medications generally progresses from initial single-drug resistance to increasing drug resistance with each episode of tuberculosis. This transition may occur in the initial individual in whom resistance developed or in his or her contacts who develop active disease. In general, the majority of simpler forms of single-drug-resistance tuberculosis respond well to the currently recommended four-drug regimens. The problems occur in cases that do not respond to therapy and go on to develop resistance to more than one drug. Of these cases, the most significant are those that develop resistance to isoniazid and rifampin, the two most effective drugs used to treat tuberculosis. A person can develop resistance to multiple drugs, but the term **multi-drug resistant** (MDR) is defined as resistance to isoniazid and rifampin with or without other drug resistance. MDR leads to much worse outcomes, with as many as 50 percent of people with MDR-TB dying. If susceptibility to isoniazid or rifampin is retained, failure of treatment, delayed responses with prolonged infectiousness, and death are much less common as compared to MDR. Worse yet is the more recently described **extremely drug-resistant** tuberculosis, or XDR-TB. This classification is defined as MDR with additional resistance to the two most important second-line tuberculosis drugs, quinolones and injectable drugs known as aminoglycosides. It is almost impossible to cure people with XDR-TB in low-resource countries, resulting in very high death rates. The first well-documented outbreak of XDR-TB that served as a global alarm to the danger posed by this form of the disease occurred in Tugela Ferry, South Africa. The outbreak was discovered among HIV-positive individuals at a health care facility and resulted in fifty-two of fifty-three patients dying from the disease, the majority within a few weeks of diagnosis and the start of therapy[23].

During the resurgence of tuberculosis in the 1990s, there were numerous outbreaks of drug-resistant tuberculosis in the United States. These cases occurred mostly in health care facilities and correctional institutions and served to highlight the price to be paid for less-than-adequate care of patients with tuberculosis[24]. Now, the focus of resistant tuberculosis is outside the United States and other high-resource countries. At the time of this writing, nearly half a million new cases of MDR occur annually around the world, constituting almost 5 percent of all new cases of tuberculosis worldwide. According to data from the WHO, of persons diagnosed with tuberculosis for the first time in 2008, 17 percent have resistance to at least one drug[25]. Among those with a previous history of tuberculosis treatment, the single most important risk factor for drug-resistant tuberculosis, 35 percent are resistant to at least one drug[25].

Infection with HIV

Nothing has changed the face of the tuberculosis epidemic more than coinfection with HIV. HIV attacks the immune system primarily by weakening and eventually destroying the immune system's cellular response to infections of various kinds. The immune response required to control tuberculosis is complicated, but the body's cellular immune response is the most critical part of a person's immune response to control tuberculosis. Without an adequate immune response, people exposed to and subsequently infected with tuberculosis develop overwhelming disease and frequently die from their infection. In fact, tuberculosis is the number one cause of death globally among people with HIV infection.

Not only is tuberculosis more common and aggressive in people with HIV, the disease itself is actually different in many ways. Much of what is seen as far as symptoms in patients with tuberculosis is the result of the body's immune reaction to the tuberculosis germ. Fevers, night sweats, and damage to the lungs or other sites of infection all occur as the body tries to rid itself of the tuberculosis germ. Clinicians, doctors, and nurses diagnosing tuberculosis are used to certain symptoms and X-ray results for TB, in reaction to which they order the appropriate tests, usually a sputum test. However, because many of the typical symptoms associated with tuberculosis are changed in the face of coinfection with HIV, clinicians will many times not suspect tuberculosis because the symptoms are unusual or the lung X-ray looks like a condition other than tuberculosis. The delays in diagnosis that occur as a result of the unusual presentation of tuberculosis in persons with HIV coinfection will lead to further spread of the tuberculosis, many times to other people with HIV.

Because the HIV epidemic is most widespread in areas of the world endemic for tuberculosis, rates of tuberculosis in some countries have skyrocketed. The burden of HIV-related tuberculosis has been so great in some areas, particularly sub-Saharan Africa, that other public health services are jeopardized because of the cost, both human and financial, associated with combating TB in the setting of widespread HIV coinfection. In fact, currently available strategies to control tuberculosis, such as DOT, are largely unable to reduce the numbers of TB cases in the setting of a widespread HIV epidemic.

The Future of Tuberculosis

Despite the many challenges outlined and discussed in this chapter, the future prospects for turning the tide against tuberculosis are better than ever. Prior to the global economic downturn in 2008, funding for global tuberculosis control reached unprecedented levels. Although the funding available for tuberculosis control remains woefully inadequate in many parts of the world, DOT, treatment for HIV, and new diagnostic tests are available to millions more every year.

One of the most active and promising areas of research is the development of new drugs to treat tuberculosis. As discussed earlier, treatment for tuberculosis usually requires between six to twelve months of a complicated regimen, and if there is any drug resistance, the duration of therapy may be extended up to two years. These regimens are burdensome for both patients and the programs administering the treatment. For this reason, new drugs are being sought. There are a number of potential new drugs to treat tuberculosis that are in the development pipeline, but remember that developing new drugs and new drug regimens is a costly and long process. It may take ten years or more to fully develop a new drug from the laboratory to the bedside (see chapter 7). That said, there are several new drugs that may lead to a significant shortening of the regimen down to two to four months, even in cases of resistant tuberculosis.

Another great area of need in which there have been significant advances in recent years is that of new diagnostic tests for tuberculosis. As outlined earlier, the gold standard for diagnosing tuberculosis has been the identification of the organism in cultures obtained from patients who are ill with symptoms consistent with tuberculosis. This process is long (taking up to eight weeks), costly, and requires highly trained personnel. Can new technology shorten the time for diagnosis without increasing the costs or need for expensive, highly trained staff that are out of reach for most low-resource countries? The answer appears to be yes. New diagnostic techniques that focus on identifying tuberculosis DNA and gene mutations leading to drug-resistant germs are finding their way to laboratories in some of the poorest countries. At the time of this writing, culture and susceptibility testing are still the gold standard for diagnosis, but the newer DNA-based tests promise to revolutionize the diagnosis of tuberculosis around the world.

The holy grail of new developments for tuberculosis would be the development of a new vaccine. No infectious disease has ever been conquered without a vaccine, and tuberculosis is unlikely to be any different in this regard. The BCG vaccine held a great deal of promise as the answer to tuberculosis in the 1920s, but it has never fully lived up to its promise. Despite being one of the safest vaccines in the world today, with billions of doses given worldwide throughout the twentieth century, its effectiveness is limited. It is most effective if given during infancy, and it seemingly protects infants from developing the most aggressive forms of tuberculosis in children: miliary tuberculosis and tuberculosis meningitis. Unfortunately, there is no conclusive proof that BCG protects older children or adults. A new vaccine would have to be as effective as the BCG vaccine in preventing tuberculosis in children, prevent tuberculosis in adults, be safe and inexpensive, and be able to be given to people with HIV. This is a tall order, but early results have been promising, and human studies of potential tuberculosis vaccines are underway. It is unclear what the outcome of these studies will be, but it is hoped that a new vaccine will be in use in the next ten to fifteen years.

Summary

Tuberculosis has been a major public health concern, causing illness and death among humans, since ancient times. Despite a shift in attention from infectious to chronic diseases during the twentieth century, tuberculosis has reminded us that infectious disease resurgence is possible when infrastructure weakens and new diseases appear. *M. tuberculosis*, the bacterium responsible for the disease, has unique properties, such as a slow generation time that makes diagnosis difficult, treatment arduous, and vaccination challenging. Nonetheless, the tuberculin skin test, sputum culture, chest X-ray, and DNA testing are all available to identify people with TB infection. Used together with clinical observation, it is possible to diagnose tuberculosis with considerable accuracy. Likewise, the four-drug treatment approach is effective in curing active TB if followed as prescribed. Direct observed therapy greatly increases the likelihood a TB patient will successfully complete his or her treatment regimen, reducing the likelihood of recurrence, transmission, drug resistance, and death. Since the advent of HIV, tuberculosis has surged and now presents challenges in both diagnosis and treatment that did not exist in the past. These new challenges often require additional resources, a requirement complicated by the fact that most of the world's HIV and TB cases occur in countries with limited resources. Because, as WHO noted, "until tuberculosis is controlled everywhere, it is not controlled anywhere," a global response to TB is necessary. New screening tools, drugs, and even a vaccine, along with increased financial and public health infrastructure support from all countries, show promise in stemming the tuberculosis epidemic.

Key Terms

acid fast, 322

attenuated, 330

BCG vaccine, 324

Calmette, Albert, 330

collapse therapy, 331

contact investigation, 328

directly observed therapy, 328

extrapulmonary disease, 325

extremely drug resistant, 340

gibbous deformity, 329

Guerin, Camille, 330

incidence rate, 332

infiltrate, 326

Koch, Robert, 330

latent tuberculosis infection, 323

miliary tuberculosis, 325

MTB complex, 323

multi-drug resistant, 339

Mycobacterium tuberculosis, 322

pulmonary tuberculosis, 325

resistant, 338

sanitarium, 331

scrofula, 329

selective pressure, 338

tuberculin skin test, 324

Review Questions

1. List and describe the various methods used to diagnose tuberculosis. What are the pros and cons of each method?
2. How does income or wealth impact tuberculosis at an individual level? At a societal level?

3. Describe how direct observed therapy (DOT) works and why it is an important public health measure in controlling tuberculosis.
4. In your own words, explain how a person's failure to follow a prescribed tuberculosis treatment regimen can lead to drug-resistant forms of the disease.
5. What steps can be taken by individuals, communities, and nations to reduce the incidence of tuberculosis?
6. Why is human immunodeficiency virus important in the spread and severity of tuberculosis?
7. What recent and current developments are likely to reduce the incidence and impact of tuberculosis?

References

1. Maher DR, Raviglione M. Global epidemiology of tuberculosis. *Clin Chest Med.* 2009;26:167–182.
2. Lawn SD, Harries AD, Anglaret X, Myer L, Wood R. (2008). Early mortality among adults accessing antiretroviral treatment programmes in sub-Saharan Africa. *AIDS.* 2008;320:1897–1908.
3. Selwyn P, Hartel D, Lewis VA, et al. A prospective study of the risk of tuberculosis among intravenous drug users with human immunodeficiency virus infection. *New Engl J Med.* 1989: 320(9):545–550.
4. Rieder H, Snider D, Cauthen G. (1990). Extrapulmonary tuberculosis in the United States. *Am Rev Respir Dis.* 1990; 141(2):347–351.
5. Pfyffer G, Brown-Elliott BA, Wallace RJ Jr. Mycobacterium: General characteristics, isolation, and staining procedures. In: Murray PR, Baron EJ, Jorgenson JH, Pfaller MA, Yolken RH, eds. *Manual of Clinical Microbiology*. 8th ed. Washington, D.C.: ASM Press; 2003:532–559.
6. Comstock G. (1999). How much isoniazid is needed for prevention of tuberculosis among immunocompetent adults? *Int J Tuberc Lung Dis.* 1999; 3(10):847–850.
7. The Committee on Bible Translation. *The Holy Bible*, New International Version. East Brunswick, N.J.: International Bible Society; 1983.
8. Bunyan J. *The Life and Death of Mr. Badman*. London: Nicholson; 1808.
9. Morse D, Brothwell D, Ucko PJ. Tuberculosis in ancient Egypt. *Amer Rev Respir Dis.* 1964; 90:524–541.
10. Daniel T. *Captain of Death*. Rochester, N.Y.: University of Rochester Press; 1997.
11. Thomas H. *Montezuma, Cortes, and the Fall of Old Mexico*. New York: Simon and Schuster; 1993.
12. Garrison F. *An Introduction to the History of Medicine*. Philadelphia: WB Saunders; 1929.
13. Enarson D, Chaing C.-Y., Murray J. Global epidemiology of tuberculosis. In: Rom W, Garay S, eds. *Tuberculosis*. Philadelphia, Pa. Lippincott, Williams and Wilkins; 2004:13–30.

14. World Health Organization. *Global Tuberculosis Control 2009: Epidemiology, Strategy, Financing.* Geneva, Switzerland: World Health Organization; 2009.

15. Centers for Disease Control and Prevention. Trends in tuberculosis United States 2008. *MMWR.* 2009; 58(10):249–253.

16. Centers for Disease Control and Prevention. Tuberculosis Web page. Targeted tuberculin testing and treatment of latent tuberculosis infection, 2005. Available at: www.cdc.gov/tb/publications/slidesets/LTBI/default.htm. Accessed February 16, 2010.

17. Bellamy R. Genetic susceptibility to tuberculosis in human populations. *Thorax.* 1998; 53(7):588–593.

18. Lienhardt C, Fielding K, Sillah J, et al. Investigation of the risk factors for tuberculosis: A case-control study in three countries in West Africa. *Int J Epidemiol.* 2005; 34(4):914–923.

19. Dormandy T. *The White Death, a History of Tuberculosis.* London: Hambledon and London; 1999.

20. World Health Organization. Tuberculosis Web page. The stop TB strategy. Available at: www.who.int/tb/strategy/en/. Accessed January 14, 2010.

21. De Cock K, Chaisson R. (1999). Will DOTS do it? A reappraisal of tuberculosis control in countries with high rates of HIV infection. *Int J Tuberc Lung Dis.* 1999; 3(6):457–465.

22. Institute of Medicine. *Ending Neglect.* Washington, D.C.: National Academy Press; 2000.

23. Gandhi N, Moll A, Sturm AW, et al. Extensively drug-resistant tuberculosis as a cause of death in patients co-infected with tuberculosis and HIV in a rural area of South Africa. *Lancet.* 2006;368:1575–1580.

24. Centers for Disease Control and Prevention. Nosocomial transmission of multi-drug resistant tuberculosis among HIV infected persons—Florida and New York 1988–1991. *MMWR.* 1991; 40(34):585–591.

25. Wright A, Zignol M, Van Deun A, et al. Epidemiology of antituberculosis drug resistance 2002–07: An updated analysis of the Global Project on Anti-Tuberculosis Drug Resistance Surveillance. *Lancet.* 2009; 373(9678):1861–1873.

HEALTH SERVICES AND SOCIAL DETERMINANTS

CHAPTER 14

HEALTH POLICY AND THE U.S. HEALTH CARE SYSTEM

Lori Bilello, MBA, MHS

LEARNING OBJECTIVES

- Understand the development and the financing of the U.S. health care system.
- Describe the history of the development of the U.S. health care system and the key forces that shaped its development into a system that is unlike any other industrialized nation in the world.
- Identify the major funding sources and reimbursement mechanisms for health care services.
- Understand the role of health policy and the process of health policy development.
- Describe major health reform initiatives, both on the national level and state level.

This chapter provides an overview of the development of the U.S. health care system and how U.S. health policy has shaped the financing and delivery of health care services across the country. The United States has a unique health care system that has emerged from a historical perspective of individual responsibility, provider autonomy, and market-based principles in the financing and delivery of health care. Health care is the largest service industry in the country. It includes medical practices, managed care and insurance corporations, hospitals, nursing homes, and many other specialized care providers and facilities operating either on a for-profit or nonprofit basis. The United States has the costliest health care delivery system in the world but ranks low among industrialized nations in life expectancy, infant mortality, and other health outcomes.

Many attempts have been made to restructure the U.S. health system in order to contain costs, improve access to care for those who are uninsured or underinsured, and to improve health outcomes. With numerous powerful **stakeholders** (interested groups and organizations) in the political process, only incremental changes on how health care services are financed and delivered in this country have been possible. The result has added even more complexity and fragmentation to the health care delivery system. This chapter will provide a brief overview of the history of the health care system, the financing of health care, and the attempts to reform the system in the United States.

U.S. Health Care System

The U.S. health system is a very complex, fragmented, and decentralized health care delivery model that has rapidly evolved during the last century as the largest service sector of the U.S. economy. In fact, the term *system* implies some unifying plan or systematic approach, and the history of health care in the United States demonstrates few cohesive planning processes. Unlike the health care systems of most industrialized nations, the United States does not have a centrally controlled universal health care system that has authority over the financing and delivery of health care to all its residents. A broad definition of **universal health care** is health care coverage for all citizens and other eligible residents in a country or governmental region that provides, at a minimum, basic health care services such as primary care and hospital services. The U.S. health system has a variety of payment and financing structures, both private and public, as well as delivery mechanisms that have little integration or coordination. **Private financing** means that health care services are paid by private health insurance companies or individuals, and **public financing** means that health care services are paid for by local, state, or federal government sources such as Medicare or Medicaid. These financing and delivery mechanisms result in a health care system that varies widely in cost, quality, and access. To get a better understanding of how the U.S. health care system is structured, we need to review the historical foundation upon which it is built.

History of the U.S. Health Care System

In colonial times in the United States, women generally provided health care services using homemade remedies. Most health care practitioners at the time were self-taught or learned their trade through an apprenticeship, especially **midwives** (women who attended and assisted births), **apothecaries** (who concocted and dispensed curative remedies), and surgeons. In 1765, the University of Pennsylvania opened the first medical school in the colonies. By 1850, there were forty-two medical schools in the United States[1, p. 42]. Medicine was still largely provided at the home during the 1800s, with physicians making house calls and midwives delivering babies in homes. However, as the nation rapidly industrialized in the mid- to late 1800s, more urban areas saw the growth of physicians' offices and hospitals as places to receive care.

The early years of formalized health care in the United States (1880–1930) saw the establishment of the medical profession, both through the expanded duties and formal education of the physician and the growth of hospitals. The rapid growth of the medical profession was accompanied by an increasing need to standardize care through the licensure of physicians and accreditation of medical schools. The **American Medical Association** (AMA), which was founded in 1847, played a major role in pushing legislation through the states for licensure of physicians and founded the Council on Medical Education, which accredited medical schools[2, p. 52]. Their goal was to legitimize and organize the medical profession. Other health care practitioners followed a similar path, including the nursing profession, which formed the American Nursing Association in 1896.

Prior to the Civil War, hospitals were mainly for the mentally ill or those who were destitute and did not have families to care for them. Following the Civil War, the number of hospitals grew from around one hundred in 1870 to more than six thousand by 1920[3, p. 73]. The Civil War brought advances in medicine and sanitary practices in military hospitals, and these practices were adopted by private hospitals. For the most part, hospitals during this period were philanthropic institutions and were sponsored by churches and other humanitarian groups or municipal governments. After World War II, there was a dramatic growth in hospitals, in large part due to the passage of the **Hill-Burton Act** in 1947, which provided funding for hospital and other health care facility construction. In the twenty-five years after its enactment, the Hill-Burton program was responsible for adding over 396,000 short-term and long-term hospital beds, 37,000 nursing home beds, and over 1,000 outpatient facilities in the United States[4].

As the population shifted from rural areas to urban centers, families lived in smaller homes with less room to care for sick family members, and more family members worked outside the home[1, p. 74]. With the decrease in the reliance on family to care for the sick and the rapid advances in medicine during the early 1900s, there was greater acceptance of visiting physicians' offices and hospitals for medical care and treatment. The increased use of physicians and hospitals also increased the cost burden on individuals in need of health care. In 1927, the Committee on the Costs of Medical Care (CCMC) was formed to investigate the medical expenses of American families. The CCMC published twenty-seven research reports, offering reliable estimates of national health care expenditures. According to one CCMC study, the average American family had medical expenses totaling $108 in 1929, with hospital expenditures composing 14 percent of the total bill[5, p. 89].

The Great Depression slowed the expansion of health care facilities and trained personnel, and many Americans had trouble paying for the medical care they needed. Doctors tried to make allowances for patients in financial straits, but hospitals, with higher fixed costs, had much less flexibility. Between 1929 and 1930, average hospital receipts plummeted from more than $200 per patient to less than $60[6]. As the demand for hospital care increased, a new payment innovation was developed in 1929: the **prepaid hospital services plan**. The primary purpose of these plans was not to protect consumers from large, unforeseen expenses, but to provide a regular source of income for hospitals, especially during those difficult economic times. The first plan was introduced at Baylor University Hospital in Dallas, Texas, when a group of fifteen hundred school teachers contracted with the hospital to provide twenty-one days of hospital care for $6 per person[1 p. 295]. Other hospitals followed suit, and eventually groups of nonprofit hospitals in several cities organized multiple prepaid hospital plans. These multiple hospital plans served as a model for the development of **Blue Cross**, which, under the auspices of the American Hospital Association, spearheaded the proliferation of these nonprofit medical plans. Even though the American Medical Association was opposed to health insurance because it reduced their authority over the health care delivery system, the first **Blue Shield** plan was formed in 1939 by the California Medical Association to help pay for physician fees. Blue Cross plans paid only for hospital services.

The rapid success of the Blue Cross/Blue Shield plans persuaded **commercial insurers** (companies that sold life and casualty insurance), who initially considered insuring health care as a losing proposition, to enter the market. By 1940, commercial insurers had about 3.7 million subscribers, and the Blue Cross/Blue Shield plans had more than 6 million subscribers[7, p. 548]. Private health insurance continued to grow in popularity and is now the predominant form of financing health care services today.

Major Initiatives in the Financing and Structure of U.S. Health Care

The health care industry is one of the largest and fastest growing sectors in the U.S. economy. In the past three decades, the total national spending on health care has more than doubled to 16.6 percent of the nation's gross domestic product (GDP). According to the **U.S. Department of Health and Human Services** (HHS), the arm of the federal government with primary responsibility for health care, total health expenditures in the United States are expected to reach $2.4 trillion in 2008: this translates to spending $7,800 per person for health care services[8] (Figure 14.1).

Figure 14.1 The Growth in Health Expenditures in the United States

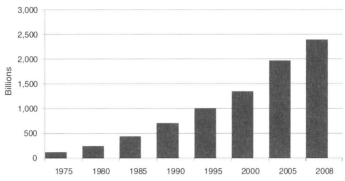

Data from CMS, National Health Statistics Group.

Of the $2.2 trillion spent on health care in 2007, private expenditures totaled $1.2 trillion, or 53.8 percent of all health spending[8]. The breakdown of private expenditures includes services paid by private health insurance at 34.6 percent, **out-of-pocket** (personal individual) payments at 12 percent, and payments by other private sources at 7.2 percent. Government sources accounted for the remaining 46.2 percent of spending, or $1 trillion, through programs such as Medicaid, Medicare, and the State Children's Health Insurance Program (CHIP), as well as health services for military service families and veterans. As the largest single payer of health care services in the country, the U.S. government is increasingly using its influence to affect how health care services are financed and delivered in the United States.

Government Programs

Before 1965, **employer-based health insurance** coverage provided through, and often paid in part by, an employer was the main source of third-party payment for health care services for most American families. Third-party payers include health insurance companies, health maintenance organizations, and other companies that receive premiums from employers or individuals to cover health care expenses. The elderly, the poor, and the unemployed had limited access to health care and relied on charity or their own personal finances to pay for care. As the cost of health care services rose, the **barriers to care**, or factors that limit a person's access to or use of health services, for these vulnerable populations increased. This led to a public debate on how to provide access to health care for these individuals, especially the elderly. After much debate in the 1950s and 1960s and strong opposition by the AMA and other health provider organizations, Congress passed Title XVIII of the Social Security Amendment

Table 14.1 Key Elements of Medicare and Medicaid

Program Features	Medicare	Medicaid
Covered population	Individuals at least 65 years old and certain disabled groups	Low-income pregnant women, children, and families, and certain disabled groups
Eligibility	No income eligibility criteria	Income eligibility criteria established by states
Administration	Federal government	Administered by states
Financing	Federal payroll tax and enrollee premiums	State funds with matching funds from the federal government; formula varies by state
Benefits	Part A: Hospitalization and short-term nursing home care Part B: Physician and outpatient services Part D: Prescription drugs	Comprehensive program: Benefits vary by state but must include hospitalization, physician services, outpatient services, prescription drugs, and nursing home care

Source: Reference 9.

of 1965 to create **Medicare**, a publicly financed health insurance program for Americans age sixty-five and older regardless of their income. They also passed Title XIX of the Social Security Amendment of 1965, which provided assistance to states to cover the eligible poor through a new program called **Medicaid**. Table 14.1 provides an overview of the key elements of Medicare and Medicaid[9].

The Department of Health and Human Services estimated that over 100 million individuals received health care coverage from the Medicaid and Medicare programs in 2008[8]. Approximately one-third of the U.S. population is receiving some portion of their health care through these government programs.

Since the creation of Medicare and Medicaid, no other major federal health care coverage initiative was enacted until 1997, when the legislation that created the State **Children's Health Insurance Program**, currently known as CHIP, was passed. This program was created through federal legislation under Title XXI of the Social Security Act for the purpose of covering children whose families make too much money to qualify for Medicaid but too little to purchase private health insurance. Within federal guidelines, each state determines the design of its individual CHIP program, including eligibility requirements, benefit packages, payment levels for coverage, and administrative procedures. In some states, the CHIP is part of the state's Medicaid program; in other states it is a separate program; and in many states, it is a combination of both. Most states offer CHIP coverage to children whose families' income is at or below 200 percent of the federal poverty level; however, it can vary from state to state. For example, a family of four would qualify if their family income were less than $44,100 (200 percent of 2009 federal poverty level). In 2008, the Department of Health and Human Services reported that over 7 million children received health care services from this program[10].

Evolution of Managed Care

Private health insurance, either through an employer or purchased individually, is a primary source of payment for health care services for those under sixty-five years of age. **Health insurance** provides a mechanism for shifting the risk from an individual to a group by pooling resources, and all members of the insured group share actual losses. Since the concept of health insurance took hold in the United States in the 1930s, it has grown into a major industry with significant influence in the way health care is delivered today. Private health insurance includes many different forms, including indemnity or conventional insurance, managed care plans, and self-insured employer plans.

Indemnity or **conventional insurance** is traditionally an insurance plan that pays a portion of the health care costs after a deductible is met. A **deductible** is the portion that an insured individual must pay first before the insurance company will begin to pay for services. Indemnity plans cover care provided by any providers and hospitals and requires filing a claim, either by the provider or the patient, to receive reimbursement for care provided. **Managed care plans** emerged in the 1980s as a predominant form of insurance in response to the rapid increase in health care costs in the 1970s and 1980s. In 2008, 90 percent of employer-based health insurance was some form of managed care (Figure 14.2).

Managed care organizations such as **health maintenance organizations (HMOs)** and **preferred provider organizations (PPOs)**, differ from conventional health insurance by using a contracted network of providers to deliver care to their enrollees and incorporate processes for the management of patients. The managed care plans negotiate reduced payment rates with providers in order to control costs. HMOs typically have tighter controls than do PPOs on how enrollees access care, including assignment to a **primary care provider (PCP)** and requiring referrals from the PCP for specialty care. HMOs typically pay providers through either a capitation arrangement or discounted fees (lower amount than the provider typically charges for their services). Under **capitation**, an enrollee is assigned to a provider, and the provider receives a fixed payment per member per month to provide an array of services to that member. Capitation shifts financial risk to providers, who are obligated to

Figure 14.2 Managed Care Versus Conventional Insurance in Employer-Sponsored Health Plans, United States 1988–2008

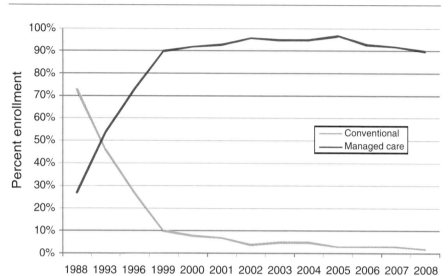

Source: Reference 11.

provide the necessary services no matter how much health care services the member consumes. Capitation incentivizes providers to actively manage the care of their assigned members. PPOs are more loosely organized than HMOs and have different levels of cost sharing with enrollees if they want to be seen by providers outside their health plan's contracted network.

HMOs gained prominence in the 1970s and 1980s due to the concerns about rising health care costs and favorable legislation that passed in 1973. The **Health Maintenance Act of 1973** provided start-up funds to establish new HMOs and added employer mandates to offer HMOs as an option if available in their community. As the HMO market matured and the backlash against HMOs became more vocal, HMO membership declined while PPO membership grew and new forms of managed care arrangements were developed. **Point-of-service (POS) plans** are a hybrid of HMO and PPO plans that have become popular in the twenty-first century. Like an HMO, POS plans have a network of providers and require members to be assigned to a primary care physician. Similar to a PPO, POS plans also offer limited coverage to members who choose to go out of network for medical care. However, out-of-network services require a deductible as well as a higher **copayment** (portion that the individual has to pay out of pocket) than in-network services.

Since the 1970s, many large employers have chosen **self insurance** and pay for their employees' health benefits directly instead of offering commercial health insurance. A major stimulus to the development of self-insurance programs was the passing of the **Employee Retirement and Income Security Act of 1974** (ERISA), which exempted employers from minimum benefit mandates under state law[12]. ERISA provided the advantage for employers to design benefit packages tailored to their employee population and theoretically allowed employers to have more control over benefit costs. Employers with self-insurance plans usually contract with another company to process claims and manage enrollment and other day-to-day operations of health benefits for their employees.

As a way to control costs and engage consumers in decisions about their health care spending, consumer-driven health plans have become a popular alternative in providing health care coverage since the creation of the **health savings account (HSA)** by the Medicare Prescription Drug, Improvement and Modernization Act of 2003. An HSA is a medical savings account that is paired with a high-deductible health plan and is used to pay for health care expenses until the high deductible is met. Individuals or their employers can make contributions to the HSA. Funds contributed to the HSA account are not subject to federal income tax at the time of deposit. In addition, any earnings on the funds accrue tax free and are not subject to tax or penalty as long as they are withdrawn to cover medical costs[13]. Proponents of HSAs believe that they will encourage more cost-conscious spending by placing more of the health care financing burden on out-of-pocket spending by the users of services, as opposed to having services incorporated in the **premium** (fixed periodic cost) component of insurance coverage, which is shared equally across all enrollees regardless of service use[14].

As policy makers continue to struggle with the high cost of health care and rising numbers of uninsured, new methods of financing and delivering health care services will continue to surface until a comprehensive health care reform strategy is adopted.

Health Policy and the Regulatory Process

Health policy and government regulation are essential to improve access to care, control costs, and provide consistent, if not high-quality, care. Health policy is a subset of public social policy, which tries to address social issues that affect human welfare, such as improving education or reducing poverty. Health policy and health regulation can be found throughout our society and our environment:

construction standards, air- and water-quality standards, food and drug standards, health professional and facility regulations, and much more. It is important for health professionals and the American public to understand how health policy works and how it affects their daily lives.

What is health policy? In the broadest sense, Beaufort Longest defines **health policy** as authoritative decisions made in the legislative, executive, or judicial branches of government that are intended to direct or influence the actions, behaviors, or decisions of others regarding health or the pursuit of health[15]. This can be at the federal, state, or local levels (see Chapter 2 for details on levels of public health). The legislative branch passes laws, provides funding, and oversees the implementation of laws. The chief executive official (the president in the federal government and the governor in the state government) sets the agenda, works closely with the legislative branch in the formulation of laws, and oversees the governmental departments that implement laws. The judicial branch determines the constitutionality of law, prosecutes violators of the law, and protects the rights of citizens. The policy-making process in the United States is a complex and dynamic process and is influenced by many groups and individuals. These groups include legislators, bureaucrats, media, social activists, and interest groups such as trade associations, all of whom may have competing interests on any specific subject matter. The policy-making process is cyclical in nature; even after legislation is passed, its impact is evaluated and oftentimes modified through additional legislation, court rulings, or regulation.

There are three major phases in policy making. The first phase is **policy formation**, which involves identifying a problem, setting a policy agenda, and developing legislation[15, p. 120]. This phase is highly dynamic and involves input and negotiation by all of the interested parties. Oftentimes, there is little resemblance to what was initially proposed compared to that which is actually passed by legislation. The second phase is **policy implementation** and involves the development of rules and regulations to guide the implementation and operationalization of the policy[15, p. 121]. The third phase is **policy modification**, which evaluates the consequences of legislation to see if it meets the original intent, or if circumstances change, what modifications are needed to more effectively address the problem. For example, the Medicare Prescription Drug, Improvement and Modernization Act of 2003 brought about major modifications to the Medicare program by adding a pharmacy benefit component that was not in the original legislation. Table 14.2 outlines some of the competing interests relevant to the policy decision to expand Medicare coverage to include a prescription drug benefit.

Federal health policy sets the national health agenda and priorities, which are implemented through the Department of Health and Human Services

Table 14.2 Competing Interests in the Health Policy Process

Example: How would different interest groups react to the expansion of the Medicare program to include a drug benefit component (Medicare Part D)?

Interest Group	Oppose or Favor	Why?
Taxpayers	Oppose	Increase tax burden and/or increase government deficits
Medicare patients	Favor	More comprehensive coverage and less out-of-pocket costs
Pharmaceutical industry	Favor	Increase in demand of pharmaceuticals when patients do not have to pay out of pocket

(HHS). HHS includes the Center for Disease Control and Prevention (CDC), the Food and Drug Administration (FDA), the National Institutes of Health (NIH), and the Center for Medicare & Medicaid Services (CMS), which provides the majority of funding for public health programs such as Medicare, Medicaid, and CHIP. Other federal departments also play a key role in providing health services, such as the Department of Veteran Affairs and the Department of Defense, and overseeing safety standards, such as the Department of Agriculture and the Department of Labor.

The state government's role in health policy and regulation include licensing and providing quality assurance oversight of health facilities and health professionals, regulating health insurance companies, ensuring public health and safety through environmental protection and public health infrastructure, and implementing programs for the poor and chronically ill (Medicaid, CHIP). State health policy and regulations vary from state to state to meet the needs of their constituents and oftentimes have more flexibility than the federal government to develop innovative approaches in organizing and delivering health services funded by the state. For instance, some states have a county health department system that provides a wide variety of primary and obstetrical care, and other states may provide only preventive services through their health departments, depending on the needs of their state's population.

Future Direction of the U.S. Health Care System

The U.S. health care system has been evolving over two hundred years and has seen great advances in medical care and health care technology. However, increasing fragmentation, lack of access and health care coverage for many

Americans, and high costs have led to a health care system in need of a major overhaul. The cost of the U.S. health system is unsustainable for the country's economy and is projected by the HHS to consume 20.3 percent of the GDP by 2018[8]. In 2008, the U.S. Census estimated that 46 million Americans are uninsured: almost one in six Americans do not have health insurance. Those in favor of government-guaranteed universal health care argue that the large number of uninsured Americans creates direct and hidden costs shared by all citizens in the form of higher costs of hospital-based care and increased insurance premiums and that extending coverage to all would lower costs and improve quality. In addition, uninsured people often clog emergency rooms. Health insurance could help them get the preventive and primary care to treat their conditions before they required urgent care. Yet emergency room visits are not entirely free to other insured users. Congress has undertaken serious health reform discussions since the passage of Medicare and Medicaid in the 1960s, but due to the many entrenched groups protecting their interests, only incremental changes have occurred.

National Health Care Reform Efforts

The United States is the only wealthy, industrialized nation that does not have universal health care or national health insurance. These programs vary from country to country with regard to their structure, covered services, and financing mechanisms. In the 1880s, Germany was the first country to develop a national health insurance program, and by the 1920s, most of the European industrialized countries, as well as Japan, had some form of national health care coverage[16, pp. 233–234]. Initiatives to try to legislate a national health insurance program in the United States began in the early 1900s with draft legislation proposed by the American Association of Labor Legislation (AALL) in 1915 for compulsory health insurance. The AMA and other powerful interest groups have strongly opposed legislation to provide universal health care coverage. Opposition is mainly focused on the impact of health reform on the private sector, the cost of a national health insurance program, and the effect of a national program on individual choice.

Prior to the Obama administration effort beginning in 2009, the most recent attempt to have a national dialogue on health care reform occurred during the Clinton administration. In 1993, President Clinton introduced the Health Security Act, which had five basic tenets: guaranteed private insurance for everyone, choice of physicians and health plans, elimination of unfair insurance practices, preservation of Medicare, and health benefits guaranteed through the worksite[17]. Even though the general public and previous administrations have supported these basic tenets, the downfall of the Health Security Act was in the details and the way it was developed. Closed door deliberations by the Task Force on National Health Reform led by First Lady Hilary Clinton brought on litigation by interest groups and opposition by the Republicans, health insurance industry, and the business community. Eventually, the lack of support from the major interest groups and some Democrats led to the plan's failure in 1994.

President Barack Obama campaigned on a platform that identified health care reform as one of the key issues his administration would tackle in order to improve access, quality, and health outcomes for Americans.

The landmark health care reform legislation, called the Patient Protection and Affordable Care Act (PPACA), was passed by Congress and signed into law by President Barack Obama on March 23, 2010. It is expected that this act will expand health care coverage to 32 million currently uninsured Americans through a combination of cost controls, subsidies, and mandates. This legislation[18]

- bars insurance companies from discriminating based on preexisting conditions, health status, and gender;

- creates health insurance exchanges, which are competitive marketplaces where individuals and small business can buy affordable health care coverage;

- offers insurance premium tax credits and cost-sharing assistance to low- and middle-income Americans;

- expands eligibility for Medicaid to include all nonelderly Americans with income below 133 percent of the Federal Poverty Level (FPL);

- encourages reimbursing health care providers on a value-based purchasing system instead of a fee-for-service system;

- tightens current health tax incentives, collects industry fees, institutes excise taxes, and increases the Medicare Hospital Insurance (HI) tax for individuals who earn more than $200,000 and couples who earn more than $250,000; and

- includes a fee on insurance companies that sell high-cost health insurance plans.

State Reform Initiatives

States have more flexibility than the federal government to develop health policy and programs and serve as the nation's testing ground for innovations in financing, coverage, regulation, and health care delivery. With the problem of the uninsured continuing to grow, states have taken the lead in developing proposals to reform their health care systems with the goal of significantly increasing the number of people with health care coverage. Three states, Maine, Massachusetts, and Vermont, have enacted and are implementing reform plans that seek to achieve near universal coverage of state residents whereas many other states are moving toward comprehensive reform[19]. The Massachusetts plan is the most well-known due to its aggressive implementation and the state's visibility in the national political arena. Massachusetts passed a health care reform law in 2006 that included the following key components:

- *The Commonwealth Care* program, which provides subsidized coverage for individuals with incomes up to 300 percent of the federal poverty level

- *The Commonwealth Health Insurance Connector* to connect individuals to insurance by offering affordable, quality insurance products

- Expansion of the Medicaid program to include children up to 300 percent of the federal poverty level

- An individual mandate that required all adults in the state to purchase health insurance by December 31, 2007

- A requirement that employers with eleven or more employees provide health insurance coverage or pay a fair-share contribution of up to $295 annually per employee.

Reducing the number of uninsured in Massachusetts has been successful with the implementation of the health care plan described above. An estimate by the Massachusetts Division of Health Care Finance and Policy showed that only 2.7 percent of Massachusetts residents were uninsured as of the spring, 2009, compared to the pre-reform level of 6.4 percent in 2006[20]. Criticisms of the Massachusetts plan include the high cost to the state for the expansion in Medicaid coverage and subsidies paid to help cover low-income individuals. The independent Massachusetts Taxpayers' Association estimated that between fiscal years 2006 and 2010, the annual incremental cost of health care reform to the state was less than $100 million (less than 0.4 percent of the state budget)[21].

Many state initiatives to improve access focus on insurance market reform, especially for small employers. Most health insurance policies for small groups or individuals are very expensive because the risk is spread among a small number of people. Many states waived mandates for specific covered services to reduce premiums or fostered cooperative purchasing pools for employers of small-sized companies to spread risk. Even with these mechanisms in place, many small business employers or employees have difficulty paying the premiums, which average $4,704 for individuals and $12,680 annually for family coverage[11]. Although voluntary efforts have resulted in limited success in improving health insurance coverage, some states, such as Massachusetts, have mandated that employers provide health insurance or pay a tax to support state-sponsored health coverage.

Some states have focused their health care reform efforts on Medicaid and the CHIP. By expanding income limits for participation, especially for pregnant women and children, these programs have been able to cover almost 60 million low-income individuals, including children and families, people with disabilities, and the elderly who are also covered by Medicare[22]. Other Medicaid reform efforts include enrolling beneficiaries into managed care plans and/or assigning them to a medical home. For example, North Carolina has implemented a medical home model of care in its Medicaid program called Community Care of North Carolina (CCNC). This program links the Medicaid beneficiary to a primary care provider who serves as a **medical home** that provides acute and preventive care, manages chronic illnesses, coordinates specialty care, and provides around-the-clock on-call assistance. The North Carolina program also incorporates care coordination, disease and care management, and quality improvement features to enhance the quality of care. Evaluations of the program have shown that it has resulted in both improved care and cost savings.

Summary

Over the last one hundred years, health care services in the United States have evolved from a small, primarily home-based cottage industry to an industry that is now the largest service sector in the country's economy. As health care services became unaffordable for the average citizen in the early 1900s, other means to finance health care were explored that led to the creation of a whole new industry, employer-based private health insurance. Even with the availability of private health insurance, many of the elderly, the poor, and the unemployed had limited access to health care. Public programs such as Medicare and Medicaid were created in 1965 to meet this need.

The rapidly changing landscape of the U.S. health system, especially in the last forty years, has led to great innovation in treatment and technology but at a significant price. As the per capita cost for health care continues to rise, new methods for delivering health services were developed to try to manage the care provided. Beginning with HMOs in the 1970s, many forms of managed care have evolved in an attempt to control costs and better organize the delivery of care. Today, managed care represents over 90 percent of the private employer-based insurance market.

Even with the growth of managed care and public programs such as Medicare and Medicaid, almost 50 million Americans do not have health care coverage. The high cost of care and the high numbers of uninsured have brought health care reform into the forefront of the political arena. Many states have attempted to reduce the numbers of uninsured through innovative programs and expansion of public programs but have seen only modest improvements. Health care reform will need to be implemented on a national basis in order to see a significant impact on the number of uninsured in the United States.

Key Terms

American Medical Association, 351

apothecaries, 350

barriers to care, 353

Blue Cross, 352

Blue Shield, 352

capitation, 355

Children's Health Insurance Program, 354

commercial insurer, 352

conventional insurance, 355

copayment, 356

deductible, 355

Department of Health and Human Services, 352

Employee Retirement and Income Security Act of 1974, 357

employer based health insurance, 353

health insurance, 355

Health Maintenance Act of 1973, 356

health maintenance organization (HMO), 355

health policy, 358

health savings account (HSA), 357

Hill-Burton Act, 351

indemnity insurance, 355

managed care plan, 355

Medicaid, 354

medical home, 363

Medicare, 354

midwives, 350

out-of-pocket payments, 353

point-of-service (POS) plans, 356

policy formation, 358

policy implementation, 358

policy modification, 358

preferred provider organization (PPO), 355

premium, 357

prepaid hospital services plan, 352

primary care provider, 355

private financing, 350

public financing, 350

self insurance, 357

stakeholders, 349

universal health care, 350

Review Questions

1. Name three characteristics of the U.S. health care system that differ from most other industrialized nations.

2. Using a national perspective, why should we worry about the rising costs of health care and its effect on the growth of the uninsured?
3. What is the difference between Medicare and Medicaid? Describe the populations they serve and who oversees these programs.
4. What is the difference between an HMO plan, PPO plan, and POS plan?
5. Looking back at the most recent national health care reform debate, name three interest groups that were influential in the debate.

References

1. Starr P. *The Social Transformation of American Medicine*. New York: Basic Books; 1982.
2. Shi L, Singh D. *Essentials of the US Health Care System*. Sudbury, Mass.: Jones and Bartlett Publishers; 2005.
3. Cassedy JH. *Medicine in America: A Short History*. Baltimore, Md.: The Johns Hopkins University Press; 1991.
4. Duncan RP. Uncompensated hospital care. *Med Care Rev*. 1992;49:3:265–330.
5. Falk IS, Rorem CR, Ring MD. *The Cost of Medical Care*. Chicago: University of Chicago Press; 1933.
6. Wasley TP. *What Has Government Done to Our Health Care?* Washington, D.C.: The Cato Institute; 1992.
7. Somers HN, Somers AR. *Doctors, Patients and Health Insurance*. Washington, D.C.: The Brookings Institution; 1961.
8. Department of Health and Human Services. Centers for Medicare & Medicaid Services. NHE Web tables. 2009. Available at: www.cms.hhs.gov/NationalHealthExpendData/downloads/tables.pdf. Accessed May 15, 2010.
9. Department of Health and Human Services. Centers for Medicare & Medicaid Services. (2005). Medicaid at a glance 2005: a Medicaid information source. Available at: www.cms.hhs.gov/MedicaidDataSourcesGenInfo/Downloads/maag2005.pdf. Accessed May 15, 2010.
10. Department of Health and Human Services. (2009). Centers for Medicare & Medicaid Services. Low cost health insurance for families & children. The Children's Health Insurance Program (CHIP). Available at: www.cms.hhs.gov/LowCostHealthInsFamChild/. Accessed May 15, 2010.
11. Kaiser Family Foundation. Employer health benefits survey, 2008 Annual survey. 2006. Available at: www.kkf.org/. Accessed May 2009.
12. Sultz HA, Young KM. *Health Care USA: Understanding Its Organization and Delivery*. Sudbury, Mass.: Jones and Bartlett Publishers; 2004.
13. Department of the Treasury. Health savings accounts [brochure]. 2007. Available at: www.treas.gov/offices/public-affairs/hsa/pdf/HSA-Tri-fold-english-07[1].pdf. Accessed May 15, 2010.

14. The Urban Institute. Health savings accounts and high deductable insurance plans: Implications for those with high medical costs, low incomes and the uninsured. 2009. Available at: www.urban.org/UploadedPDF/411833_health_saving_account.pdf. Accessed May 2009.

15. Longest BB. *Health Policymaking in the United States*. Chicago, Ill.: Health Administrative Press; 2002.

16. Jonas S, Goldsteen RL, Goldsteen K. *An Introduction to the U.S. Health Care System*. New York: Springer Publishing Company; 2007.

17. Goldfield NI. *National Health Reform American Style: Lessons from the Past*. Tampa, Fla.: American College of Physician Executives; 2000.

18. Speaker of the House. Affordable Healthcare for America: Summary. 2010. Available at: http://docs.house.gov/energycommerce/SUMMARY.pdf. Accessed May 29, 2010.

19. Kaiser Family Foundation. The Kaiser Commission on Medicaid and the uninsured, Web page. 2009. States moving toward comprehensive health care reform. Available at: www.kff.org/uninsured/kcmu_statehealthreform.cfm. Accessed May 15, 2010.

20. Massachusetts Division of Heathcare Finance and Policy. Estimates of health insurance coverage in Massachusetts from the 2009 Massachusetts Health Insurance Survey. 2009. Available at: www.mass.gov/Eeohhs2/docs/dhcfp/r/pubs/09/his_policy_brief_estimates_oct-2009.pdf.

21. Massachusetts Taxpayers Association. *Massachusetts Health Reform: The Myth of Uncontrolled Costs*. 2009. Available at: www.masstaxpayers.org/files/Health%20care-NT.pdf. Accessed May 15, 2010.

22. Kaiser Family Foundation. Medicaid: A Primer 2009. Available at: www.kff.org/medicaid/upload/7334-03.pdf. Accessed May 15, 2010.

CHAPTER 15

HEALTH SERVICES RESEARCH

Lori Bilello, MBA, MHS

LEARNING OBJECTIVES

- Describe the variables that affect access to health care.
- Measure the quality of health care and identify methods to improve health care services.
- Recognize the many cost-containment strategies that have been employed in the United States.
- Understand the role of health information technology in improving the cost, quality, and accessibility of health services.

Health services research has emerged as a field of study in response to the increasing complexity of our health care system and the need to improve the efficiency and effectiveness of the delivery and financing of health services. This chapter will provide an overview of the key concepts of cost, quality, and accessibility of health services and how to measure them.

Health Services Research

AcademyHealth, the professional society for health services researchers, defines **health services research** as the multidisciplinary field of scientific investigation that studies how social factors, financing systems, organizational structures and processes, health technologies, and personal behaviors affect access to health care, the quality and cost of health care, and ultimately our health and well-being[1]. The primary goals of health services research are to identify the most effective ways to organize, manage, finance, and deliver high-quality care. Findings from health services research inform the health care policy-making process, lead to improvements in clinical practice, and help shape how health care will be delivered and paid for in the future.

The elements of health services research include the following:

- Understanding the relationships between a population's need of and demand for health services, as well as the access and supply of health services

- Examining the processes and structures of health services, including quality and effectiveness

- Evaluating the cost and efficiency of health services interventions.

Health services research differs from clinical research because it focuses on the health system, whereas clinical research focuses on the patient, especially the diagnosis and treatment of disease or injury.

Access to Health Care

The growing number of uninsured in the United States continues to fuel the health policy debate on access to health care. Many local, state, and federal programs have been put into place to improve access to care for certain populations such as the elderly (Medicare) and low-income uninsured (Medicaid), but these programs address only one part of the access issues found in this country today: cost. Individuals without health insurance oftentimes do not have a primary care provider, do not receive appropriate preventive care, and use the emergency department as their usual source of care. Lack of insurance also affects access to care for relatively serious medical conditions. Evidence suggests that lack of insurance over an extended period significantly increases the risk of premature death and that death rates among hospitalized patients without health insurance are significantly higher than among patients with insurance[2].

Access to care involves more than having health insurance and can be affected by socioeconomic factors, such as education or geography, or health system factors, such as shortages in ambulatory or hospital services in a community. Other barriers to care, such as lack of transportation or language difficulties, can make gaining access to needed health care services difficult. The Institute of Medicine Committee on Monitoring Access to Medical Care[3] defined access as timely use of personal health services to achieve the best possible outcomes. Defining and measuring access to care has been a key focus of health services researchers, and several models or frameworks have been developed.

The dominant theoretical approach to evaluating access and use is based on a conceptual framework developed by Ronald Andersen in 1968[4] and further refined with his colleague Lu Ann Aday, as well as other colleagues over the years, and is widely used as a model to analyze access-to-care issues. The **Andersen framework** viewed access as a function of three categories of variables: (1) **predisposing factors**, such as personal resources, education, race, and age; (2) **enabling factors**, such as the availability of providers in a community, an individual's insurance coverage, and existence of a regular source of care; and (3) an individual's need for health care, as indicated by health status and symptoms. His framework measured access to care as the actual use of health care services.

The Institute of Medicine adopted a variation of Andersen's framework in their 1993 report, *Access to Health Care in America*[3]. This framework (Figure 15.1) not only looks at service use as a measure of access but also whether the services received were appropriate. In addition, the framework considers whether the services lead to improved health status and equity across groups. Barriers to care are categorized in three major groups: structural, financial, and personal/cultural barriers. **Structural barriers** are impediments to medical care

FIGURE 15.1 Model of Access to Personal Health Care Services

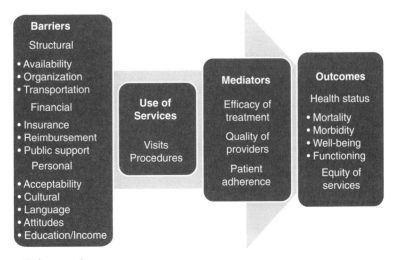

Source: Reference 3.

directly related to the number, type, concentration, location, or organizational configuration of health care providers. **Financial barriers** may restrict access either by patients' inability to pay for needed medical services or by discouraging physicians and hospitals from treating patients of limited means. Personal and **cultural barriers** may inhibit people who need medical attention from seeking it or, once they obtain care, from following recommended posttreatment guidelines.

Using this framework, the effects of these barriers on access to care can be observed through measurement of health status or health outcomes. Studies using this framework have demonstrated that variation in the use of services and health outcomes can be explained by differences in health status, sociodemographic factors, and characteristics of the health care market. To determine **equity of access**, you need to identify if there are **systematic differences** (regular, measured differences) in use and outcomes among groups in society and whether these differences are the result of certain barriers to care.

Another approach widely cited as a framework for understanding access to care uses a multidimensional concept developed by Penchansky and Thomas. Their definition of access is to measure the degree of fit between the clients and the health care system across five dimensions: availability, accessibility, accommodation, affordability, and acceptability[5]. Their definitions of these dimensions are as follows:

- **Availability:** the relationship of the volume and type of existing services or resources to the clients' volume and types of needs. It refers to the adequacy of the supply of physicians, dentists, and other providers; of facilities such as clinics and hospitals; and of specialized programs and services such as mental health and emergency care.

- **Accessibility:** the relationship between the location of supply and the location of clients, taking into account client transportation resources and travel time, distance, and cost.

- **Accommodation:** the relationship between the manner in which the supply resources are organized to accept clients (including appointment systems, hours of operation, walk-in facilities, telephone services); the clients' ability to accommodate to these factors; and the clients' perception of their appropriateness.

- **Affordability:** the relationship of prices of services and providers' insurance or deposit requirements to the clients' income, ability to pay, and existing health insurance.

- **Acceptability:** the relationship of clients' attitudes about personal and practice characteristics of providers to the actual characteristics of existing providers, as well as provider attitudes about acceptable personal characteristics of clients. Characteristics include provider attributes such as age, sex, ethnicity, type of facility, neighborhood of facility, and religious affiliation of facility or provider. In turn, providers have attitudes about the preferred attributes of clients and may be unwilling to serve certain types of clients (e.g., welfare patients) or, through accommodation, such as the availability of interpreters or the presence of ramps and automatic doors, make themselves more (or less) available. In general, it has been found that patients are more comfortable with providers who are more like them in socioeconomic terms and vice versa.

Access Indicators

Monitoring access to care is important in the identification of problems within the health care delivery system and society as a whole. Access indicators are often used to measure problems over time and are essential for health planning and health policy development. Key indicators for access include utilization measures and outcome measures. Some common **utilization measures** are visits to medical providers and number of medical procedures, hospitalizations, and emergency department visits. For example, examining the number of avoidable emergency department visits and hospitalizations is a good indicator of lack of access to primary care services. National surveys from the National Center for Health Statistics (NCHS) are good tools for exploring detailed information about health services utilization combined with detailed patient demographic and socioeconomic data (see Chapter 3 for more on national data). Surveys attempting to explore the nature of access have investigated various properties of utilization: who provided the care (physician, dentist); the care setting (doctor's office, outpatient department); the purpose of the visit (preventive, curative, custodial); and the frequency and continuity of use[6]. The shortcoming of using utilization indicators as a measure of access is the absence of information about the efficacy of the care addressed by the measures.

Utilization measures alone do not provide the full picture on access to care. It is also important to know that the care an individual received was appropriate for that patient's condition and if the patient's health improved after receiving treatment. **Outcome measures** such as death rates, disease incidence, complications due to treatment, disability, and patient satisfaction are often used to measure access to care. For instance, infant mortality is often used as an indicator of poor access to care. Oftentimes, poor birth outcomes are due to the mother not receiving adequate prenatal care during her pregnancy, especially when she

Table 15.1 Selected Access Measures from *Healthy People 2010*

Measure	2010 Target
1–1. Increase the proportion of persons with health insurance.	100%
1–5. Increase the proportion of persons with a usual primary care provider.	85%
1–6. Reduce the proportion of families that experience difficulties or delays in obtaining health care or do not receive needed care for one or more family members.	7%
1–9. Reduce hospitalization rates for three ambulatory-care-sensitive conditions—pediatric asthma, uncontrolled diabetes, and immunization-preventable pneumonia and influenza.	17.3 admissions per 10,000 population
16–1. Reduce fetal and infant deaths.	4.5 per 1,000 live births
16–8. Increase the proportion of very low birth weight (VLBW) infants born at level III hospitals or subspecialty perinatal centers.	90%
21–1. Reduce the proportion of children and adolescents who have dental caries in their primary or permanent teeth.	11%
21–2. Reduce the proportion of children, adolescents, and adults with untreated dental decay.	9%
25–1. Reduce the proportion of adolescents and young adults with *Chlamydia trachomatis* infections.	3%
25–7. Reduce the proportion of childless females with fertility problems who have had a sexually transmitted disease or who have required treatment for pelvic inflammatory disease (PID).	15%

Source: Reference 7.

may have an underlying health condition that can affect the pregnancy. Many of the leading health indicators outlined in the Centers for Disease Control and Prevention's (CDC's) *Healthy People 2010* are indicators of access, as illustrated in Table 15.1[7]. As noted in Chapter 14, these kinds of indicators paint an unflattering picture of the quality of U.S. health care.

Quality of Health Care

The quality of health care services provided in the United States has been a major concern for several decades but came to the forefront of national attention with the release of the Institute of Medicine's report *To Err is Human: Building a*

Safer Health System in 2000[8]. The report cited two large studies that found adverse events occurred in 2.9 and 3.7% of hospitalizations. When extrapolated over the 33.6 million admissions to U.S. hospitals in 1997, the results of these studies imply that at least 44,000 Americans die each year as a result of medical errors[8]. The quality of health care should not focus strictly on how well the care was delivered but also if the care provided was the most appropriate and effective given the patient's health condition. This section will discuss how to improve health care processes and patient safety as well as clinical effectiveness of health care services.

It is often noted that the U.S. health care system is complex due to its decentralized and fragmented nature, which makes it difficult to provide coordinated, patient-focused care. With multiple settings and providers involved in the care of a patient, this often leads to duplication of services, silos of patient's clinical information (for example, independent pharmacy and medical/clinical procedures data systems), and difficulties in the implementation of best practices across settings. The addition of multiple payers (health insurance companies, Medicare, Medicaid) in the U.S. health system further complicates these issues because each payer may have requirements for how care is delivered and what services are covered under its plan.

Licensure and accreditation of health providers and health facilities by state and voluntary accrediting agencies were the initial step in defining the minimum quality standards for the U.S. health care infrastructure (see also Chapter 14 for an overview of these state functions). In the 1980s, the concept of **continuous quality improvement** (CQI) took hold in the health care industry, largely due to the work of Avedis Donabedian, who developed a model to help define and measure quality in health care organizations. **Donabedian's quality model** focused on three domains in which health care quality can be examined and measured: structure, process, and outcomes. Donabedian defined structure as "the relatively stable characteristics of the providers of care, of the tools and resources they have at their disposal, and the physical and organizational settings in which they work."[9] Structure means the basic resources needed to deliver care, including the availability and acceptability of facilities, staff, and equipment. Quality measures of structure include licensure of staff, staffing ratios, types of equipment available, and the condition of the physical plant/facilities.

Process is how care is delivered to the patient. It specifically looks at the procedures of how the diagnosis and treatment of patients are carried out as well as the interpersonal relationships between the staff and the patient. Most of the quality improvement activities in hospitals focus on improving the process of care, such as reducing wait times in the emergency department or improving the accuracy of dispensing medications. Several quality improvement initiatives have become popular over the years, including Total Quality Management (TQM) and Six Sigma. These quality improvement methodologies each use a systematic process to identify areas for improvement and reduce variation in the delivery of services. Clinical practice guidelines are also an important tool in the diagnosis and treatment of patients, and they provide a systematic process based on evidence-based medicine for clinicians to follow in the delivery of health care services. For example, clinical practice guidelines in the management of diabetes patients includes a recommended schedule of laboratory testing and follow-up exams for the management and control of the disease in patients who are receiving insulin.

Process focuses on how health care is delivered, but **outcomes** refer to the effects of that care on the patient's health status (positive or negative). Both structure and process can have an effect on outcomes as well as patients' individual characteristics. Some examples of outcome measures include mortality rates, postoperative infection rates, and improved patient functioning. Health outcomes can be measured at the individual level (clinical outcomes) as well as at the population level. Population health indicators include age-adjusted death rates, disease-specific death rates, and life expectancy measures such as **quality-adjusted life years** (QALY), **disability-adjusted life years** (DALY), and **years of potential life lost** (YPLL). QALY is a measure of health care outcomes that adjusts gains (or losses) in years of life after a health care intervention and considers the quality of life during those years, whereas DALY measures the years of potential life lost due to premature mortality and the years of productive life lost due to disability[10]. QALY and DALY measures are often used in cost-effectiveness analysis of health interventions. YPLL is defined as the number of years of potential life lost by each death occurring before a predetermined end point, such as age sixty-five or seventy years. Certain diseases may have low mortality (death rate) but high morbidity (disability), such as depression or chronic fatigue syndrome, and will have a negative impact on the quality of life.

Quality Indicators

The collection and analysis of data to monitor the quality of health care has become commonplace in both the inpatient (hospitals, nursing homes) and outpatient (clinic) setting. For hospitals and other health care facilities, organizations such as the Joint Commission for the Accreditation of Healthcare Organizations (JCAHO) provide standards that address patient safety, patient rights, infection control, staffing, and a multitude of other areas that may affect the quality of care provided by a health care organization (go to www.jointcommission.org).

An example of a JCAHO quality measure for hospital care is the provision of antibiotics within six hours of patient arrival in the hospital for individuals diagnosed with pneumonia[11]. The accreditation of managed care plans is performed by the National Commission on Quality Assessment (NCQA), which also tracks quality indicators focusing on outpatient care and provision of prevention. The Healthcare Effectiveness Data and Information Set (HEDIS) is the tool developed by NCQA to measure the performance of health plans across many dimensions of care, including patient satisfaction, proper use of health care services, and access to care. Many of the HEDIS measures focus on whether providers meet standards for prevention and early intervention services, such as immunizations and cancer screenings (www.ncqa.org).

Medicare, as the largest single payer of health care in the United States, also plays a significant role in measuring the quality of services that are provided to its beneficiaries. The **Centers for Medicare & Medicaid Services** (CMS) has developed an extensive array of quality measures for hospitals, nursing homes, home health care agencies, physicians, and other professionals. Many of these measures can be found using the CMS search tools, such as Hospital Compare at www.Medicare.gov, where they compare quality indicators for hospitals as well as other health care organizations in local areas. You may find it interesting to see how your area providers rate.

To increase the adoption of quality measures, CMS is moving toward **value-based purchasing** of health services, which ties reimbursement to providers based on their reporting of quality measures[12]. For instance, CMS will not reimburse hospitals for care provided to a patient due to a hospital-acquired infection or for care of a patient fall in the hospital, both of which are considered preventable with high-quality care. Many other health plans have also tied reimbursement to the provision of quality care, and these programs are often referred as **pay-for-performance** programs. Under these programs, providers are rewarded for meeting preestablished performance measures for quality and efficiency, such as following clinical practice guidelines (such as timely mammograms for women) or adopting the use of electronic medical records.

Cost of Health Care

As reviewed in Chapter 14, health care costs in the United States are the highest in the world, and health care expenditures continue to rise at rates exceeding the general inflation rate of the U.S. economy. As health care expenditures exceeded 16 percent of the gross domestic product (GDP) in 2008 and continue to grow, there is a growing urgency for policy makers and payers to control costs and improve the efficiency and effectiveness of health care services. The rapid expansion of health care technology and pharmaceutical advances has fueled increased costs but with only some evidence that these advances have a major impact on health outcomes commensurate with their costs.

An important goal of health services research is to assess and ultimately improve how health care is delivered. Evaluating the efficiency of how health care is delivered and if the care provided is effective in improving the health status of a patient will lead to controlling costs and increasing quality of health services.

Efficiency and Effectiveness

The current structure of the U.S. health care system is very complex and fragmented and therefore does not make the best use of its resources. There are great inefficiencies in our health care system and wide variation in the use of health services across the country, as illustrated by the Dartmouth Atlas, which uses Medicare data to analyze the variation in spending and medical practices of local markets (Figure 15.2). Mapping the variation in health care use suggests there are areas where there are too many or too few of some health care services and wide variability of cost.

After adjusting for differences in severity of patients' medical conditions and pricing among different markets, Dartmouth still found significant geographic differences in the overall cost of care, which they mainly attribute to the volume of services received by similar types of patients. They found that areas with an abundant supply of physicians, hospitals, and other health care resources tend to have higher use of resources; however, patients did not tend to have better outcomes due to the increased use of resources[13]. Receiving more medical care does not necessarily mean better medical care, and there is substantial evidence documenting that overuse of many services can lead to a situation in which the potential risk of harm outweighs the potential benefits[14]. For instance, overuse of medications such as antibiotics for nonbacterial infections can lead to damage to the normal flora in the intestines as well as an increase in antibiotic resistance of some strains of bacteria.

To address this variation and overuse of health services, we need to do a better job of analyzing the effectiveness of treatment options and to standardize care by using clinical practice guidelines founded on evidence-based medicine. In 2009, as part of the American Recovery and Reinvestment Act, Congress approved a $1.1 billion effort to improve the quality and efficiency of health care through comparative effectiveness research[15]. **Comparative effectiveness**

FIGURE 15.2 Total Rates of Reimbursement for Noncapitated Medicare per Enrollee

By hospital referral region (2006)

■ $9,000 to 16,352 (57)
■ 8,000 to < 9,000 (79)
■ 7,500 to < 8,000 (53)
□ 7,000 to < 7,500 (42)
□ 5,310 to < 7,000 (75)
□ Not populated

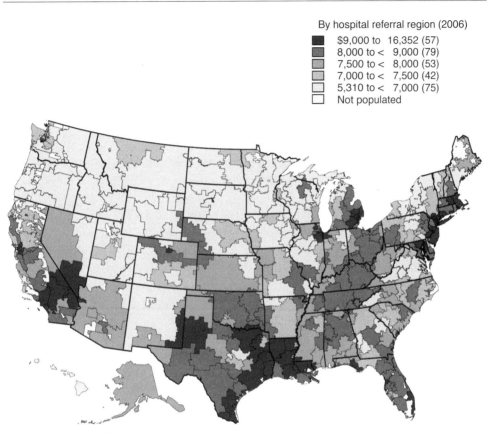

Source: Reference 13.

research (CER) evaluates the impact of the different treatment options available for a given medical condition for a particular set of patients. In these clinical questions, there may be two apparently good treatments, and CER asks if one of them provides better patient outcomes (or saves money given equally good outcomes). Studies may compare similar treatments, such as competing drugs, or they may analyze very different approaches, such as surgery versus drug therapy for heart disease. The analysis may focus only on the relative medical benefits and risks of each option, or it may also weigh both the costs and the benefits of those options[16]. Methods for analyzing costs as well as benefits include cost-effectiveness analysis, cost-utility analysis, and cost-benefit analysis. These studies are often based on clinical research trials and use some form of quality of life measure such as QALY or DALY to assign a value to the impact of treatments.

As part of the American Recovery and Reinvestment Act (ARRA) of 2009, the Institute of Medicine (IOM) was asked to recommend national priorities for research questions to be addressed by comparative effectiveness research. The panel recommended twenty-nine categories, including both primary and secondary care research areas. The top ten categories and examples of recommended research are listed in Table 15.2.

Cost Containment

Over the last three decades, many payment methodologies and strategies have been implemented in the health care industry to try to control the rapid growth of health care costs.

The oldest form of payment, and one that is still common for physicians and other health professionals, is the **fee-for-service** payment system in which providers are paid a fee for each service provided. This gives an incentive for health care providers to provide more care than needed and, coupled with their concerns of malpractice lawsuits, overuse health care services for patients who have health insurance (e.g., unnecessary laboratory tests or MRIs). In response to these concerns, Medicare and other payers have developed other payment methodologies to control the overuse of services such as per case payment methods (DRGs) and per patient payment methods (also called capitation).

Initially, efforts were focused on controlling hospital costs through rate setting by government payers. In 1984, Medicare implemented a new payment methodology called the **prospective payment system** (PPS) through which hospitals are paid a predetermined rate for each Medicare admission. Each patient is classified into a **diagnosis-related group** (DRG) based on clinical information from his or her medical record. DRG classification includes the principal diagnosis (why the patient was admitted), complications and comorbidities (other secondary diagnoses), surgical procedures performed, age of patient, and discharge disposition (whether they went home, transferred to another facility, or expired). Except for certain patients with exceptionally high costs, called **outliers**, the hospital is paid a flat rate for the DRG regardless of the actual services provided.

During this time period, managed care companies implemented capitation as a method to pay hospitals and, especially, primary care physicians for health care services provided to their enrollees. **Capitation** provides a fixed amount of money, paid in advance, per patient per month to providers for the delivery

Table 15.2 Institute of Medicine (IOM) Priority Research Areas

Priority Research Area	Example
1. Health delivery	Compare the effectiveness of the various delivery models (e.g., primary care, dental offices, schools, mobile vans) in preventing dental caries in children.
2. Disparities	Compare the effectiveness of interventions (e.g., community-based multilevel interventions, simple health education, usual care) to reduce health disparities in cardiovascular disease, diabetes, cancer, musculoskeletal diseases, and birth outcomes.
3. Disabilities	Compare the effectiveness of different residential settings (e.g., home care, nursing home, group home) in caring for elderly patients with functional impairments.
4. Cardiovascular	Compare the effectiveness of treatment strategies for atrial fibrillation, including surgery, catheter ablation, and pharmacological treatment.
5. Geriatrics	Compare the effectiveness of primary prevention methods, such as exercise and balance training, versus clinical treatments in preventing falls in older adults at varying degrees of risk.
6. Psychiatry	Compare the effectiveness of wraparound home and community-based services and residential treatment in managing serious emotional disorders in children and adults.
7. Neurology	Compare the effectiveness of therapeutic strategies (e.g., behavioral or pharmacological interventions or the combination of the two) for different autism spectrum disorders (ASD) at different levels of severity and stages of intervention.
8. Pediatrics	Compare the effectiveness of school-based interventions involving meal programs, vending machines, and physical education, at different levels of intensity, in preventing and treating overweight and obesity in children and adolescents.
9. Endocrinology	Compare the effectiveness and cost-effectiveness of conventional medical management of type 2 diabetes in adolescents and adults versus conventional therapy plus intensive educational programs or programs incorporating support groups and educational resources.
10. Musculoskeletal	Compare the long-term effectiveness of weight-bearing exercise and bisphosphonates in preventing hip and vertebral fractures in older women with osteopenia and/or osteoporosis.

Source: Reference 17.

of health care services. Capitation rates are determined by the types of services that are provided, the number of patients involved, and the period of time during which the services are provided. Capitation and per case payment methods for physicians and hospitals have raised concerns about potential underuse in order to stay within payment limits. For example, a family practice physician may receive $20 per month ($240 per year) to provide primary care services for a patient in the office. He or she may discourage office visits and try to manage the patient's health concerns by phone to reduce costs and stay within the $240 payment.

No payment method perfectly aligns financial incentives with the goal of high-quality, efficient health care delivery. As a result, other payment methodologies are being tested, such as blended or bundled payments and value-based purchasing. With **bundled payments**, hospitals and physicians are paid a combined fee for all the care associated with a given patient episode. For example, a single payment would be provided for coronary artery bypass graft (CABG) surgery, including preadmission diagnostic services, facility and physician fees for the surgery, and follow-up care, including rehabilitation. The goal of bundled payments is to increase coordination among providers and decrease duplicated and unnecessary services. Value-based purchasing links payment to performance by rewarding providers who meet efficiency and quality benchmarks. Bonus or incentive payments are paid to providers who meet certain clinical quality measures and resource utilization measures for a broad array of health conditions and procedures. The goal of value-based purchasing is to foster clinical and financial accountability in the delivery of health care services by physicians, hospitals, and other types of providers. Although each payment method discussed above may address certain problems in our current system, they are unlikely to slow the overall growth of health care spending unless major health care system reforms are implemented.

Information Technology

It is widely recognized that improvements in **health information technology** (HIT) and **health information exchange** (HIE) will allow improvements in the cost, quality, and efficiency of health care. Information technology in health services delivery can be categorized into two major areas: clinical information systems and administrative information systems. **Clinical information systems** or applications provide tools for managing health care data and guide clinical decision making. Table 15.3 provides definitions of key HIT applications used in the delivery of health care services.

Table 15.3 Health Information Technology (HIT) Applications

Product or Functionality	Description
Electronic health record (EHR)	An electronic record of health-related information for an individual that conforms to nationally recognized interoperability standards and that can be created, managed, and consulted by authorized clinicians and staff across more than one health care organization.
Electronic medical record (EMR)	An electronic record of health-related information for an individual that can be created, gathered, managed, and consulted by authorized clinicians and staff within one health care organization.
e-Prescribing (eRx)	Enables a physician to transmit a prescription electronically to the patient's choice of pharmacy. It also enables physicians and pharmacies to obtain information about the patient's eligibility and medication history from drug plans. Often comes with built-in alerts for drug–drug, drug–allergy, and drug–disease interactions.
Personal health records	An electronic record of health-related information for an individual that conforms to nationally recognized interoperability standards and that can be drawn from multiple sources while being managed, shared, and controlled by the individual.
Computerized physician order entry (CPOE)	Refers to a computer-based system of ordering medications and often other tests. Physicians directly enter orders into a computer system that can have varying levels of sophistication. Basic CPOE ensures standardized, legible, complete orders, and thus primarily reduces errors due to poor handwriting and ambiguous abbreviations.
Clinical decision support (CDS)	Any system designed to improve clinical decision making related to diagnostic or therapeutic processes of care. CDS addresses activities ranging from the selection of drugs (e.g., the optimal antibiotic choice given specific microbiological data) or diagnostic tests to detailed support for optimal drug dosing and support for resolving diagnostic dilemmas. Often incorporated as part of CPOE or EMR/EHR systems.
Disease registries	A database feature that includes key clinical data for a subset of chronically ill patients for the purpose of tracking their condition and managing treatment.

Source: Reference 18.

Administrative information systems are used to assist in managing financial and administrative data within an organization, including billing, resource management, budgeting, and cost control. Administrative decision support systems provide tools for forecasting patient volume and project staffing requirements, analyzing the use of services and resources consumed, and collecting and monitoring quality indicators.

The potential of health information technology to improve patients' health and the functioning of the health care system has been recognized as a priority for health care reform. A significant financial commitment has been made by the U.S. government for health information technology and health information exchange as evidenced by the $19 billion allocated in the American Recovery and Reinvestment Act of 2009. Of this amount, $17 billion includes incentive payments to physicians and hospitals participating in the Medicare and Medicaid programs to implement and meaningfully use certified electronic health records applications by 2014. The remaining $2 billion was allocated to establish the Office of the National Coordinator for Health Information Technology (ONCHIT) within the Department of Health and Human Services (HHS) to promote the development of a nationwide interoperable HIT infrastructure and work with states to implement this process. The goals of the HIT infrastructure are to ensure protection and privacy of health care information; improve patient care by reducing medical errors; reduce costs by removing administrative barriers that result in duplicative claims and services; and improve care coordination among health care providers[15]. Interestingly, the idea of better and portable electronic medical records surfaced in the Clinton health care debate and was dismissed as unfeasible. Improvements in electronic data systems, experiments showing reduced medical errors, and legislation about record privacy and patient rights all combine to increase the interest in information technology in health care. Nationwide, the Department of Veterans Affairs health care system has been a leader in applying information technological innovation.

An important aspect of HIT adoption includes the use of clinical decision support tools to alert providers of the need for screenings and other preventive care for their patients, as well as drug interactions, especially if the provider is e-prescribing (sending prescriptions electronically to pharmacies). By e-prescribing, physicians have access to a national pharmacy database that allows them to see if their patients have multiple providers and prescriptions and will allow them to see what drugs are covered under the patient's health plan. Finally, the development of **personal health records** (PHR), which will allow patients to have access to and add to their health information, will empower patients to take a more active role in their health care and overall well-being.

Summary

The aim of health services research is to produce valid research to aid in the decision-making process to improve access, efficiency, and quality of health care services. Understanding some of the issues behind the lack of access for millions of Americans will aid in developing public policy in addressing this critical problem. The lack of health insurance is only one major component of access: other factors include socioeconomic factors, supply of health care services, and personal or cultural barriers to health care.

With increasing scrutiny of how health care services are delivered, analyzing and documenting the quality of health services and developing methods to improve quality has become a major focus in the health care industry. Quality improvement strategies have focused on both the structural aspects of the health care system as well as the clinical practices of health care providers. By examining the structure and process of how health care is delivered, inefficiencies can be identified and improvements made to the health care system. Improving clinical effectiveness and patient safety will, in part, require more research of evidence-based practices and the development and adoption of clinical practice guidelines.

Having timely and accurate data is paramount in improving the health care system. Health information technology and health information exchange has become a national priority and will allow greater efficiencies in the delivery of health services by improving coordination of care, reducing duplication of services, and minimizing errors in the transfer of patient information. This will help control some of the unnecessary costs within the health care system, but until major payment reforms are adopted and the issue of the uninsured is addressed, the United States will continue to struggle with the burgeoning costs of the most expensive health care system in the world.

Key Terms

acceptability, 371

accessibility, 370

accommodation, 370

administrative information systems, 382

affordability, 370

Andersen framework, 369

availability, 370

bundled payments, 380

capitation, 378

Centers for Medicare & Medicaid Services, 375

clinical information systems, 380

comparative effectiveness research (CER), 376

continuous quality improvement, 373

cultural barriers, 370

diagnosis-related group, 378

Review Questions

1. Describe the three main barriers to access to health care as defined in Andersen's framework and give examples for each barrier.
2. What is the difference between a utilization measure and an outcome measure? Provide an example of each type of measure.
3. What is continuous quality improvement (CQI)? Describe Donabedian's model for quality improvement in health care settings.
4. What is the difference between a QALY and a DALY and why would you use these measures?
5. What is the Joint Commission for the Accreditation of Healthcare Organizations (JCAHO), and are all health care facilities required to be accredited?
6. What was the motivation for Medicare and private insurance companies in the development of value-based purchasing or pay-for-performance programs?
7. What is Medicare's prospective payment system and how does it reimburse hospitals for inpatient care?
8. How many hospitals and how many doctors' offices are currently using electronic medical records at their facilities? *Hint:* Check HHS government Web sites or medical journals for latest statistics.

References

1. AcademyHealth. What is HSR. Available at: www.academyhealth.org/About/content.cfm?ItemNumber=831&navItemNumber=514. Accessed May 16, 2010.

2. Reinhardt UE. Coverage and access in health care reform. *New Engl J Med.* 1991;330:1452–1453.

3. Institute of Medicine, Committee on Monitoring Access to Personal Health Care Services. *Access to Health Care in America.* Washington, D.C.: National Academy Press; 1993.

4. Andersen RM. *A Behavioral Model of Families' Use of Health Services.* Research Series, No. 25. Chicago, Ill.: Center for Health Administration Studies, University of Chicago; 1968.

5. Penchansky R, Thomas JW. (1981). The concept of access: Definition and relationship to consumer satisfaction. *Med Care.* 1981;19(2):127–140.

6. Aday L., Anderson R, Fleming G. (1980). *Health Care in the U.S.: Equitable for Whom?* Newbury Park, Calif.: Sage Publications; 1980.

7. U.S. Department of Health and Human Services, Office of Disease Prevention and Health Promotion. Healthy people 2010. Volumes 1 and 2. Available at: www.healthypeople.gov/Document/. Accessed May 16, 2010.

8. Institute of Medicine. *To Err Is Human: Building a Safer Health System.* Washington, D.C.: National Academies Press; 2000.

9. Donabedian A. *Explorations in Quality Assessment and Monitoring: The Definition of Quality and Approaches to Its Assessment.* Vol. 1. Ann Arbor, Mich.: Health Administration Press; 1980.

10. National Information Center on Health Services Research and Health Care Technology (NICHSR). (2004). HTA 101: Glossary. Available at: www.nlm.nih.gov/nichsr/hta101/ta101014.html. Accessed May 16, 2010.

11. Joint Commission on Accreditation of Healthcare Organizations. (2008). Current specifications manual for national hospital inpatient quality measures. Vers. 2.6. Available at: www.jointcommission.org/PerformanceMeasurement/Performance Measurement/Current+NHQM+Manual.htm. Accessed May 16, 2010.

12. Centers for Medicare & Medicaid Services. *Road Map for Quality Measurement in the Traditional Medicare Fee-for-Service Program.* 2009. Available at: www.cms.hhs.gov/QualityInitiativesGenInfo/downloads/QualityMeasurementRoadmap_OEA1–16_508.pdf. Accessed May 16, 2010.

13. Dartmouth Institute for Heath Policy and Clinical Practice. February 2009. *Healthcare Spending, Quality and Outcomes: More Isn't Always Better.* A Dartmouth Atlas Project Topic Brief. Available at: http://www.dartmouthatlas.org/downloads/reports/Spending_Brief_022709.pdf. Accessed June 3, 2010.

14. Schuster MA, McGlynn EA, Brook RH. How good is the quality of health care in the United States? *Milbank Q.* 76(4):517–563, 1998.

15. The American Recovery and Reinvestment Act of 2009 (ARRA), Public Law 111–5, 111th Cong., 1st sess. 2009. Available at: http://frwebgate.access.gpo.gov/cgi-bin/getdoc.cgi?dbname=111_cong_bills&docid=f:h1enr.pdf. Accessed May 16, 2010.

16. Congressional Budget Office. *Research on the Comparative Effectiveness of Medical Treatments: Issues and Options for an Expanded Federal Role.* 2007. Available at: www.cbo.gov/ftpdocs/88xx/doc8891/12–18-ComparativeEffectiveness.pdf. Accessed May 16, 2010.

17. Institute of Medicine. (2009). Report brief: Initial national priorities for comparative effectiveness research. Available at: http://www.iom.edu/Reports/2009/ComparativeEffectivenessResearchPriorities.aspx. Accessed June 3, 2010.
18. Moiduddin A, Moore J. (2008). The underserved and health information technology: issues and opportunities. Prepared for the Office of the Assistant Secretary for Planning and Evaluation, U.S. Department of Health and Human Services. Available at: http://aspe.hhs.gov/sp/reports/2009/underserved/report.html#_edn10. Accessed May 16, 2010.

CHAPTER 16

HEALTH DISPARITIES

Amy B. Dailey, PhD, MPH
Allyson G. Hall, PhD, MBA/MHS

LEARNING OBJECTIVES

- Define health disparities and describe examples of health disparities that are currently impacting the United States.
- Understand the major social determinants of health disparities.
- Recognize how the social-ecological model is a useful framework for understanding the social determinants of health disparities.
- Identify current initiatives to reduce health disparities and the subsequent policy implications.

Health disparities have been a subject of much concern and discussion over the past few decades. In response to this concern, The Centers for Disease Control and Prevention (CDC) established an Office of Minority Health in the 1980s (now the Office of Minority Health and Health Disparities) (www.cdc.gov/omhd/). The mission of this office includes eliminating health disparities "for vulnerable populations as defined by race/ethnicity, socioeconomic status, geography, gender, age, disability status, risk status related to sex and gender, and among other populations identified to be at-risk for health disparities." In this chapter we will describe some of the health disparities that exist in the United States. Although we will not be including other countries in our discussion, it is important to recognize that health disparities also occur on a broader, global scale (see Chapter 3 for health differences by geographic regions). Health disparities have been observed for myriad diseases and health outcomes, and in this chapter we will review in detail observed disparities in cancer, cardiovascular diseases, obesity, and HIV/AIDS. Many of the examples draw attention to racial/ethnic disparities, but we will also discuss disparities by other subgroups. We will then discuss the major social determinants of health disparities, including differential access to opportunities and resources, the role of discrimination, disproportionate exposure to environmental contaminants, and the social factors that influence health behaviors that may contribute to health disparities. Finally, we will conclude by discussing some of the current efforts underway to reduce health disparities.

What Are Health Disparities?

Health disparities are defined in many different ways, but in general, disparities are differences in health between populations or between subgroups in populations. What distinguishes health disparities from health differences is that the term *disparities* refers to disproportionate disease burden or adverse health outcomes experienced by disadvantaged social groups when compared with more advantaged social groups. Health disparities are measured by assessing differences between populations using epidemiological calculations, including incidence, prevalence, morbidity, mortality or survival of diseases, and other health outcomes (see Chapter 4). Related terms, such as *inequalities* or *inequities* are sometimes used interchangeably, but have slightly different meanings. The term **inequality**, like disparity, refers to populations being unequal on a particular measure of health, with disadvantaged populations faring worse than more advantaged populations, whereas **inequity** is usually reserved to specifically refer to the ethical considerations underlying health disparities and social justice[1,2]. In public health, there is a long history of using principles of social justice and the belief that the burdens and benefits of society should be fairly and equitably distributed[3] as a framework for understanding the harmful effects of "economic exploitation, oppression, discrimination, inequality, and degradation of natural resources."[4] Ultimately, all segments of society should be able to achieve the highest levels of health status, regardless of social status. Throughout this chapter we will use the term *disparities* and *inequalities* interchangeably.

Measuring Health Disparities

Two of the most common ways used to describe disparities is by socioeconomic conditions and race or ethnicity. Many terms have been used to describe socioeconomic conditions, including social class, socioeconomic status, and social stratification. We will use the term **socioeconomic position** (**SEP**) throughout the chapter, which is a term that encompasses social and economic factors that influence the positions that individuals in groups hold within a society[5]. Here we will describe how health disparities are measured by SEP and race/ethnicity.

Socioeconomic Position

Three of the most common measures of SEP are education, income, and occupation. Education, often the most conveniently measured of the socioeconomic concepts, attempts to capture the knowledge-related assets that people have acquired, generally completed by young adulthood. This variable is usually measured by self-reported information on the years of education completed or by milestones completed (e.g., high school graduate). Education is thought to influence other aspects of SEP, such as income and employment opportunities. In addition to contributing to access to economic resources, education may influence other factors, such as knowledge of health issues, reception to health education messages, or health communication skills. Some of the limitations of using education as a measure of SEP include variability in quality of education or prestige of institutions, small range in the data, and variation in education levels due to age of cohorts (i.e., education levels may differ by generation). In addition, being ill as a child may influence the level of education achieved, which is an example of reverse causality, or temporal sequence (see Chapter 5), whereby health affects SEP rather than SEP impacting health.

Income is another regularly used measure of SEP, often measured as self-reported annual household or family income. Income is thought to have an effect on health by directly influencing access to material resources, such as food and shelter, and access to services, such as health care. Some of the limitations associated with using income as a measure of SEP include instability (may not have stable levels of income over time), failure to include other sources of income besides employment-based earnings, and failure to take into account differences in values of goods across different geographies and circumstances (i.e., $10 in one community may allow you to buy more goods than in another community). Income is also vulnerable to reverse causality, whereby having an illness can influence the ability to earn income. Wealth, an additional indicator related to income, is also used in health studies. Wealth includes additional material resources such as the value of houses, cars, investments, and inheritance.

Related to both income and education, occupation is the other major individual-level variable used in characterizing SEP. Most measures ask about current occupation or longest-held job. Occupation is strongly related to income and is directly related to access to material resources. Occupation also can reflect social-standing privileges and social networks. Occupation-based measures may influence health through additional mechanisms such as work-based stress, job strain, or feelings of control. An additional element that occupation measurement may capture is exposure to physical or environmental hazards. Some of the limitations of using occupation as a measure of SEP arise from the inability to differentiate jobs into meaningful categories useful to examining differences in health. Some measures, for example the United States Census occupational classification (www.census.gov/hhes/www/ioindex/overview.html), can be divided into simple distinctions such as manual and nonmanual labor or more detailed categories designated by coding specialists. The usefulness of these kinds of categories has been a source of much debate. Other limitations include inability to capture differences in pay equity and gender issues, such as using a husband's occupation to classify a wife's SEP. As with education and income, occupation can also be influenced by health status.

There is increased recognition that SEP encompasses more than the individual socioeconomic measures of education, income, and occupation. The socioeconomic conditions of where people live are also important indicators used in health disparities research. These measures are often calculated by aggregating individual-level indicators up to a specific area of interest, such as a neighborhood. Many studies of neighborhood have used U.S. Census boundaries to define neighborhoods. For example, neighborhood SEP has been calculated using **census tracts**, small, relatively permanent statistical subdivisions of a county of 1,500 to 8,000 people each (www.census.gov/geo/www/cen_tract.html), as neighborhood boundaries. Neighborhood SEP can include multiple measures of socioeconomic conditions using aggregated Census data on indicators such as mean income, mean education, and mean unemployment of the area. Often, the purpose of collecting information on neighborhood SEP is to determine if where people live influences their health above and beyond their individual SEP. One of the major limitations with measuring neighborhood SEP is that using administrative boundaries to define neighborhoods may not translate into meaningful definitions of neighborhoods for residents.

Race and Ethnicity

In addition to examining health disparities by SEP, in the United States we are also concerned with examining differences by racial and ethnic groups. We regularly examine differences in health, comparing racial/ethnic minorities (e.g., non-Hispanic Blacks or Hispanics) to the majority racial/ethnic group (non-Hispanic Whites). Measurement of race and ethnicity has become increasingly complex as we try to understand health issues affecting our diverse populations. Later in the chapter we will describe social factors that contribute to differences in health by race and ethnicity, but here we focus on how to *measure* race and ethnicity. The United States has been collecting information on race as part of each decennial Census since 1790, and many changes have occurred over this time period[6]. The Office of Budget and Management (OMB) first released a directive on creating federal standards for the collection of race and ethnicity in 1977, creating the four mutually exclusive single-race categories of White, Black, American Indian/Alaska Native, and Asian/Pacific Islander, followed by a yes/no ethnicity question (Hispanic or not Hispanic). This directive was changed two decades later in three ways: (1) Native Hawaiians and other Pacific Islanders were separated from the Asian and Pacific Islander category, (2) individuals can identify themselves as belonging to more than one racial group, and (3) the placement of the Hispanic origin question precedes the race question. The OMB race/ethnicity classifications (and variations of these classifications) are widely used nationally, including use by federal agencies, the U.S. Census, and many of the large population-based surveys.

Although changes provided opportunities for individuals to classify themselves more accurately and have likely improved the ability to classify rarer populations, there have been some major challenges to using the OMB classification system. Most notably, the multiracial option has made analyzing racial/ethnic disparities in health more complex. In order to compare across time periods, increase statistical power, or create more meaningful classifications, data are frequently reclassified back into single-race categories. Some surveys such as the National Health Interview Survey (NHIS) have asked multiracial persons which one race best represents them in order to estimate single-race counts.

Regardless of the method chosen to measure race and ethnicity, there is still much debate over the constructs we are measuring when classifying by these categories. The large heterogeneous categories most often used to classify race and ethnicity do not reliably relate back to genetic classifications, thus most researchers agree that race and ethnicity represent social factors in some manner. We will discuss some of these factors in the section Social Determinants of Health Disparities below.

Examples of Health Disparities

Every decade the U.S. Department of Health and Human Services (HHS) initiates ten-year national health objectives that provide a framework for addressing risk factors, determinants of health, and the diseases and disorders that affect our communities[7]. The initiative, **Healthy People**, is a collaborative effort between scientific experts and public participants. Although we are embarking on a new decade and plans for Healthy People 2020 are underway[8], this chapter will review the efforts of Healthy People 2010. One of the two primary goals of the Healthy People 2010 initiative is to eliminate health disparities. Before we can begin to determine ways to eliminate health disparities, diseases and health outcomes must be monitored and evaluated (one of the core public health functions: assessment), paying close attention to differences by population subgroups. As noted in Chapter 3, this core public health function helps drive the functions of policy development and assurance. To this end, much of the Healthy People 2010 documentation is focused on describing the current state of health status for the U.S. population, with specific goals for reaching particular outcomes by the year 2010 that will lead to reductions in the currently observed disparities by race/ethnicity, gender, disability, and other subgroups. In this section, we will describe some of the major health disparities that have been targeted by the Healthy People 2010 initiative. We will discuss disparities in the following four topics in detail: cancer, cardiovascular diseases (CVD), obesity, and HIV/AIDS. We will then discuss some of the major social and behavioral determinants of disparities.

Cancer

We have made great strides in increasing rates of survival from cancer, but disparities in cancer outcomes remain, particularly by socioeconomic status and race/ethnicity categories. Although it is difficult to generalize about cancer because there are many different types, we highlight some of the major cancer disparities that have been observed in incidence, mortality, and survival rates. According to statistics published by the American Cancer Society, and despite overall decreasing trends in cancer incidence and mortality, significant disparities persist (varying by cancer type) by race/ethnicity, education status, and geographic location[9]. For all cancer sites combined (2000–2004), African American men have both higher incidence of cancer (19 percent higher) and mortality due to cancer (37 percent higher) than do White men. However, African American women have lower incidence rates than do White women, yet experience higher overall cancer mortality rates. In general, for most cancers incidence and mortality rates have been consistently higher in African Americans than Whites. Notable exceptions include higher incidence and mortality rates due to lung cancer for Whites compared to other racial/ethnic groups and higher kidney cancer mortality rates for Whites compared to other racial/ethnic groups. Sometimes we observe disparities in cancer mortality or survival rates, but not in incidence rates. For example, although breast cancer incidence is lower for African American women than White women, mortality due to breast

PUBLIC HEALTH CONNECTIONS 16.1

RACIAL/ETHNIC DISPARITIES IN BREAST CANCER

Despite lower incidence rates, African American women continue to die of breast cancer at significantly higher rates than do White women. In fact, although the overall death rates due to breast cancer have been on the decline, the disparity in mortality between African American women and White women has widened over time (see Figure 16.1). Although there are many factors that contribute to this disparity, the stage of the cancer at diagnosis remains a major contributor to these differences. African American women continue to be diagnosed at later, or more advanced, stages than White women. Researchers have examined the role that early detection such as mammography screening plays in this disparity[11]. Although survey data show that African American women have similar rates of *ever* having a mammogram as White women, they may not receive *regular* screening. Socioeconomic differences in access to primary health care and mammograms may be impeding the full benefit of mammography, particularly for minority women. There is also evidence that the socioeconomic characteristics of neighborhoods influence adherence to mammography screening guidelines[12]. In addition, health system factors such as communication issues involving understanding results of mammograms and problems with adequate follow-up of abnormal mammograms may also contribute to mammography not being as effective for African American women as compared with other women[13,14].

cancer is significantly higher for African American women than White women (see Figure 16.1). This figure shows that although breast cancer mortality rates have been decreasing for many years, the racial gap has not decreased (see Public Health Connections 16.1).

There are also racial/ethnic disparities in cancer survival. Cancer survival statistics represent the proportion of individuals that remain alive after having been diagnosed with cancer[15]. These statistics incorporate deaths from all causes, not solely cancer-related causes of death. For nearly every cancer site, African Americans have poorer survival than do Whites. This disparity is observed across all **stages of diagnosis**, which measures how advanced the cancer was at the time of diagnosis. Thus while some of the racial/ethnic cancer mortality disparity is explained by presenting to the health care system at later stages of diagnosis overall, racial/ethnic disparities are observed *within* each stage of diagnosis stratum, suggesting that additional factors are involved. African

FIGURE 16.1 Age-Adjusted Mortality Rates Due to Breast Cancer Among Women in the United States by Race/Ethnicity, 1975–2005

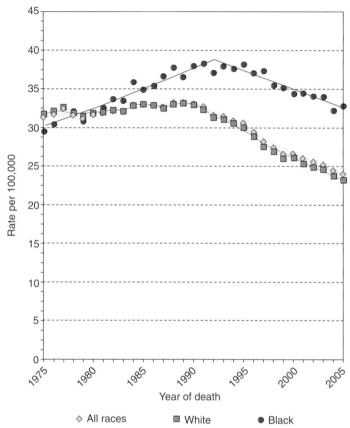

◇ All races   ▣ White   ● Black

Cancer sites include invasive cases only unless otherwise noted.

Mortality source: US Mortality Files, National Center for Health Satistics, CDC. Rates are per 100,000 and are age-adjusted to the 2000 US Std Population (19 age groups – Census P25-1130). Regression lines are calculated using the Joinpoint Regression Program Version 3.3, April 2008, National Cancer Institute.

Source: Reference 10.

Americans, however, are not the only minority group to experience lower survival rates after cancer diagnosis. All minorities, with the exception of Asian American/Pacific Islander women, have lower survival rates than non-Hispanic Whites, even after accounting for stage at diagnosis.

In addition to racial/ethnic cancer disparities, there are also considerable disparities by education status. Individuals with twelve years of education or less have significantly higher death rates for all cancers combined than do those with more than twelve years of education. For example, among White men, the ratio of death rates comparing those less-educated to more-educated was 3.36, suggesting that less-educated White men have cancer death rates more than three times higher than White men with more education. Because socioeconomic status is highly correlated with race/ethnicity in the United States, sometimes it is difficult to fully understand the independent effects of socioeconomic status and race/ethnicity. Although many times racial/ethnic disparities can be partially explained by socioeconomic status, there is often a residual effect of race/ethnicity on health outcomes, even after accounting for socioeconomic status.

Cardiovascular Diseases

Cardiovascular diseases (CVDs) include the following conditions: high blood pressure, coronary heart disease (including myocardial infarction and angina pectoris), heart failure, and stroke. CVD can also include congenital cardiovascular defects, but they will not be discussed here. It has been estimated that approximately 80 million American adults (nearly 1 in 3) have one or more of these cardiovascular conditions. Although CVD is common across all populations, there are some notable disparities. The death rates due to CVD in 2005 were highest for Black males (438.4 per 100,000), followed by White males (324.7 per 100,000), Black females (319.7 per 100,000), and White females (230.4 per 100,000)[16]. In general, men have higher rates of CVD overall, but there are some gender differences by age and also in treatment of CVD. For example, in younger ages (under seventy-five years of age), a higher proportion of CVD events due to coronary heart disease occur in men than in women, yet a higher proportion of events due to stroke occur in women than in men.

It is difficult to fully understand the differences in CVD rates between men and women without considering additional variables, as well as other issues such as **detection bias** (men may be diagnosed more often simply due to greater awareness of CVD conditions in men). There is also evidence that women express different CVD-related symptoms then men, complicating diagnoses. For example, with respect to heart attacks, women are more likely than men to express symptoms such as shortness of breath, vomiting, sweating, fatigue, and neck, shoulder, back, or abdominal discomfort. Although these differences in symptoms may reflect biological differences between men and women, there is also evidence that men and women do not receive equal treatment, unrelated to biology. For example, analyses of the 2005 National Ambulatory Medical Care Survey and the National Hospital Ambulatory Medical Care Survey have shown that among patients with hypertension, women were less likely than men to receive aspirin and beta-blockers for secondary prevention of CVD[17]. As with most health outcomes with racial/ethnic or gender disparities, there are also disparities in CVD by socioeconomic position (SEP). For example, coronary heart disease (CHD) and stroke were more common in groups with lower education, income, and higher poverty status.

While it is difficult to generalize about disparities in CVD because of the many component conditions involved, high blood pressure (defined as systolic blood pressure greater or equal to 140 mm Hg or diastolic blood pressure greater or equal to 90 mm Hg, or taking antihypertensive medicine, or having been told at least twice by a physician or other health professional that one has high blood pressure) is of particular concern for Blacks living in the United States. The

FIGURE 16.2 Age-Adjusted Prevalence Trends for High Blood Pressure in Adults 20 Years of Age or Older in the United States by Race/Ethnicity, Sex, and Survey (NHANES: 1988 to 1994, 1999 to 2004, and 2005 to 2006)

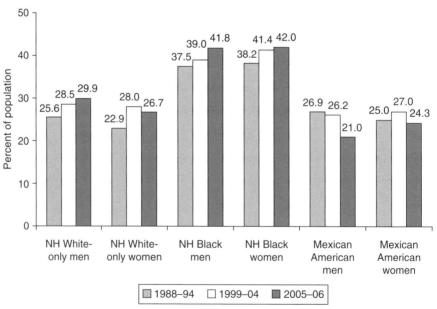

Source: Reference 16.

prevalence of high blood pressure in the U.S. Black population (regardless of sex or educational status) is among the highest in the world, and there is evidence that the rates continue to increase. American Indian/Alaska Native adults also have higher rates of high blood pressure than do Whites.

There are many factors that are associated with higher risk of CVD, including high lipid values (high cholesterol), diabetes, overweight/obesity, cigarette smoking, and physical inactivity. These risk factors are often distributed unequally by social status. For example, according to Behavioral Risk Factor Surveillance Survey (BRFSS, see Chapter 3) data, the prevalence of having two or more risk factors for CVD was highest among African Americans and American Indians/Alaska Natives compared to other races/ethnicities. Individuals reporting the lowest annual household income levels ($10,000 or less) and those who reported being unable to work had the highest rates of having two or more risk factors, compared to higher SEP groups. Thus not only are low-SEP individuals more likely to have higher prevalence of one risk factor (e.g., smoking or physical inactivity), they are at higher risk of having multiple risk factors, further compounding the risk. There are also significant geographic differences in risk factor prevalence, with many states in the South faring the worst (Alabama, Arkansas, Georgia, Kentucky, Louisiana, Mississippi, North Carolina, Oklahoma, Tennessee, and West Virginia). Indiana, Ohio, Guam, and Puerto Rico also reported high risk factor prevalence.

Obesity

Nearly two-thirds of adults in the United States are overweight, and almost one-third are obese[18]. Body mass index (BMI), measured as weight (kg) divided by height [(m)^2] is a common way to measure overweight (greater than 25 kg/m^2) and obesity (greater than 30 kg/m^2) and is a useful indicator of current or future health problems. Obesity is a major concern for the general population but is of particular concern in terms of disparities in health[19]. Overweight and obesity are known risk factors for myriad health outcomes, including diabetes, CVD, gallbladder disease, osteoarthritis, sleep apnea (breathing problems), cancer, pregnancy complications, psychological disorders, and increased mortality.

The prevalence of obesity has increased over the years across all ages, racial/ethnic groups, educational levels, smoking levels, and gender. Although obesity is a problem for the United States population as a whole, there are some populations that suffer from obesity more than others. According to the CDC, in the years 2006–2008, Blacks had 51 percent higher prevalence of obesity than Whites, and Hispanics had 21 percent higher prevalence of obesity than Whites. Large racial/ethnic differences are also observed among adolescents and

FIGURE 16.3 Prevalence of Obesity (Body Mass Index ≥30 kg/m²) Among Adolescents in the United States by Ethnicity, Using National Longitudinal Survey of Adolescent Health, 1994–1996 Data

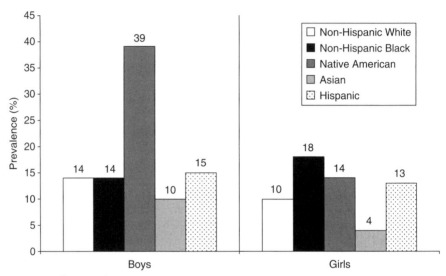

Source: Reference 20.

children. Studies have shown that non-Hispanic White children and adolescents have lower rates of obesity than non-Hispanic Blacks and Mexican-Americans[20]. Among boys, Mexican Americans aged six to eleven had the highest prevalence of obesity, and among girls, non-Hispanic Black adolescents (aged twelve to nineteen) had the highest prevalence of obesity. Marked geographic disparities in obesity are also observed in the United States. For both non-Hispanic Blacks and non-Hispanic Whites there was greater prevalence of obesity in the South and the Midwest than in the Northeast or West, whereas for Hispanics, the prevalence of obesity in the West region was similar to the prevalence in the South and Midwest regions.

There are well-documented SEP differences in rates of obesity, showing that individuals of lower SEP are more likely to be obese. However, some studies have come to the conclusion that that there is racial/ethnic variation in the association between SEP and obesity and that observed ethnic/racial differences in obesity are not fully explained by individual SEP[20]. Given that obesity may adversely affect socioeconomic opportunities, it is also possible that SEP and obesity share a bidirectional causal relationship. In other words, low SEP may increase the risk of being obese, but obesity may also cause a person to have low

SEP. The relationships between race/ethnicity, SEP, and gender are complex. For example, there is a general trend showing that with decreased SEP there is increasing obesity prevalence. However, for reasons not well understood, a notable exception has been observed for Black women. Black women in the United States with less than a high school education had the lowest prevalence of obesity compared with Black women who had higher educational levels.

HIV/AIDS

HIV/AIDS is a disease marked by disparities by race/ethnicity, sexual orientation, gender, and socioeconomic position. Over half of newly diagnosed HIV/AIDS infections in the years 2001 to 2004 occurred in the Black population, despite the fact Blacks accounted for only 13 percent of the total population[21]. Hispanics have also been shown to have HIV diagnosis rates significantly higher than that of Whites.

More than three-fourths of people living with AIDS are men, but there are some alarming and increasing trends for some women. In 2005, the rate of AIDS diagnosis was nearly twenty-three times higher for non-Hispanic Black women and five times higher for Hispanic women than that for non-Hispanic White women[22]. In fact, in 2004 HIV infection was the leading cause of death for Black women aged twenty-five to thirty-four years. HIV/AIDS is also heavily influenced by SEP. In addition to reduced access to health care resources, lack of socioeconomic resources, including unstable housing, is linked to riskier health behaviors associated with HIV/AIDS[23]. Some of these HIV risk behaviors that have been linked to SEP include earlier initiation of sexual activity, less frequent use of condoms, and intravenous drug use.

Although there have been some shifts in population trends, HIV/AIDS continues to disproportionately impact men who have sex with men (MSM). The number of HIV diagnoses for MSM decreased in the 1990s, but there is evidence that HIV diagnoses are once again on the rise in this group. In 2005, the number of new HIV/AIDS cases among MSM was 11 percent more than the number of new cases in 2001. Furthermore, there are racial disparities in HIV infection within the MSM population. For the years 2001 to 2004, Black and Hispanic MSM not only had higher rates of HIV/AIDS diagnoses across all age groups compared to White MSM, but they also progressed into AIDS more quickly[24]. While racial/ethnic and SEP differences in HIV risk behaviors among MSM may explain some of the poorer outcomes, Black and Hispanic MSM are also more likely than White MSM to be diagnosed at late stages of infection, suggesting access to testing and health care services is more limited in this group.

Social Determinants of Health Disparities

Health disparities by social status are primarily the result of social influences embedded within historical, geographic, sociocultural, economic, and political contexts[25]. The following discussion focuses on some of the major social determinants of health disparities, including differential access to resources, racial/ethnic discrimination, racial residential segregation, environmental justice, and lifestyle factors that are influenced by social circumstances. In order to better understand these social determinants of health, we will first describe the social-ecological model and the conceptual framework that this model provides in examining social determinants of health disparities. Chapters 2 and 11 also examine this model.

In the 2003 report, *The Future of the Public's Health*, the Institute of Medicine (IOM) describes the **social-ecological model** as a guide to conceptualizing determinants of population health[26]. We will not examine every element in detail, but it is a useful framework for taking a critical look at the various levels of exposure and interaction that have given rise to disparities in health by race/ethnicity, social status, and other social strata.

In Chapter 2, the innermost circle in Figure 2.3 represents the individual innate traits, such as age, sex, race, and biological factors, that are important in determining population health. For example, many diseases increase with age, such as arthritis and heart disease, and some genes have strong influences on individual's risk of disease. Until recently, much of epidemiology has focused on trying to better understand the causes of disease by focusing on individual characteristics. However, we are now recognizing that diseases (both chronic and acute) and health disparities are not only related to individual characteristics, but the other levels represented in this figure. It is important to note that each of these levels does not influence health separately from the other, but rather by interacting across levels. We can readily observe how these different levels influence each other. For example, the next level after innate individual traits is individual behavior. We know that individual behavior is not just a function of one's individual characteristics, but that behavior is influenced by the other levels, including social, family, and community networks; living and working conditions; and the broad social, economic, cultural, health, and environmental conditions and policies (Chapter 11 explores health behavior in detail). In short, all of these levels of the social-ecological model are important to recognize to fully understand the determinants of health and health disparities.

When health disparities in the United States are discussed, undoubtedly racial/ethnic disparities receive the most attention. Race/ethnicity is a **social**

construct (that is, culturally defined rather than biologically defined) that is often a marker for differential exposures to social circumstances, which then give rise to disproportionate exposures that influence health. These exposures can include reduced access to economic, material, or physical resources, or increased exposure to social stressors and/or environmental hazards that can have direct biological consequences. Here we will focus on three major sources of health disparities: (1) access to resources, (2) discrimination and historical discriminatory policies, and (3) exposure to environmental hazards. We will also discuss how these social factors influence individual behaviors that also contribute to health disparities.

Access to Resources

Differential access to resources, whether they are material or social resources, is a major source of socioeconomic and racial/ethnic disparities in health outcomes. **Material resources** include economically based assets such as access to goods and services, and **social resources** are assets associated with relationships with others, such as social networks or social support. Access to health care is an important contributor to disparities in health. Access to care refers to the ability to obtain needed, affordable, convenient, acceptable, timely, and effective health care services[27]. There are a number of factors that influence whether a person can get medical care easily or not. These include having the financial means to pay for care, the degree to which the health care delivery system has enough capacity (such as physicians and hospitals), and whether an individual is able to obtain transportation to a medical care visit. Chapters 14 and 15 provide detailed discussion of the determinants of access to health care.

Perhaps the most often discussed barrier to health care services is the lack of health insurance. In the United States, nearly 47 million people do not have health insurance, severely limiting their access to medical care given the immense financial burden associated with most preventive care and treatments. People without health insurance are more likely to report not having a usual source of medical care, to have not received preventive care, to have unmet dental care needs, and to postpone care due to cost[28,29]. The uninsured may also be sicker when they do access medical care[28]. The quality of care is also different for individuals without insurance compared to those with insurance. For example, one study showed that among individuals who recently experienced a heart attack, patients who were uninsured were statistically significantly less likely to receive invasive procedures relative to individuals with health insurance[30].

FIGURE 16.4 Relationship Between Access to Care and Use of Preventive Care and Chronic Disease Management Services

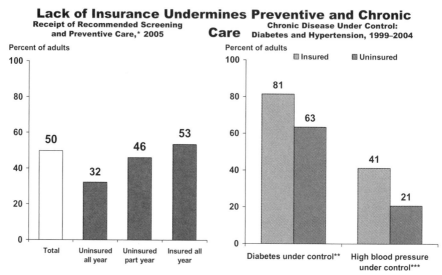

Lack of Insurance Undermines Preventive and Chronic Care

Receipt of Recommended Screening and Preventive Care,* 2005

Chronic Disease Under Control: Diabetes and Hypertension, 1999–2004

*Recommended care includes: blood pressure, cholesterol, Pap, mammogram, fecal occult blood test or sigmoidoscopy/colonoscopy, and flu shot within a specific time frame given age and sex. **Refers to diabetic adults whose HbA1c is <9.0 ***Refers to hypertensive adults whose blood pressure is <140/90 mmHg.

Data: Preventive care–B. Mahato, Columbia University analysis of Medical Expenditure Panel Survey; Chronic disease–J. M. McWilliams, Harvard Medical School analysis of National Health and Nutrition Examination Survey.

Source: Commonwealth Fund National Scorecard on U.S. Health System Performance, 2008.

Source: Reference 31.

Not having health insurance varies by sociodemographic characteristics, including race/ethnicity, education, gender, and income. Those without coverage are disproportionately poor, young, and a member of a racial or ethnic minority group. For example, among people below age sixty-five, about 12 percent of Whites do not have health insurance compared to 34 percent of Hispanic and 21 percent of African Americans[32]. Similarly, about 20 percent of children who live below the poverty level (level set by the federal government) have no health care coverage compared to 4 percent of children who are in families who live at 300 percent or more of the federal poverty level (FPL) (poverty level multiplied by 3)[33].

Efforts to increase access to medical care are needed, but access to health care also encompasses the idea of quality of health care. Some studies have shown that African Americans, compared with Whites, experience lower quality care. Examples include less timely emergency transportation for assault victims, poorer quality emergency room care, and lower rates of preventive, diagnostic, treatment, and rehabilitation services for cancer. There is also evidence that minorities are less likely than Whites to have continuity in their health care providers or a usual place they go for health care and are more likely to use emergency rooms for acute care needs. Additional factors that may impact quality of care, and thus health disparities, include patient and provider communication, health literacy, cultural competency, and discrimination in the health care setting[25].

In addition to access to quality health care, we are now beginning to consider how access to other kinds of material and social resources influence health in the United States. A large amount of evidence has accumulated in the last decade linking where one lives with health outcomes. Neighborhoods can directly influence disease via environmental contaminants, for example. There is mounting evidence that neighborhoods influence health in other ways, as well. Major pathways by which neighborhoods are important to health is through lower crime rates, recreational and green spaces, transportation, and high-quality food. These resources have direct impacts on health behaviors, which can range from diet, exercise, and smoking to cancer screening behavior.

Access to healthy, nutritious food can be a major barrier for some populations. For example, according to the Robert Wood Johnson Commission to Build a Healthier America (www.commissiononhealth.org), in Detroit, Michigan, there are only five grocery stores in a 139-square mile area with nine hundred thousand residents. It is well-documented that low-income neighborhoods often do not have access to affordable, fresh foods. Furthermore, people living in these neighborhoods may not have access to reliable transportation, which limits their ability to travel to grocery stores outside their immediate residential area. Transportation obstacles may also make it difficult for individuals to seek medical care or seek employment far from where they live. Neighborhoods and physical locations can also be related to social resources such as social networks. Social networks, described also in Chapter 11, have been shown to exert significant influence on risky health behaviors, particularly related to unhealthy substance use such as tobacco and sexual behaviors.

Education and employment opportunities also greatly influence health and disparities in health. For centuries we have observed that rates of disease increase with decreases in SEP. Studies have shown that individuals who are unemployed are more likely to view their health as fair or poor[34]. Job loss can be a highly stressful event that can also lead to adverse health consequences. In addition to direct effects of socioeconomic status on health, differential access to education and employment opportunities for minority groups also perpetuate racial/ethnic disparities in health. Education and employment directly influence access to health insurance; for example, discrimination (which will be discussed in more detail below) in education can influence literacy skills, possibly making health promotion messages less accessible. Furthermore, discriminatory practices in employment can restrict access to high-paying jobs or jobs that offer health insurance benefits.

Discrimination and Racial Residential Segregation

As we started to discuss above, differential access to material and social resources is intertwined with discrimination and racial residential segregation. In the United States, when we characterize individuals by their race or ethnicity (usually self-reported), we are measuring a variable that is likely a **marker** for social circumstances and/or stressors that have arisen out of discriminatory practices. These discriminatory practices are rooted in **racism**, which is the system of structuring opportunity and assigning value based on the social interpretation of phenotype (race)[35]. Racism can take many forms, including institutionalized, interpersonal, and internalized. Institutionalized racism includes differential access to, for example, housing, education, employment, medical facilities, clean environments, and information. *Personally mediated* racism is differential assumptions about the abilities, motives, and intents of others by race. This type of racism can result in discrimination that leads to police brutality, heightened vigilance by store clerks, or devaluation of student abilities by teachers, for example. *Internalized racism* refers to the acceptance of negative messages about their own abilities and worth by individuals in the stigmatized group. This kind of racism can lead to self-devaluation or feelings of hopelessness that can have direct impacts on health. The term racial (or ethnic) **discrimination** refers to the differential *actions* toward others that are a result of racism . Although difficult to measure, researchers have begun to quantify experiences of racial/ethnic discrimination and their subsequent health effects. Racial/ethnic discrimination has been shown to be associated with mental health outcomes, such as psychological distress, and physical health outcomes, including cardiovascular diseases. Discrimination can range from everyday hassles to unfair practices in hiring, school-related activities, the judicial system, and other major race-related experiences. Perceived race-based unfair treatment has also been shown to influence quality of health care and compliance with recommendations, including lower use of preventive health screenings and delays in filling prescriptions.

Discrimination can also manifest in very broad social and economic policies and subsequently have an impact on access to resources (as described above) and health. For example, housing policies have been a major contributor to racial residential segregation, which has also led to isolation from resources and increased concentration of poverty, with direct implications for racial/ethnic and socioeconomic disparities in health. Some examples of U.S. policies that have led to discrimination and segregation include original Social Security policies (1935), rights to unionize (1935 Wagner Act), federal housing programs, and loan lending practices[36]. When the U.S. Social Security program (the federal government–funded financial benefits available to U.S. workers and families that provides retirement, disability, and death benefits) first began, it excluded agricultural workers and domestic servants, who were predominantly African American, Mexican American, and Asian American. Thus the protections offered to most White Americans through Social Security excluded populations that were most vulnerable to the effects of economic recessions. The Wagner Act of 1935 (right to unionize) was designed to protect wages, medical care, and job security for individuals in unions. Yet the Wagner Act did not include all Americans; the final version permitted unions to exclude non-Whites. Even after the laws changed in the late 1950s, many unions remained all White into the 1970s. The federal housing programs of the 1930s and 1940s also posed unequal opportunities by race/ethnicity. The national appraisal system used to assign property values and loan eligibility was tied to race. Because minority and mixed-race neighborhoods received the lowest ratings, minorities were often denied loans under the housing programs. Less than 2 percent of the $120 billion in housing subsidies went to non-White families. All of these policies are examples of institutional factors that lead to social and economic inequalities. Ultimately, economic inequalities lead to poorer health through reduced access to resources and increased exposure to social stressors.

Many of these policies have also contributed to racial residential segregation, which also leads to isolation from resources. The residential segregation of African Americans is high at all levels of income in the United States[20]. Thus regardless of individual-level SEP, African Americans live in poorer areas than Whites. Furthermore, the most affluent African Americans actually experience higher levels of residential segregation than the poorest Latinos and Asians[25]. However, residential segregation in and of itself is not the problem. It is the isolation from resources and being excluded from opportunities that has given rise to segregation-related problems. Residential segregation directly influences access to education and employment opportunities (e.g., transportation, urban inner city schools, proximity to businesses).

Although racial/ethnic discrimination is salient to our discussion of racial/ethnic disparities in health, other groups also experience discrimination. For example, stigma associated with HIV/AIDS has proven to be an important barrier to receiving adequate health care. Sexual minorities, including MSM, often experience higher rates of mental health issues and may engage in risky health behaviors as a result. Stigma associated with being a sexual minority can lead to increased experience of social stressors and can also influence health-seeking behaviors, such as seeking testing or health care for HIV/AIDS. There is evidence that sexual orientation-based discrimination may exist in the health care system, but stigma associated with homosexuality and cultural influences may also inhibit some individuals from seeking care. Furthermore, because Black and Hispanic MSM are less likely than White MSM to live in gay-identified neighborhoods, minorities may have reduced exposure to prevention programs that have targeted these areas[37].

Exposure to Environmental Hazards

Exposure to overt or hidden environmental hazards and contaminants may also be a major contributor to health disparities. Also related to some of the issues discussed above with respect to discrimination and segregation, hazardous waste sites are disproportionately located in minority communities. Other communities that have more political and economic resources can lobby for waste sites to be located outside their communities, but poorer communities often do not have the same political capital to resist. There are also often economic incentives in the form of jobs that may increase if communities are willing to accept these kinds of facilities into their communities[38].

Although exposure to environmental contaminants is a contributor to health disparities, exposures to other kinds of hazards is also important to consider. In addition to being at higher risk of exposure to environmental contaminants, low-income, minority neighborhoods are also at higher risk of exposure to marketing campaigns of harmful substances, such as alcohol and cigarette advertisements.

Health Behaviors

It is well-documented that health behaviors are a major contributor to disease, particularly the conditions we highlighted above (cancer, CVD, obesity, and HIV/AIDS). Therefore, there is great interest in addressing health behaviors as a way to improve health (Chapter 11 describes aspects of research and theories about health behaviors in detail). Although health behaviors are individual-level factors, there is strong patterning by social factors across most health behaviors that we track in public health. In fact, many of the social determinants of health detailed above influence health partly through their impact on health behaviors.

Cigarette smoking is one example of a health behavior that is influenced by social determinants. There is a very large disparity in cigarette smoking between socioeconomic groups. Although the price of cigarettes has increased in many areas, individuals that can least afford to smoke are the ones most likely to smoke, least likely to stop smoking, and most likely to suffer the health consequences of smoking. Although some of the uptake of smoking in disadvantaged areas may be due to smoking-related norms, in other words, being in an environment where smoking is accepted, there are other factors that contribute to the socioeconomic disparity. Nicotine dependence has been shown to significantly increase with increases in economic deprivation. Thus quitting smoking may be difficult for disadvantaged groups, particularly in light of increased social stressors and daily hassles associated with living in deprived areas. Smoking (and other health behaviors) may also serve as a way to cope with the increased stressors experienced by disadvantaged populations. Furthermore, disadvantaged neighborhoods are more likely to be targeted for alcohol and cigarette advertisement campaigns[39].

As we described in our discussion of access to resources, other ways that the social environment influences health behaviors is through living and working conditions, access to affordable nutritious foods, and disproportionate exposure to alcohol and tobacco marketing. For example, if individuals do not feel safe in their neighborhoods or do not have access to recreational facilities or green spaces, they may have fewer opportunities to engage in physical activity. As noted earlier in this chapter, there is also evidence that access to affordable, nutritious foods is limited in low-income areas, and this lack has an impact on diet.

Actions to Address Health Disparities

To solve health disparities we need to determine what caused them and design appropriate interventions that take into account the multiple levels of causality. At the federal government level, in 1986 the Office of Minority Health was established by the U.S. Department of Health and Human Services. The mission of this office is to improve and protect the health of racial and ethnic minority populations through the development of health policies and programs that will eliminate health disparities. In addition, in 2000 the **Minority Health and Health Disparities Research and Education Act** was passed, which authorizes many programs and initiatives to address particular disparities[40].

You may recall that one of the two major goals of the Healthy People 2010 initiative is to eliminate health disparities. In 2005 the Healthy People 2010 initiative conducted a midcourse review to evaluate progress toward the goals. There were reductions in disparity among racial and ethnic populations for twenty-four objectives and subobjectives and reductions in disparity between gender groups for twenty-five objectives and subobjectives. Although we observed reductions in disparity for some outcomes, such as reductions in new AIDS cases for non-Hispanic Blacks, unfortunately we also observed increases in disparity between racial and ethnic populations for fourteen objectives and subobjectives and between men and women for fifteen objectives and subobjectives. For example, there were significant increases in prostate cancer deaths, fire arm–related deaths, and smoking during pregnancy among non-Hispanic Blacks compared to non-Hispanic Whites. There were also significant increases in new cases of tuberculosis, exposure to environmental particulate matter, and physical assault for Hispanics compared to non-Hispanic Whites. Furthermore, there were no changes in disparities among populations by education level, income level, geographic location, and disability status for the majority of indicators. Thus, although there have been widespread improvements in health status for the general population as a whole, there is little evidence that we have systematically improved disparities for any group[41].

There are countless studies on disparities in health. Yet, as we just reviewed, we have made relatively few major advances in the elimination of health disparities, despite the attention they receive in the public health literature. Many of the efforts put forth to eliminate health disparities have focused on improving access, coverage, quality, and the intensity of health care[42]. But it is possible that current efforts to reduce disparities in health have not been effective because we are not focusing on addressing the social determinants (as depicted in the social-ecological model in Figure 2.3) of health. Although there have been preventive health care interventions that show promise, medical care system interventions primarily focus on factors associated with poor outcomes after a disease or other health outcome has already occurred. But because we now know that health begins much farther upstream (where we live, learn, work, and play), health care interventions are not likely to eliminate disparities. Williams and colleagues suggested that in order to reduce gaps in health, greater attention needs to be paid to the social determinants of health, such as housing, neighborhood conditions, and SEP[36]. Furthermore, there is need for systematic evaluation of social and economic policies that likely have great impacts on social status and subsequent health outcomes. In order to make sustainable changes that are likely to reduce health disparities, it is important to engage not only health researchers and health care providers, but also policy makers, leaders, and communities. Unfortunately, the onus often falls upon the populations experiencing disproportionate health problems to solve their own problems while in isolation from the more advantaged groups. However, disparities are a problem of society as a whole and cannot be ignored by more advantaged populations. Moreover, society as a whole stands to benefit from the elimination of health disparities. By one estimation, if all adult Americans experienced the level of illness and mortality of college graduates, the annual economic benefit would equal at least $1 trillion dollars[43].

A U.S. Task Force on Community Preventive Services[42,44] highlighted six key areas that influence health: (1) neighborhood living conditions; (2) opportunities for learning and capacity for development; (3) employment opportunities and community development; (4) prevailing norms, customs, and processes; (5) social cohesion, civic engagement, and collective efficacy; and (6) health promotion, disease prevention, and health care opportunities. Although more than two hundred community-based interventions were identified by the task force, it concluded that there was very little information available on how effective these programs were for improving health outcomes and reducing disparities. Nonetheless, there is some evidence that interventions aiming to target these six areas have been successful. For example, some studies suggest that improvements in the infrastructure of communities can lead to improvements in health. Interventions, which can be as simple as providing income supplements to families, can also impact health outcomes. Programs that enhance academic enrichment for children have been shown to have large impacts on improving health in some populations. There is some evidence that large social movements and social policies can also have broad socioeconomic and health impacts. For example, the civil rights movement and the War on Poverty had a significant impact on the economic and health outcomes for African Americans. Although some promising interventions have been identified, it remains unclear whether these programs should be implemented at local, state, or national levels. Furthermore, in order to make the necessary policy changes, both the political will and collaboration among many stakeholders must occur.

The Robert Wood Johnson Commission to Build a Healthier America (www.commissiononhealth.org) has also made recommendations for addressing social determinants of health. One area on which they have focused is nutrition, recommending increased funding for federal programs that support the nutritional needs of families in need, feeding children only healthy foods in schools, and creating public-private partnerships to open and sustain full-service grocery stores in communities without access to healthy foods. In addition to recommendations on required physical activity in schools, the elimination of smoking nationwide, and early childhood educational opportunities, the commission also focuses on healthy places, recommending the creation of healthy community demonstration programs, development of a health impact rating for housing and infrastructure projects, and the integration of safety and wellness into every aspect of community life. Finally, the commission recommends ensuring that decision makers in all sectors have the evidence they need to build health into public and private policies and practices.

Summary

Health disparities refer to the disproportionate disease burden or adverse health outcomes experienced by disadvantaged social groups when compared with more advantaged social groups. Health disparities are well-documented across many health outcomes, including cancer, cardiovascular diseases, obesity and HIV/AIDS, and continue to be a major population health concern. Disparities in health largely occur because of social factors such as differential access to resources and opportunities, discrimination, or differential exposure to environmental contaminants. Although there are many efforts underway to address health disparities, we have made relatively little headway, particularly in terms of racial/ethnic and socioeconomic disparities. It is likely that the most expeditious way to address the elimination of health disparities is through multifaceted interventions that can address multiple levels of the social-ecological model, with particular attention to the broad social, economic, cultural, health, and environmental conditions and policies.

Key Terms

cardiovascular diseases, 395

census tracts, 390

detection bias, 395

discrimination, 404

health disparities, 388

Healthy People, 391

inequality, 388

inequity, 388

marker, 404

material resources, 401

Minority Health and Health Disparities Research and Education Act, 408

racism, 404

social-ecological model, 400

social construct, 400

social resources, 401

socioeconomic position (SEP), 388

stage of (cancer) diagnosis, 393

Review Questions

1. Describe the variables used in measuring SEP. Discuss some of the advantages and disadvantages associated with the measures. Does it matter which variables you choose?
2. Choose a type of cancer (e.g., breast, prostate, kidney) to investigate with respect to disparities. Use the Internet and/or other resources to report any current disparities in incidence, prevalence, survival, or treatment of this cancer.
3. Explain how the social-ecological model can be used to understand social determinants of health disparities.
4. What is the difference between racism and discrimination?
5. How does SEP influence health behaviors? Describe a specific example.
6. At what level of the social-ecological model are the initiatives to address disparities that are described in the chapter?

References

1. Braveman P. Health disparities and health equity: Concepts and measurement. *Annu Rev Public Health*. 2006;27:167–194.
2. Braveman P, Gruskin S. Defining equity in health. *J Epidemiol Community Health*. 2003;57(4):254–258.
3. Beauchamp D. Public health as social justice. *Inquiry*. 1976;13(1):3–14.
4. Krieger N. A glossary for social epidemiology. *J Epidemiol Community Health*. 2001;55(10):693–700.
5. Galobardes B, Lynch J, Smith GD. Measuring socioeconomic position in health research. *Br Med Bull*. 2007;81–82(1):21–37.
6. Mays VM, Ponce NA, Washington DL, Cochran SD. Classification of race and ethnicity: Implications for public health. *Annu Rev Public Health*. 2003;24:83–110.
7. U.S. Department of Health and Human Services. Healthy People Web page. Available at: www.healthypeople.gov. Accessed May 6, 2009.
8. U.S. Department of Health and Human Services. Developing Healthy People 2020 Web page. Healthy People 2020: The road ahead. Available at: www. healthypeople.gov/HP2020/. Accessed May 6, 2009.
9. Jemal A, Siegel R, Ward E, et al. Cancer statistics, 2008. *CA Cancer J Clin*. 2008;58(2):71–96.
10. Ries LAG, Melbert D, Krapcho M, et al., eds. SEER Cancer Statistics Review, 1975–2005, National Cancer Institute. Bethesda, Md. Based on November 2007 SEER data submission, posted to the SEER Web site, 2008. Available at: http:// seer.cancer.gov/csr/1975_2005/.

11. Jones B, Patterson EA, Calvocoressi L. Mammography screening in African American women: Evaluating the research. *Cancer.* 2003;97:258–272.

12. Dailey AB, Kasl SV, Holford TR, et al. Neighborhood-level socioeconomic predictors of nonadherence to mammography screening guidelines. *Cancer Epidemiol Biomarkers Prev.* 2007;16:2293–2303.

13. Jones BA, Dailey A., Calvocoressi L., Kasl SV, Lee CH, Hsu H. Inadequate follow-up of abnormal screening mammograms: Findings from the race differences in screening mammography process study (United States). *Cancer Causes Control.* 2005;16:809–821.

14. Jones BA, Reams K, Calvocoressi L, et al. Adequacy of communicating results from screening mammograms to African American and White women. *Am J Public Health.* 2007;97:531–538.

15. National Cancer Institute. Cancer Control and Population Sciences. Surveillance research Web page. Available at: http://surveillance.cancer.gov/statistics/types/survival.html. Accessed May 6, 2009.

16. Lloyd-Jones D, Adams R, Carnethon M, et al. Heart disease and stroke statistics—2009 update: A report from the American Heart Association Statistics Committee and Stroke Statistics Subcommittee. *Circulation.* 2009;119(3):480–486.

17. Keyhani S, Scobie JV, Hebert PL, McLaughlin MA. Gender disparities in blood pressure control and cardiovascular care in a national sample of ambulatory care visits. *Hypertension.* 2008;51(4):1149–1155.

18. U.S. Department of Health and Human Services. Weight-control Information Network. Statistics related to overweight and obesity page. Available at: www.win.niddk.nih.gov/STATISTICS. Accessed May 6, 2009.

19. Ogden CL, Carroll MD, Curtin LR, McDowell MA, Tabak CJ, Flegal KM. Prevalence of overweight and obesity in the United States, 1999–2004. *JAMA.* 2006;295(13):1549–1555.

20. Wang Y, Beydoun MA. The obesity epidemic in the United States—gender, age, socioeconomic, racial/ethnic, and geographic characteristics: A systematic review and meta-regression analysis. *Epidemiol Rev.* 2007;29:6–28.

21. The Centers for Disease Control and Prevention. Racial/ethnic disparities in diagnoses of HIV/AIDS—33 states, 2001–2005. *MMWR.* 2007;56(9):189–193.

22. The Centers for Disease Control and Prevention. HIV/AIDS, health disparities Web page. Available at: www.cdc.gov/nchhstp/healthdisparities/HIV_AIDS.htm. Accessed May 6, 2009.

23. American Psychological Association. Fact sheet: HIV/AIDS and socioeconomic status. Available at: http://www.apa.org/pi/ses/resources/publications/factsheet-hiv-aids.aspx. Accessed June 1, 2010.

24. Hall HI, Byers RH, Ling Q, Espinoza L. Racial/ethnic and age disparities in HIV prevalence and disease progression among men who have sex with men in the United States. *Am J Public Health.* 2007;97(6):1060–1066.

25. Williams DR, Jackson PB. Social sources of racial disparities in health. *Health Aff.* 2005;24(2):325–334.

26. Institute of Medicine. *The Future of the Public's Health in the Twenty-First Century.* Washington, D.C.: National Academies Press; 2002.

27. Shi L, Singh D. *Delivering Health Care in America: A Systems Approach.* 4th ed. Sudbury, Mass.: Jones and Bartlett; 2008.

28. Hadley J. Sicker and poorer—the consequences of being uninsured: A review of the research on the relationship between health insurance, medical care use, health, work, and income. *Med Care Res Rev.* 2003;60(2 Suppl):3S–75S; discussion 76S–112S.

29. Institute of Medicine. *Coverage Matters: Insurance and Health Care.* Washington, D.C.: National Academy Press; 2001.

30. Canto JG, Rogers WJ, French WJ, Gore JM, Chandra NC, Barron HV. Payer status and the utilization of hospital resources in acute myocardial infarction: A report from the National Registry of Myocardial Infarction 2. *Arch Intern Med.* 2000;160(6):817–823.

31. The Commonwealth Fund. Commission on a high performance health system. National Scorecard on U.S. Health System Performance, 2008, New York, NY. Available at: www.commonwealthfund.org/~/media/Files/Publications/Fund%20Report/2008/Jul/Why%20Not%20the%20Best%20%20Results%20from%20the%20National%20Scorecard%20on%20U%20S%20%20Health%20System%20Performance%20%202008/Scorecard_Chartpack_2008%20pdf.pdf. Accessed June 2, 2010.

32. The Henry J. Kaiser Family Foundation. Key health and health care indicators by race/ethnicity and state. 2009 update. Available at: www.kff.org/minorityhealth/upload/7633–02.pdf. Accessed May 20, 2010.

33. Schwartz K, Howard J, Williams A, Cook A. Health insurance coverage of America's children. The Henry J. Kaiser Family Foundation, The Kaiser Commission on Medicaid and the Uninsured; 2009. Web page. Available at: www.kff.org/uninsured/7609.cfm. Accessed June 1, 2010.

34. Bartley M, Ferrie J, Montgomery S. Health and labour market disadvantage: Unemployment, non-employment, and job insecurity. In: Marmot M, Wilkinson R, eds. *Social Determinants of Health.* New York: Oxford University Press; 2006.

35. Jones CP. Levels of racism: A theoretic framework and a gardener's tale. *Am J Public Health.* 2000;90(8):1212–1215.

36. Public Broadcasting System. What is race? Web page. Available at: www.pbs.org/race/001_WhatIsRace/001_00-home.htm. Accessed May 6, 2009.

37. The Centers for Disease Control and Prevention. Fact sheet. HIV and AIDS among Gay and Bisexual Men. Available at: www.cdc.gov/hiv/topics/msm/resources/factsheets/msm.htm. Accessed May 6, 2009.

38. U.S. Environmental Protection Agency. Environmental Justice Web page. Available at: www.epa.gov/oecaerth/environmentaljustice. Accessed May 6, 2009.

39. Jarvis M, Wardle J. Social patterning of individual health behaviors: The case of cigarette smoking. In: Marmot M, Wilkinson R, eds. *Social Determinants of Health.* New York: Oxford University Press; 2006.

40. U.S. Department of Health and Human Services. The Office of Minority Health Web page. Available at: www.omhrc.gov. Accessed May 6, 2009.

41. U.S. Department of Health and Human Services. Midcourse review, Healthy People. Executive summary. Goal 2: Eliminate health disparities. Available at: www.healthypeople.gov/data/midcourse/html/execsummary/Goal2.htm. Accessed May 6, 2009.

42. Williams DR, Costa MV, Odunlami AO, Mohammed SA. Moving upstream: How interventions that address the social determinants of health can improve health and reduce disparities. *J Public Health Manag Pract.* 2008;14 (Suppl):S8–17.

43. Braveman P, Egerter S. *Overcoming Obstacles to Health: Report from the Robert Wood Johnson Foundation to the Commission to Build a Healthier America.* Princeton, N.J.: Robert Wood Johnson Foundation; 2008.

44. Anderson L, Scrimshaw S, Fullilove M, Fielding J. Task Force on Community Preventive Services. The community guide's model for linking the social environment to health. *Am J Prev Med.* 2003;24(35):12–20.

FORECASTING PUBLIC HEALTH

CHAPTER 17

FUTURE OF PUBLIC HEALTH

Barbara A. Curbow, PhD
Stephanie L. Hanson, PhD

LEARNING OBJECTIVES

- Discuss major global challenges facing humanity.
- Discuss four health-related trends that are likely to impact the focus of future public health priorities in the United States.
- Identify specific factors impacting the success of disaster response.
- Describe the six areas of change the Institute of Medicine believes are central to ensuring population health.
- Describe how your individual choices contribute to the health of the public and identify specific actions you can take to contribute to the public's health.
- Describe how surveillance systems and data banks aid public health planning.
- Name four principles that are important for you to maintain a public health perspective.
- Describe the eight WHO Millennium Development Goals.

Suppose you are one of ten thousand fans watching State University's basketball team playing its biggest rival for the conference championship. You get a call on your cell phone, and a friend asks you, "What are Janie and Anna up to?" You look around and see them and report back to your friend, "They are in the stands twittering." Not too long ago, if Janie or Anna had overheard you, they may have taken offense that you had made a sexist comment putting down their manner of speaking to each other. Now, however, they would just assume that you were talking about their use of technology to report back on the game to friends outside the gym. Your generation, more than any other, has been caught up in the rushing currents of technological change. Over the past decade, you have grown to use, expect, and take for granted technologies that were never imagined by the bulk of the world's citizenry, including new ways to communicate (Skype, BlackBerrys, smartphones, webcams), to express who you are (Facebook, MySpace, YouTube), to gain information (Google, Wikipedia), and to entertain yourself (PlayStation, Wii Fit©, iTunes).

This explosion in technology has not come without a price, and researchers and policy makers have found that new public health and social issues have been created. Some of these issues have come about as a direct result of the use of new technology, for example, cyber bullying, "sexting," cyber child predators, and identity theft. For other issues, new technologies have helped to spread both the prevalence of new products and behaviors and instructions on how to perform them; this is often called **diffusion of innovations**[1] (see Public Health Connections 17.1). For example, over the past year or two some tobacco companies, in an attempt to find new markets for their products, have first test-marketed and then widely marketed a product called *snus* (rhymes with *loose*). Snus is a sachet-type pouch filled with flavored tobacco that is placed between the lip and gum; the pouch absorbs the liquid generated and so there is no need to spit out excess "juices," as with regular chew or dip tobacco. Therefore, it allows individuals to use tobacco in virtually any setting, mostly without detection. On the Internet you can learn about products associated with snus (e.g., attractive carrying containers) and view instructional videos on YouTube. A third way that technology has raised new issues is through both the creation of new health problems (e.g., Wii knee problems[2]) and opportunities to address old problems (e.g., among teenagers, playing Wii expends much more energy than sedentary games, thus helping combat adolescent obesity[3]).

There are several key points to be made from this discussion that concern the future of public health. First, as noted in Chapter 1, because public health must "[fulfill] society's interest in assuring conditions in which people can be healthy"[4], public health is a "fluid discipline." As social and environmental conditions change, so do the problems and issues that are important to the public's health. Second, oftentimes the changes that we live through are not planned changes; they come about because of technological advances, natural disasters, or human negligence and/or ignorance. Third, even when changes are planned, they may bring unexpected consequences, either positive or negative. For example, over the past decade states have created **safe haven laws** such that infants can be dropped off at hospitals or other approved sites without penalties to parents. In July 2008, Nebraska created such a law, but the legislators who created it did not define an age limit; thus, legally, it covered "children" up to age eighteen. The result was that some parents dropped off older children, including teenagers, and expected that the state would care for

PUBLIC HEALTH CONNECTIONS 17.1

DIFFUSION OF INNOVATIONS

Have you ever wondered why some products, technologies, or ideas spread through our culture quickly and some never seem to catch hold? This question has fascinated social scientists for over one hundred years, but the science behind the question became fully developed with the work of Everett Rogers in the 1960s. Rogers defined diffusion as "... the process by which an innovation is communicated through certain channels over a period of time among the members of a social system"[1, p. 79]. One of the interesting contributions that Rogers made to the field was to identify what makes an innovation diffuse more quickly.

What makes an innovation diffuse quickly?

1. **Relative advantage:** The innovation is seen to be superior to what it is replacing (for example, a cell phone is more portable than a landline phone).

2. **Compatibility:** The innovation is perceived to be consistent with existing values, past experiences, and needs of potential adopters (both telephones and cameras are consistent with past experiences, so a cell phone that takes pictures diffused quickly).

3. **Complexity:** The innovation is perceived to be easy to understand and use (my cell phone walks me through the steps to do the things I need to do).

4. **Trialability:** An innovation can be experimented with on a limited basis (thus all phone stores allow you to try their products).

5. **Observability:** The results of an innovation can be observed by others (gee, that's a cool cell phone).

their children and that the parents would not be charged with child abandonment. In fact, parents of teens from neighboring states attempted to take advantage of the law. This **unintended effect**, or change brought about by an action that was not planned for, could only be reversed by identifying a reasonable age limit; the state changed the law to apply to infants up to three days old. (And note, this did not resolve the issue of parents who want a respite from their teenagers.) A final point is that public health is a science-based discipline. As such, public health scientists want to go beyond *describing* relationships between phenomena; they want to be able to *predict* what will happen when key individual, social, and environmental factors are changed. Also pointed out in Chapter 1 is that a hallmark of public health is its focus on prevention. All forms of prevention are important, but primary prevention, or preventing a problem before it occurs, is associated with the least amount of disability and suffering. If we are always *reacting* to changes after they occur, we will always be scrambling to catch up, and we will not be able to engage fully in primary prevention.

Can We Plan for the Future?

When we think of the word *future*, we think of a time period, of any length, that has not yet happened. Thus we can think of increments of the future ranging from the most minute (an attosecond) through the very long-term (a millennium). In most cases, both ends of this spectrum would not be useful to us in preparing for public health changes. Oftentimes in public health, we are concerned with planning in increments of time (for example, in the Healthy People goals, we plan in ten-year increments such that we are now concerned with Healthy People 2020,[5]) around visible trends (such as the developed world's aging population), around trends supported by available data (such as climate change), around potential events (including flooding due to a tsunami), and around identified needs (for example, health care for the uninsured).

Have you ever wished you could foresee the future? There is a cadre of scientists, strategists, and policy makers whose work is just that: understanding possible trends that may occur over time. Names for this area of study include *futurist*, *futurology*, and *future studies*. (Of course, you can think of others who support this as their craft, such as fortune-tellers and marketers.) **Futures research** uses a variety of methodological tools such as trend analysis and trend extrapolation (examining trends over time and then projecting where they might go in the future based on different possible scenarios), cyclical pattern analysis (looking for cycles over long periods of time, such as with climate), environmental scanning (keeping sight of events going on around you on a constant basis), and the Delphi (or polling) technique (gathering data from groups of experts until consensus is reached)[6]. For example, in his book, *The Next 100 Years: A Forecast for the 21st Century*, George Friedman[7] paints the geopolitical landscape for the next one hundred years by starting with one important trend, the end of the population explosion, which in turn leads to a shortage of labor in developed countries. This demographic trend can then be seen as being a component contributing to a variety of future scenarios. Next, we discuss trends that may influence the future of public health.

PUBLIC HEALTH CONNECTIONS 17.2

2008 STATE OF THE FUTURE INDEX

The **Millennium Project**[8] is a "global participatory futures research tank of futurists, scholars, business planners, and policy makers who work for international organizations, governments, corporations, nongovernmental organizations (NGOs), and universities." For the past twelve years, they have engaged hundreds of participants in an analysis of evidence concerning the state of the future; they use trends from the past twenty years to predict the next ten years. Their overall assessment for 2008 is in Table 17.1. Additionally, they list yearly fifteen global challenges facing humanity. For 2008, these were sustainable development, clean water, population and resources, democratization, long-term perspectives, global convergence of Internet technology, the rich–poor gap, health issues, capacity to decide (better decision-making processes), peace and conflict, status of women, transnational organized crime, energy, science and technology, and global ethics.

Table 17.1 Millennium Project: Where Is Humanity Winning and Losing?

Where we are winning	Where we are losing
Life expectancy (increasing)	CO_2 (increasing)
Infant mortality (decreasing)	Terrorism (increasing)
Literacy (increasing)	Corruption (increasing)
Gross domestic product (GDP) per capita (increasing)	Global warming (increasing)
Conflict (decreasing)	Voting population (decreasing)
Internet users (increasing)	Unemployment (increasing)

Source: Reference 9.

How Can We Think About the Future of Public Health?

As noted earlier, in thinking about and planning for the future in public health, we can segment situations into categories such as those based on trends we know about, those based on trends we think will happen, and those trends for which we can plan but not precisely predict. Here we give examples of each of these situations.

Trends We Know About

Here we will review four important trends that can affect public health priorities. These include the aging population, the rise in obesity and chronic diseases, inequitable health care access and delivery, and the reemergence of infectious diseases.

The Aging Population

Perhaps the most obvious trend that has the potential to affect health care in the United States is the aging population. Life expectancy in the United States has increased approximately thirty years over the past century[10]. Between 1982 and 2004, the elderly population, defined as people age sixty-five years or older, increased by 34.6 percent, rising to 36.2 million people. It has been commonly assumed that the aging population would mean increased disability, resulting in increases in health care costs associated with rising demand for services in sectors such as rehabilitation and long term care. Recent elderly disability prevalence data do not support this assumption. In fact, the prevalence of disability has been declining among the elderly across the twentieth century, and the rate of decline has been accelerating in recent years, especially between 1999 and 2004[11,12]. These declines have been associated with significant Medicare cost savings[13].

However, there is variability within the broad spectrum of the elderly. Manton and colleagues[14] found that the younger elderly cohort (ages sixty-five to seventy-four) was healthier than the older cohort, and Freedman and coworkers[12] reported inconclusive findings regarding whether severe disability is declining. In addition, prevalence data are not the same as disease burden or demand placed on other types of services, and 20 percent of the elderly still have chronic disabilities[12,14]. In addition, the health care costs associated with the rise in obesity in the United States are likely to offset any potential cost savings associated with declining disability among older adults.

Obesity and Chronic Diseases

The Centers for Disease Control and Prevention (CDC)[15] reported an alarming increase in the prevalence of obesity in the past twenty years in the United States. In 2007, for example, **obesity** (defined as body mass index [BMI] greater than 30 kg/m^2) prevalence ranged from 18.7 percent in Colorado to 32 percent in Mississippi. Collectively, more than 25 percent of the U.S. population meets the criteria for obesity. Obesity is of particular concern because of its interrelationships with other diseases such as type 2 diabetes and heart disease. These chronic diseases are linked to additional morbidity and mortality. Ford and colleagues[16], using data from the National Health and Nutrition Examination Surveys

(NHANES), found that the prevalence of obesity among people with hypertension almost doubled in twenty-five years (from 25.7 to 50.8 percent). During the same time, the prevalence of obesity among people without high blood pressure also increased by 16.7 percent. Because weight management is an important means of preventing or reducing comorbidities associated with obesity, this trend raises concerns regarding the future demand for chronic disease services because people who are obese are more likely to have a disability.

Perhaps more alarming is the finding that the prevalence of childhood obesity has also risen, with the largest increases in BMI among six to seventeen-year-old Black children[17]. Similar to adults, obesity in children is linked to risk factors for cardiovascular disease and diabetes[18], as well as an array of other health problems, such as renal (kidney) disease[19]. Obesity in adolescence has also been linked to obesity in adulthood. For example, the CDC reported that 80 percent of overweight children were obese at age twenty-five. This finding is particularly important because the length of time one is obese may be a critical factor in morbidity. Obesity exposes children to its metabolic consequences over a much longer period of time, creating increased risk for disease complications in adulthood[19]. In addition, specific BMI ranges are associated with risk of subsequent disability in the elderly. For example, using data from the Established Populations for Epidemiologic Studies of the Elderly, Snih and colleagues[20] found that disability-free life expectancy was greatest for those with a BMI between 25 and less than 30. However, more research is required for us to understand the complexity of BMI distribution on health and overall quality of life. It is also important to note that obesity is not just a significant health risk in wealthy countries, such as the United States; the World Health Organization (WHO) indicated obesity is an intermediate risk factor for chronic disease globally[21].

Although public health interventions have contributed to decreases in both cardiovascular disease and stroke-related deaths, chronic diseases remain prevalent across the globe. WHO, in providing the main causes of death on a worldwide scale, indicated chronic diseases accounted for 60 percent (or 36.56 million) deaths in 2007[22]. Another 30 percent was attributed to communicable and maternal diseases and nutritional deficiencies and 9 percent to injuries. Only in low-income countries was infectious disease the largest cause of death. From lower-middle-income to high-income countries, chronic disease represented the largest categorical cause of death (Chapter 1 covers the transitions in types of disease in more detail). In China alone, the yearly economic impact of chronic disease is estimated to be over $500 billion. Chronic disease is also expected to be a long-term public health challenge. By 2030, it is likely the top three causes of disease burden will be HIV/AIDS, depression, and heart disease[23].

WHO estimates that 80 percent of premature heart disease, stroke, and type 2 diabetes is preventable[24]. However, preventive care does not appear to be part of routine health care. The Commonwealth Fund's 2008 International Health Policy Survey in eight countries revealed that in only three countries were more than half the patients with diabetes recommended for four routine care procedures (hemoglobin check, feet and eyes examined, and cholesterol check)[25]. WHO suggests using a stepwise framework of providing core desirable services to address the complex constellation of issues associated with chronic disease, and Shoen and Osborn[25] recommend more integrated systems with a stronger focus on engaging patients, preventative care, broader consideration of alternative provider payment options, and use of technology to enhance information access.

Inequitable Health Care Systems

Access to high-quality care is critical to health optimization. Unfortunately, as you learned in the health disparities chapter (Chapter 16), there are inequities in access and delivery of health care services, as well as socioeconomic, racial, and educational differences in health outcomes. (For example, see Peters and Muraleedharan's[26] description of India's health care sector.) In low-income countries, access to quality care can be limited based on shortages of health professionals and lack of infrastructure or quality monitoring. Perceived satisfaction with care can also directly impact services use[27,28]. However, health disparities are not restricted to developing countries. Over 45 million people in the United States lack health insurance, including 8.1 million children[29]. In addition, coverage varies by ethnicity (higher percentage of uninsured among Latinos and Blacks compared to non-Hispanic Whites). Disparities between urban and rural health care delivery systems are also well documented[30]. Lack of health insurance leads to delayed diagnosis, life-threatening complications, and eighteen thousand premature deaths in the United States each year[31]. Improving access and patient satisfaction could help shift costs away from expensive emergency and tertiary care toward lower cost preventive care. Health care is an interesting paradox: lower use does not mean lower costs; in fact, less use can be the most costly choice of all.

Infectious Disease

Yellow fever and cholera are examples of diseases that re-emerged in the last quarter of the twentieth century. In general, infectious diseases are both appearing and spreading more quickly than in previous generations. The overuse of antibiotics has also made some diseases more resistant to pharmacological intervention. Severe acute respiratory syndrome (SARS), avian influenza, and the appearance of other viral agents such as Ebola have all required significant public health response early in the twenty-first century. The CDC estimates that the swine flu (novel H1N1 influenza) infected approximately 22 million people between the beginning of the outbreak in April and October 17, 2009[32]. Food-processing plants have also become a renewed concern in the spread of food-borne disease, as exemplified in recent illnesses associated with contaminated peanuts and tomatoes. This concern is exacerbated by the global distribution of agricultural products as well as the need to dispose of a host of by-products from consumer consumption. WHO[33] indicated that between 2002 and 2007 over 1,100 epidemic events occurred. SARS, in particular, had the potential to threaten health worldwide given its characteristics. It transmitted person to person; symptoms took more than a week to develop; and it required no vector or particular environment to incubate. (See Chapter 8 for more detail on infectious disease methods.) Public health efforts limited its transmission, but SARS also raised awareness of broken or weak links in infection control efforts. For example, Toronto developed a response plan including communication, infection control, potential quarantine sites, and resource allocation to address the needs of the homeless during an outbreak[34]. Clearly, infectious diseases will remain a threat that requires vigilance in early identification and containment practices.

Trends We Suspect Will Occur

In addition to trends that are already evident, specific global changes are occurring that will likely have even greater influence in future public health planning. Three trends that transcend national borders will be discussed in this section: water shortages, climate change, and technological advances that may affect future health.

Water Shortages

The twentieth century may become known as the century in which dams were the primary means used to capture and control the flow of water. The unintended consequence of such an approach has been that the earth's natural means of managing water, such as flood plains, have been seriously compromised. In many countries, the end result has been contaminated or unavailable water. In addition, water rights agreements across state and country borders are often outdated, reflecting neither current demand nor supply. Did you know that it takes three thousand gallons of water to produce a quarter-pound hamburger based on the grain it takes to feed a cow[31]? Lack of water and contaminated water sources, if not addressed, will contribute to a dramatic rise in illness from the direct effects of contamination and the secondary nutritional effects of depletion of healthy food supplies. The consequences of contaminated water for Bangladesh have already been severe. Water accessed by wells that were set up to compensate for ground level pollution contained unacceptably high levels of arsenic, resulting in health problems associated with arsenic poisoning. Millions of that country's citizens may be affected. In the United States, the Rio Grande has been all but drained near the mouth of the river because of overuse. Damming also increases the chances of a catastrophic flood. For example, if the Three Gorges Dam in China were to break, it could create "the worst manmade disaster in history."[35] There are 350 million people living downstream on the Yangtze River.

It has been only recently that officials cleaning up water supplies and negotiating water rights have begun returning to traditional strategies for water management, such as restoring flood plains and turning to ancient traditions to reinvigorate polluted waterways. One such project is the cleanup of Lake Apopka in Florida using aluminum sulfate, an approach used by ancient Romans. More than a million gallons of polluted water flow into the county waterways from the lake, and this cleanup project (in which aluminum sulfate, used to remove phosphorus, is placed into the water as it flows through a water treatment canal) is considered the largest of its type in the world[36].

Climate change

Similar to illnesses associated with polluted drinking supplies and water shortages, **climate change** has been linked to adverse health outcomes. Also similar to water concerns, climate change is inextricably linked to human consumption. Population growth and our resulting appetite for car and air travel and burning of fossil fuels coupled with deforestation practices have resulted in carbon dioxide emissions that trap solar heat in the earth's atmosphere, warming the earth's surface. The resulting climate change is expected to include rising sea levels and more severe weather, such as floods, droughts, and extreme heat. These unpredictable events can tax the limits of a community's adaptability, psychologically and economically. Although predictions regarding the rate at which warming will continue are controversial, the National Climatic Data Center reported that the last decade of the twentieth century has been the warmest on record[37]. If scientists' predictions are right, the long-term effects of climate change on health could be far reaching unless public health interventions counteract its progression. These public health interventions might include public education and behavioral adaptations, such as managing deforestation, controlling vector-borne disease transmission, and developing drought-resistant crops. The long-term effects of climate change include (1) escalating risk of insect and waterborne diseases; (2) heat stroke, cardiovascular problems, and other serious health consequences for already vulnerable populations; (3) increased respiratory problems from pollution; (4) malnutrition secondary to food shortages as a result of lost agricultural and ocean food productivity; and (5) injury and death from extreme weather events[38,39]. Other secondary effects include displaced people, changed migration patterns, and political conflicts as a result of resource depletion and intolerable regional climate changes. Even though industrialized countries produce the most greenhouse gases, the negative effects are likely to be felt most gravely in developing countries that lack the infrastructure and technology to efficiently manage such threats[38]. However, it should be noted that if the warming trends are mild, positive health effects, such as reduced mortality in winter, are possible[40].

New Technology

The impact of emerging trends will depend in part on technological advances that can be used to improve health operations, prevent and treat disease, and control risk factors. Peters and colleagues[41] illustrated the potential of computer technology as a diagnostic and treatment aid for nonphysician practitioners in poor countries. They showed that patients' satisfaction and visits increased with the implementation of a computer-based decision support program. Other advances directly impact disease outcome. Fewer cardiac deaths in the elderly have been the result of surgical advances[42]. Similarly, the promise of **genomics** to allow manipulation at the intracellular level to cure and prevent the spread of disease is breathtaking. Consider the immediate global impact of a genetic discovery that could prevent HIV infection, which has already led to the deaths of over 20 million people[43].

Although technological advances can clearly move health care forward in unexpected ways, the ethics of these advances sometimes lag behind our technical understanding. Existing screening programs (such as newborn hearing screens and prenatal ultrasound) are predicated on the fundamental belief that knowledge helps aid future decision making, but not everyone desires that knowledge. The ethical complexities of genomics are ambiguous at best. You should worry, for example, about potential discrimination against those who test positive for specific genetic markers in areas such as employment, in social circles, and in health insurance. Scully[44] discussed the ethical considerations of genomics as these relate to how one views disability. For example, does genetic testing for a disability devalue those who have that disability?

Technological advances have also created an increasingly mobile world, which poses unique challenges for managing the public's health. Global travel increases risks for infectious disease transmission, provides easier access to targets for bioterrorists, and taxes infrastructure systems unable to manage significant population shifts or changes in migration patterns. Ease of mobility has demanded attention to policies created to ensure the public's health. Classic examples include limitations to global travel when attempting to contain disease outbreaks, the establishment and enforcement of policies controlling the transportation of plants and animals, and country-specific immigration requirements. However, country-specific policies to manage public health issues cannot be the norm. Merely attempting to control one country's border falls short of the type of comprehensive planning needed to address global concerns. Countries must work collaboratively for successful management of public health issues, not only because we operate in a global economy but also because technology has made it possible to cross any border, thus ensuring the interconnectedness of all people.

Finally, technical advances are not always beneficial to health. The use of iPods is just one behavioral example of technology setting the stage for future health problems, in this case hearing loss. Similarly, the use of the Internet as a health communication tool is a mixed opportunity. The ability to quickly reach across the world to deliver critical health information is being realized, but it is coupled with our inability to control the accuracy or coerciveness of material being presented, potentially creating misperceptions regarding safe health behavior and inappropriately influencing critical decision making. In addition, the availability of technology does not mean people will take advantage of it. For example, in the first comprehensive U.S. study on cancer screening for women with and without diabetes, both groups fell below the recommended Healthy People 2010 screening guideline objectives[45]. Technology clearly represents only one piece of the puzzle in solving pressing public health concerns. A broad-based **social-ecological model** that integrates multiple system considerations will be critical to substantially moving forward on meeting core needs (this model also is discussed in Chapters 2, 11, and 16).

Events We Can Plan But Not Predict

Although sobering, we know that events requiring a comprehensive public health response, such as wars, hurricanes, floods, and infectious disease outbreaks, will all occur. The probable direct outcomes resulting from catastrophic events include economic losses, such as those associated with infrastructure damage, and human losses, including psychological and physical injuries and loss of life. Although the impact of disasters is not totally predictable, the success of disaster response can in large measure be attributed to how refined our layers are within our social-ecological model (including communication links across the system, supply access and mobilization, identified and trained personnel, etc.).

So how do we go about planning to address realized or anticipated problems, especially on a global scale? A core set of tools is emerging to help us understand the magnitude of events, which in turn can help us respond more efficiently and effectively. There are two categories of tools that assist public health professionals in prioritizing resources: datasets that provide information after events have occurred, such as the **Spatial Hazard Event and Loss Database for the United States (SHELDUS)**, and data analyses that attempt to predict the likelihood of future occurrence of events. SHELDUS is one of the most comprehensive data banks for tracking natural disasters, encompassing eighteen different types of hazards by county. Borden and Cutter[46] made analysis adjustments to these data and found that heat/drought was the most likely natural disaster to result in death, causing 19.6% of total hazard-related fatalities in the United States. Severe summer and winter weather ranked second and third, causing 18.8% and 18.1% of total hazard-related deaths, respectively, followed by floods (14%), tornadoes (11.6%), and lightning (11.3%). Natural hazard mortality statistics such as these help us understand where and under what circumstances resources are likely to be most needed in the future. This information can assist local governments in mitigating the effects of such events. They also help public health efforts aimed at educating people living in hazard-prone zones about preparedness and ensuring adequate training of emergency responders for likely events. Currently, however, there is no standardized global classification system for counting hazard-related fatalities such as that used in the United States.

Prediction models commonly use previous datasets to help predict future occurrences or use a set of variables considered predictive of future events based on the empirical literature. For example, knowing that cardiovascular disease is a leading cause of death, and also knowing that hypertension is a major risk factor for cardiac death, you might reasonably include hypertension prevalence data and known costs associated with its prevention and treatment in a model predicting future costs of heart disease.

Similarly, those of us who live in Florida are acutely aware of the predictions made by the National Weather Service regarding the type of hurricane season we are likely to expect each year. This prediction is based on a complex model that accounts for previous years' hurricane frequency and magnitude, weather currents, etc. The importance of this modeling is tied to a state's ability to set aside appropriate resources to mobilize equipment and train personnel who can then effectively respond when a crisis occurs. Underestimating the expected occurrence and likely damage can strain or even deplete emergency response funds; overestimating can unnecessarily delay resource allocation to other public health priorities. This type of delay may ultimately result in a higher cost burden to the state. That said, prediction models go only so far in helping to plan and respond to catastrophic events. The models are only as good as their assumptions, probability is not certainty, and there are many uncontrolled variables that make predictions difficult. Perhaps more importantly, even under the best of circumstances, if these models are not part of a comprehensive approach to addressing risk, systems failure is a likely outcome. Consider the lessons learned from Hurricane Katrina in 2005. Disaster management involves multiple levels of planning and organized response. (The Council on School Health[47] provides a discussion of a coordinated school disaster plan, including preparedness, response, and recovery components.) If these are not based on a coordinated ecological system, the depths of the disaster can tragically result in even more far-reaching consequences, some of which are preventable.

Emergency preparedness is critical to ensuring the health of the population, whether locally or globally. Thus the real value of prediction models is in the ability of public health professionals to use the data provided to ultimately reduce the burden of disease and disability and maximize positive health outcomes either in specific populations or on a more global scale. In essence, these models can influence health policy, aid in the prediction of changes in illness and mortality patterns over time to help plan for future health needs, and track the potential success of public health interventions.

Is It Always Possible To Plan?

The essence of this question assumes that we know how to not only define but also anticipate all of the public health issues in the world, which is not possible. That said, we can anticipate needs and prioritize these based on what we already know from a significant number of individuals and organizations that have experience with different parts of the public health interface. Public health is a wonderful example of the sum being greater than its parts, and many organizations provide core systems to aid in public health efforts, locally to globally. However, we have much we can improve, as identified in the Institute of Medicine reports on the future of public health and keeping the public healthy[31]. These will be discussed later in the chapter.

Being Ready to Meet the Future: What Do We Need?

You have probably thought a lot about the type of future that you want to have, and like most college students, you have probably thought about what you will need to realistically attain that future. Many successful people will tell you that planning and preparing for their lives were essential, but other things, such as being in the right place, being connected to the right person, having a particular skill or interest, or just being lucky, also contributed to attaining their goals. Just as you have envisioned the type of future you want and what you need to do to attain it, public health professionals have engaged in this process at multiple levels, institutional (for example, our imaginary State University), city, county, state, national, and global, to plan for the future of the public's health. It would take an entire book to discuss planning across all of these levels in any amount of detail, so we will briefly discuss two levels, national and global, and some key areas of planning and preparation.

The National Level

In Chapter 2, you read about the agencies at the federal level that are involved in protecting the nation's health; this involves both active involvement in current issues and planning for future events. One prestigious organization, the **Institute of Medicine** (IOM) of the National Academies, plays a key role in tracking the nation's health, recognizing emerging trends, and planning for the future. The IOM is a nonprofit organization whose mission is "to serve as adviser to the nation to improve health."[48] To do this, the IOM "provides unbiased, evidence-based, and authoritative information and advice concerning health and science policy to policy makers, professionals, leaders in every sector of society, and the public at large." In 2003, the IOM published a major statement on health, *The Future of the Public's Health in the 21st Century*. Findings and suggestions from this report continue to make an important contribution to planning for public health across an array of federal agencies. The authors of the report proposed "six areas of action and change to be undertaken by all who work to assure population health."[49, p. 4] These proposed areas are listed in Public Health Connections 17.3.

Let's look briefly at each of these areas of actions and change. The first action should, by now, seem familiar. This action suggests the use of an ecological framework (as in the social-ecological model we discussed) to view the determinants of health. Although on the surface this may seem simple, it actually brings up many ethical, political, and economic issues. For example, if, as we believe, poverty and racism are major contributors to health disparities, to adequately address health issues we must think about solving these systemic problems rather than seeing the solutions as being simply at the individual level.

The second action is based on findings that identified several major issues concerning the infrastructure. Among them are the following:

1. Public health law at the federal, state, and local levels "is often outdated and internally inconsistent."[49, p. 4]

2. A majority of governmental public health workers have little or no training in public health.[49, p. 5]

3. There is a need to harness and better use information and communication technologies.

4. The information-exchange networks among agencies are difficult to use and impede surveillance, reporting, and responding to threats.

5. There is no system for routinely assessing the state of the infrastructure.

6. The state of the nation's laboratories (for rapid identification of potentially harmful substances, for example) needs to be evaluated.

PUBLIC HEALTH CONNECTIONS 17.3
SIX AREAS OF ACTION AND CHANGE

The IOM in *The Future of the Public's Health in the 21st Century,* suggested these areas of action and change:

1. Adopting a population health approach that considers the multiple determinants of health

2. Strengthening the governmental infrastructure, which forms the backbone of the public health system

3. Building a new generation of intersectoral partnerships that also draw on the perspectives and resources of diverse communities and actively engage them in health action

4. Developing systems of accountability to assure the quality and availability of public health services

5. Making evidence the foundation of decision making and the measure of success

6. Enhancing and facilitating communication within the public health system (for example, among all levels of the governmental public health infrastructure and between public health professionals and community members)

Source: Reference 49

These findings depict problems in the infrastructure that need urgent attention.

The third action pertains to the need to build new partnerships to address public health issues, not just the agencies listed in Chapter 2, but beyond those to include providers, communities, the media, employers, and others. The fourth action focuses on the need to be held accountable for the outcomes of our public health programs: Are they actually improving the health of the nation? The fifth action is compatible with a growing trend in health, the use of scientifically sound evidence to make decisions about medical treatments and preventive health measures; that is, when deciding between multiple treatments (for example, for breast cancer), what does the scientific literature say is most effective (and most cost-effective)? This same thinking can be applied to other types of interventions, such as deciding the best way to reduce smoking initiation in middle school students. There is clearly a need to more effectively link research to policy decisions[50]. Finally, the sixth action focuses on the need to improve all forms of communication across agencies and with those outside the public health establishment. Oftentimes, there are so many players involved that efforts are either duplicated or go unnoticed (and unused) because communication is lacking.

This list of actions and changes suggests there is much to accomplish to improve public health efforts on a national basis; remember, these are the suggestions of one agency only. Clearly, however, these actions point to specific structural and policy changes, and they also suggest the types of skills future public health workers might need to cultivate, including communications skills, verbal, written, and visual; the ability to think about systems and the interrelatedness of actions; data analysis skills, including the ability to merge and analyze large datasets; ability to read and interpret the scientific literature; ability to develop and execute evaluation plans; and perhaps most important, creativity to see old problems in new ways and flexibility to adapt to crises and new public health issues.

The Global Level

The World Health Organization (WHO) is an agenda-setting organization at the global level. WHO is the "directing and coordinating authority for health within the United Nations system. It is responsible for providing leadership on global health matters, shaping the health research agenda, setting norms and standards, articulating evidence-based policy options, providing technical support to countries and monitoring and assessing health trends."[51] In 2000, WHO released eight **Millennium Development Goals** to be achieved by 2015, and

PUBLIC HEALTH CONNECTIONS 17.4

HEALTH IN THE MILLENNIUM DEVELOPMENT GOALS

Goal 1: Eradicate extreme poverty and hunger.
Goal 2: Achieve universal primary education.
Goal 3: Promote gender equality and empower women.
Goal 4: Reduce child mortality.
Goal 5: Improve maternal health.
Goal 6: Combat HIV/AIDS, malaria, and other diseases.
Goal 7: Ensure environmental sustainability.
Goal 8: Develop a global partnership for development.

Source: World Health Organization, 2005.

the compact to achieve these goals was signed by 189 countries. In 2005, WHO updated these goals and released a statement on the progress that had been made[52]. The eight goals are presented in Public Health Connections 17.4. At first glance, it may appear that some of these goals have more to do with economics and politics than with public health. However, researchers have found that some of these key indicators are indeed found in countries with higher levels of health. WHO also considers other types of threats to global health; in 2007, they released a report on the major threats to global health security[53]. Security threats include: epidemic-prone diseases (e.g., cholera, yellow fever, Ebola), foodborne diseases, accidental and deliberate outbreaks (e.g., toxic chemical accidents, radionuclear accidents), and environmental disasters.

As with national goals noted above, these global goals call for a workforce that is diverse in skills and abilities. Described below are two examples of interdisciplinary work to solve problems.

Enhancing Data Systems

Clearly critical to successful planning for public health resource allocation are functional approaches to assessment, surveillance, and data analysis. For example, the Global Burden of Disease Studies offered one of the first comprehensive views of global health by attempting to quantify **disability-free life expectancy (DFLE)** and **disability-adjusted life expectancy (DALE)** by variables such as age, sex, and geographic region[54,55]. Such a broad undertaking involved struggles with consistency of definitions and measurements. Nevertheless, the approaches undertaken have had substantial collective value in delineating priorities by identifying significant contributors to morbidity and mortality over time that are potentially responsive to public health intervention.

Consistency across data banks would enhance the utility of data needed to plan public health initiatives. For example, vital statistics registries would significantly aid in global policy decisions. Although WHO has worked to improve these systems in developing countries, consistency of data entry (i.e., extent of coverage in a country) and the comprehensiveness and timeliness of data provided are highly inconsistent. Mathers et al.[56] found that only 23 of 115 countries produced high-quality death registration data (see Chapter 3 for an example of Turkey's vital statistics). Given the cost of implementing such a system, it is not surprising that many low-income countries lack adequate data tracking abilities. However, even higher income countries, such as France and Greece, are producing lesser quality data than are desired. Not having reasonable data on who dies from what and at what age compromises public health planning. Needed changes to existing systems include broader coverage, use of physicians to certify cause of death, and avoidance of ill-defined cause of death codes. For countries without infrastructure, implementing sampling techniques at representative surveillance sites at different geographical locations rather than the more costly countrywide data registries would still provide useful information. WHO continues to address the need to more effectively measure variables associated with mortality[56].

Innovative Partnerships to Address Health Disparities

There are multiple examples of projects around the world addressing health disparities. Social franchising is an example of a partnership that can be used to create more equitable health care access for people living in poverty compared to that provided by private markets. In **social franchising**, small provider groups organize into units under a particular business contract that provides business support, training, and quality monitoring. The providers gain economies of scale for loans, purchases, and brand recognition under the franchised name while maintaining user fees at their local operation. Patients accessing family planning and reproductive services in Pakistan reported higher quality under this model compared to other private or public providers[57].

Another type of partnership focusing on health care delivery is **Future Health Systems**: Innovations for Equity (also known as its abbreviated name, future health systems, or FHS), a research consortium that is working with six low- and middle-income countries to better understand specific health system factors that contribute to a significant health problem within each country[57].

The ultimate goal is to translate findings on how decisions are made into policy that improves health delivery. For example, a project in Afghanistan addresses factors that influence women's decisions to use maternal health services given maternal health in Afghanistan is one of the worst in the world. A project in Nigeria addresses factors that contribute to the vulnerability of people living in poverty to malaria. The goal is to develop an intervention that will guide health system changes[58]. These partnerships incorporate an evidence-policy framework that recognizes the complexity of policy making and the importance of key stakeholders, decision-making processes, and developmental context (e.g. poverty, vulnerability, capability) in health outcomes. This type of model is particularly compelling because it addresses an important criticism of public health interventions: that strategies are implemented without adequate evidence. Peters et al.[41] argued that we do not know what health care delivery strategies work best in low-income countries because our research base is weak, and even when it does exist, it is not linked to decisions. They suggest several basic principles to improve the quality of information being used: (1) define the strategy/intervention in detail; (2) identify uncontrollable factors that can bias results; (3) use a sufficient sample size and systematic methodology for data collection; (4) measure other potential causal factors beyond the strategy of interest, preferably over time and with a comparison group, and (5) draw conclusions based on the data, not the opinions of involved parties.

Being Ready to Meet the Future: Public Health Workforce

State of the Workforce

If you are beginning to think that public health might be a good career choice for you, there is good news, at least from the perspective of a future public health employee; there is widespread consensus that there is a shortage of public health workers[59]. It is anticipated that this shortage will increase as older workers retire and as the demand for public health services increases. How urgent is the situation? The Association of Schools of Public Health presented a policy brief on the issue in 2008[60]. They concluded that by 2020 there would be a national shortfall of 250,000 public health workers. This need is not easily met, and in fact, a finding listed in the brief is that schools of public health would have to train three times the number of workers they now train to catch up. Shortages are predicted to be especially large among public health physicians, public health nurses, epidemiologists, health care educators, and administrators[60].

Now you may be wondering, because public health is an exciting and critical field, why is there a shortage of workers? Think about your own pathway to taking this course. How much did you know or think about public health before you started the course? Did you take the course because you knew it would be interesting to you or for some other reason? In many respects, public health is a hidden field; it encompasses many different types of careers and places to work, and yet it is not often discussed routinely. It is usually during crises such as a natural disaster or an emergent infectious disease that we hear groans about our public health infrastructure! Beyond this, there are other barriers, including inadequate funding at all levels (local, state, national)[59]. This shortage of workers can be felt in concrete ways, as the quote to the right from a report authored by Draper and colleagues illustrates.

Instead, communities have chosen to forgo what would be seen as essential services in many locales. They face delays in getting basic services or having them provided by persons with questionable qualifications. They routinely accept greater risks of health problems arising because of insufficient surveillance or inadequately trained workers. They also may lack the leadership needed to take charge and provide direction in the event of a serious public health crisis. All of these problems will likely worsen as recruitment difficulties persist, retention challenges grow and the wave of approaching retirement crests.[59]

Training and Education Needs

A second issue that has been raised about the public health workforce is that many of the current workers do not have formal training in the field[59] or they may lack important skills that have recently emerged as being necessary to meet new public health threats. Public Health Connections 17.5 lists some of the challenges, according to the American Schools of Public Health, that the public health workforce must meet in the future[60]. Unlike some professions that may require a narrow set of skills, public health professionals need to have a breadth of skills, even those who specialize in a particular area, such as epidemiology or social and behavioral science. During the past few years, **public health competencies**, skills and knowledge that someone trained in public health should be able to demonstrate, have been developed for students receiving the master's of public health (MPH) and doctor of public health (DrPH) degrees. As you might imagine, there are specific competencies for each of the core areas of public health. What might be surprising is that there are cross-cutting competencies as well those that are more general in nature. These competencies fall into the following categories: communication, diversity and cultural proficiency, leadership, professionalism and ethics, program planning and assessment, and systems thinking[61]. What these cross-cutting competency areas illustrate is that public health workers of the future will be challenged to meet complicated health issues that affect diverse groups of people. To meet these challenges requires not only knowledge of the field but also interpersonal skills and sensitivities, a broad view of the interconnectedness of health with other aspects of our society, and a global, multicultural view.

PUBLIC HEALTH CONNECTIONS 17.5

CHALLENGES THE PUBLIC HEALTH WORKFORCE MUST BE PREPARED TO MEET

- Confront emerging communicable diseases such as Ebola virus and avian influenza.

- Meet environmental challenges, including food security and climate change.

- Tackle chronic diseases, including the myriad health consequences of tobacco use and obesity.

- Assist communities in preparing for emergencies such as natural disasters and biological chemical attacks.

- Advocate for policies designed to promote health, for example, increasing access to care and reducing health disparities.

- Promote an emphasis on public education and disease prevention and wellness.

- Conduct research and build evidence for interventions that work.

Source: Reference 60

Being Ready to Meet the Future: Educated Citizens

Congratulations, you have nearly accomplished the first step in becoming an educated citizen in public health: finishing this course. Some of you, through this course, may have found that public health is your future career, some may have found that public health is interesting and important but not the career for you, and some may be saying, "let me out of here!" Whether your future career involves public health or not, we hope that you can see that public health touches virtually every aspect of your life. As you go about your everyday life, we encourage you to see the world through a public health lens so that you are aware of how events and actions around you affect the health of all. Each of the trends we discussed earlier in the chapter illustrates different factors that can impact the public's health. Significant evidence supports the concept that the health of our population has benefited from both clinical advances and risk factor management from a micro to macro level. Consider, for example, that the increased life expectancy in the United States between 1970 and 2000 resulted in an estimated economic value of $3.2 trillion per year, or a total of $95 trillion (yes, trillion)[10]. Although you cannot change your chronological age, you can change how you age by the choices you make continually throughout your lifetime. If you are committed to a healthy life, you must make healthy choices for yourself and your environment today. In addition, as a consumer of health services, you need to be aware of your interrelationship with society and the impact your choices have on your community's ability to help others, whether that community is your hometown or the world. Your choices affect how resources are used and thus the national and global priorities that can be addressed through resource allocation. Understanding what it means to become a globally educated citizen, and doing so, can make a real difference, one person at a time.

Public Health Actions We Can All Take

In 2006, according to the CDC[62], the leading causes of death in eighteen- to twenty-four-year-olds were, in order of frequency of occurrence, unintentional injuries (primarily vehicular crashes), homicide (primarily by guns), and suicide (primarily by guns and suffocation). The next decade in age (twenty-five to thirty-four years old) sees the same three causes but in a slightly different order (unintentional injury, suicide, and homicide); but by ages thirty-five to forty-four, the causes change substantially to unintentional injury, cancer, and heart disease. What is the point of presenting these leading causes of death? There are three. First, it is important to know, statistically, the most important causes of death as you age so that you can think about protective behaviors for yourself, such as not drinking and driving, and for those around you, such as being alert for warning signs of suicide. Second, it is to show that within a scant twenty years, the causes of death in today's college students begin to resemble those of the entire population. Third, it is important to note that all of these causes of death have a large behavioral component. You are part of the public, part of the statistics, and at the most basic level, you can affect public health by leading a healthy lifestyle. This will make you live longer and healthier, you may serve as a role model to others, and you will do your part to lower health care costs.

There are also simple measures to help curb the spread of infectious diseases: wash your hands often (especially when you or those around you are sick), always practice safe sex (especially using a condom), take all prescribed doses of antibiotics or stop only with the direct permission of your physician (to reduce drug-resistant strains of diseases), stay current on your age-appropriate vaccinations, and when you are sick with a virus, stay home and away from others. Obviously, these practices protect your own health, but they also protect the public's health. Here is a way to improve the public's health that you may not have thought about. Did you know that one of the leading causes of disability within our country[63] and worldwide[64] is depression? Even though depression is multi-causal, we can all be agents of public health by treating others with kindness and by being sensitive to the struggles of those around us: be a source of social support within your network.

Finally, it is important to be aware of public health issues that emerge, to think through these issues, develop an informed opinion, and then take actions to support your opinions. These issues might involve the environment (Should plastic bags be banned? How should green space in my community be used? Should certain pesticides be banned?); your community (Should we limit the number of fast food restaurants? Should we fund after-school programs?); at-risk populations (Should we have universal health insurance? Should we fund more drug treatment centers?); and you personally (What is the role of employers in paying for health care?). The key is to stay informed and to take actions to support your beliefs.

Maintaining a Public Health Perspective

Throughout this book, you have learned important concepts and principles related to public health. There are four of these principles that are most central to having a public health perspective. The first is that health is a right not a privilege; every person is entitled to the same opportunities for leading a healthy life. Second, the word *public* applies to everyone; we are all part of the public. Thus when you take on a public health perspective, you are interested in the welfare of all human beings and in the factors that sustain them (e.g., a clean environment, a peaceful nation, high rates of literacy and employment). Third, the social-ecological framework can be used both to frame the causes of problems and to build interventions for their solutions. When we frame problems at a single level, we are being overly simplistic. Not only are most public health problems complex, their causes can be found at multiple levels that often interact with each other. Thus when we think of solutions, it is usually not enough to work at a single level. For example, teaching children living in poverty that they should eat fruits and vegetables (an individual-level intervention) when they have no access to them (a community-level problem) likely will not address the public health issue of poor nutrition in low-income children. And fourth, our lives are interconnected; we interact within social networks, live within communities, have interactions with institutions, are citizens of nations, and increasingly, we mingle with groups globally. These relationships have the potential to sustain us through providing valuable emotional, social, economic, and political resources, but they also have the potential to put us at risk, through exposure to biological, environmental, economic, and political hazards. Protecting the quality of our interconnectedness is critical to protecting public health.

Maintaining an Ethical Perspective

You are probably familiar with the term *ethics* (recall Chapter 1), but maybe you have not thought about how it ties to maintaining a public health perspective in your life and career. At the core of ethical thinking are three principles: **justice** (resource fairness), **beneficence** (facilitating good), and **nonmaleficence** (not harming). At the personal or professional level, we might think of the application of these principles to the individuals with whom we come in contact; for example, we might strive toward treating others fairly in a way that facilitates what is in their best interest (not our own) and in a way that poses no harm. **Public health ethics** has been defined as "the principles and values that help guide actions designed to promote health and prevent injury and disease in the population."[65] This means that instead of thinking about how actions affect individuals, we think about how actions affect the population as a whole. Remember, we can think about a population as representing everything from a relatively small group (e.g., all the students at State University) all the way up to the world's population. At the population level, it is easy to see that sometimes actions taken to help one group may come into conflict with what might help another group; in fact, ethical issues at a population level may include multiple **stakeholders**, the people who have an interest in the outcome of a decision. For example, say there is an outbreak of a highly infectious disease at State University, which is located five miles outside of Central City. Central City health officials decide to place a ten-day quarantine on State University: no one can go on or off campus. Who might be the stakeholders in such a decision? Would there be competing views on what is ethical? Oftentimes it is difficult to gain clarity on what is best for the population's health. Acknowledging this, Bruce Jennings[66] developed a set of steps called an **ethical analysis** to use when trying to clarify and resolve an ethical problem (see Public Health Connections 17.6).

PUBLIC HEALTH CONNECTIONS 17.6
ETHICAL ANALYSIS

Jennings[66, p. 11] suggests that the following steps can be used to analyze public health ethical problems:

1. Identify the ethical problem.

2. Identify the information needed before a responsible decision can be made: What is this information and from whom should it come?

3. Identify the stakeholders in the decision.

4. Articulate the values relevant to this problem.

5. Identify the available options and assess them in light of feasibility (e.g., financial, political, organizational constraints).

6. Discuss the process by which the decision should be made and who should be involved in making it.

Apply these steps to an analysis of this situation between two hypothetical countries.

Centura, a small country in South America, has an infectious disease outbreak. Not having the capacity to manufacture its own supply of vaccines, it quickly drains all available vaccine provided by external agencies. The vaccine was used preventively to stop the spread of the disease, which is nonfatal but creates flulike symptoms lasting a week. Bravera, also a small country, is located adjacent to Centura on its western border. Officials and citizens from Bravera call for Centura to close it borders for at least ten days so that the outbreak can die down and not spread to neighboring regions. Before this can be accomplished, a citizen from Centura, who has contracted the disease but is asymptomatic, travels to Bravera, which sets off a massive outbreak there. Because there is no vaccine, thousands of people contract the disease, resulting in millions of dollars in lost work productivity, cancellation of vacations by foreign travelers, and a few deaths from associated complications. Bravera demands restitution from Centura for the losses incurred.

Summary

In this chapter we have provided some ways to think about the challenges public health professionals and citizens might face in the future. We have discussed challenges that are likely to happen and challenges that we need to be ready to face in case they happen. We have also discussed your role in public health, whether that be as an informed citizen or as a future professional in the field. Although discussing the future raises many uncertainties, there are several things we can count on. First, as we pointed out in the introduction to this chapter, the speed with which technology and social trends emerge and diffuse is unprecedented in human history, and there is no reason to think that these changes will slow down. This guarantees that although many current public health issues will continue to be of concern (obesity, an aging population), new emerging issues will force us to be vigilant and prepared for action. Second, it is likely that no matter where you live or how you live, you will be touched by critical public health issues. Your level of involvement with and understanding of these issues will have a profound effect on your own life, the lives of those close to you, and the lives of all other citizens of the world. Third, there are actions that you can take as a citizen and skills that you can gain as a public health professional that can help address old and new public health challenges and find solutions to them. Finally, if you choose a career in public health, it is likely to never be boring! As we become more interconnected and global in our perspectives, we will be challenged to deal effectively with complex and evolving health issues; this will require commitment, creativity, and flexibility.

Key Terms

beneficence, 441

climate change, 426

diffusion of innovations, 418

disability-adjusted life expectancy (DALE), 434

disability-free life expectancy (DFLE), 434

ethical analysis, 442

Future Health Systems, 435

futures research, 420

genomics, 427

Institute of Medicine, 431

justice, 441

Millennium Development Goals, 433

Millennium Project, 421

nonmaleficence, 441

obesity, 422

public health ethics, 441

public health competencies, 437

safe haven laws, 419

Review Questions

1. Considering the factors that make an innovation diffuse quickly, identify a new product, idea, or technology that you predict will diffuse quickly. Explain your reasoning, touching on the five factors listed in Public Health Connections 17.1.

2. Think about a time in your own life when a new rule or policy had an unintended effect. Describe the rule or policy, what unintended effect occurred, and what was (or should be) changed to make the rule or policy work correctly.

3. Look back over the Millennium Project's fifteen global challenges facing humanity in 2008 (Public Health Connections 17.2). Which of the challenges listed are most strongly related to public health?

4. Select one of the trends we know about (aging population, obesity and chronic diseases, inequitable health care systems, and infectious disease) and write about the extent to which that trend has touched you or someone close to you. What resources were needed to cope with this trend?

5. Use your library, the Internet, or other reliable sources to identify which natural disaster caused the most fatalities in the United States during the past decade. Describe the nature of this disaster and why so many lives were lost.

6. What is climate change and how does it affect the public's health? What actions can individuals and countries take to combat it?

7. If genetic testing were available that would definitely confirm you would develop a chronic disease, would you take that test? Why or why not? What other factors would you consider in making that determination?

8. Discuss the pros and cons of having a career in public health.

9. In your opinion, what would it take to be an educated citizen in relation to public health issues?

10. Describe an issue or situation that you believe is deserving of an ethical analysis. Why did you choose this issue or situation? Is an ethical resolution possible?

References

1. Rogers EM. The diffusion of innovations perspective. In: Weinstein, ND, ed. *Taking Care: Understanding and Encouraging Self-Protective Behavior*. Cambridge: Cambridge University Press; 1987:79–94.

2. Robinson RJ, Barron DA, Grainger AJ, Venkatesh R. Wii knee. *Emerg Radiol.* 2008;15:255–257.

3. Graves L, Stratton G, Ridgers ND, Cable NT. (2008). Energy expenditure in adolescents playing new generation computer games. *Br J Sports Med.* 2008; 42:592–594.

4. Institute of Medicine. *The Future of Public Health*. Washington, D.C.: National Academy Press; 1988.

5. U.S. Department of Health and Human Services. Developing Healthy People 2020 Web page. Healthy People 2020: The road ahead. Available at: www.healthypeople .gov/HP2020/. Accessed May 23, 2010.

6. World Future Society. Methods. Available at: http://beta.wfs.org/methods. Accessed November 6, 2009.

7. Friedman G. *The Next 100 Years: A Forecast for the 21st Century*. New York: Doubleday; 2009.

8. The Millennium Project. Global Studies and Research. Home page. Available at: www.millennium-project.org/index.html. Accessed November 6, 2009.

9. Glenn JC, Gordon TJ, Florescu E. 2008 State of the Future. Executive summary. 2008. Available at: www.millennium-project.org/millennium/SOF2008-English .pdf. Accessed November 6, 2009.

10. Murphy KM, Topel RH. The value of health and longevity. *J Polit Econ.* 2006;114(5):871–904.

11. Manton KG. Recent declines in chronic disability in the elderly U.S. population: Risk factors and future dynamics. *Annu Rev Public Health.* 2008;29:91–113.

12. Freedman VA, Martin LG, Schoeni RF. Recent trends in disability and functioning among older adults in the United States: A systematic review. *JAMA.* 2002;288(24):3137–3146.

13. Manton KG, Lamb VL, Gu, X. Medicare cost effects of recent U.S. disability trends in the elderly: Future implications. *J Aging Health.* 2007;19(3):359–381.

14. Manton KG, Gu, X, Lowrimore GR. Cohort changes in active life expectancy in the U.S. elderly population: Experience from the 1982–2004 National Long-Term Care Survey. *J Geronotol B Psychol Sci Soc Sci.* 2008;63B(5):S269–S281.

15. Centers for Disease Control and Prevention. Overweight and Obesity Web page. U.S. obesity trends: 1985–2007. July 24, 2008. Available at: www.cdc.gov/ nccdphp/dnpa/obesity/trend/maps/index.htm. Accessed January 30, 2009.

16. Ford ES, Zhao G, Li C, Pearson WS, Mokdad AH. Trends in obesity and abdominal obesity among hypertensive and nonhypertensive adults in the United States. *Am J Hypertens.* 2008;21(10):1124–1128.

17. Freedman DS, Khan LK, Serdula MK, Ogden CL, Dietz WH. Racial and ethnic differences in secular trends for childhood BMI, weight, and height. *Obesity*. 2006;14(2):301–308.

18. Centers for Disease Control and Prevention. Overweight and Obesity Web page. Childhood overweight and obesity. November 25, 2008. Available at: www.cdc .gov/nccdphp/dnpa/obesity/childhood/index.htm. Accessed January 30, 2009.

19. Bakker SJL, Gansevoort RT, de Zeeuw D. Metabolic syndrome: A fata morgana? *Nephrol Dial Transplant*. 2007;22:15–20.

20. Snih SA, Ottenbacher KJ, Markides KS, et al. The effect of obesity on disability vs mortality in older Americans. *Arch Intern Med*. 2007;67:774–780.

21. World Health Organization. Obesity. Available at: www.who.int/topics/obesity/en. Accessed November 6, 2009.

22. World Health organization. Face to face with chronic disease. Available at: www.who.int/features/2005/chronic_diseases/en/. Accessed November 6, 2009.

23. Mathers CD, Loncar D. Projections of global mortality and burden of disease from 2002 to 2030. *PLoS Med*. 2006;3(11):2011–2030.

24. World Health Organization Regional Office for Europe. Available at: www.euro.who.int/mediacentre/PR/2006/20060908_1. Accessed November 6, 2009.

25. Schoen C, Osborn R. The Commonwealth Fund. 2008 International Health Policy Survey in eight countries. Available at: www.commonwealthfund.org/ Search.aspx?search=2008+INternational+Health+Policy+Survey+in+Eight+ Countries. Accessed May 23, 2010.

26. Peters DH, Muraleedharan VR. Regulating India's health services: To what end? what future? *Soc Sci Med*. 2008;66:2133–2144.

27. Hansen PM, Peters DH, Niayesh H, et al. Measuring and managing progress in the establishment of basic health services: The Afghanistan health sector balanced scorecard. *Int J Health Plan Manage*. 2008;23:107–117.

28. Peters DH, Kohli M, Mascarenhas M, Rao K. Can computers improve patient care by primary health care workers in India? *Int J Qual Health Care*. 2006;18(6): 437–445.

29. U.S. Bureau of the Census. Income, Poverty, and Health Insurance Coverage in the United States: 2007. Current Population Reports No. P60–235. Washington, D.C.: Government Printing Office; 2008.

30. Reynolds W, Page S, Johnston M. Coordinated and adequately funded state streams for rehabilitation of newly injured persons with TBI. *J Head Trauma Rehabil*. 2001;16(1):34–46.

31. Institute of Medicine. *Insuring America's Health: Principles and Recommendations*. Washington, D.C.: National Academies Press; 2004.

32. Centers for Disease Control and Prevention. CDC estimates of 2009 H1N1 influenza cases, hospitalizations, and deaths in the united states, April-October 17, 2009; Reported November 12, 2009. Available at: www.cdc.gov/h1n1flu/estimates_2009_ h1n1.htm. Accessed November 23, 2009.

33. World Health Organization. The world health report 2007: A safer future. Global public health security in the 21st century. Overview. Available at: www.who.int/whr/2007/overview/en/print.html. Accessed May 23, 2010.

34. Leung CS, Ho MM, Kiss A, Gundlapalli AV, Hwang SW. Homelessness and the response to emerging infectious disease outbreaks: Lessons from SARS. *J Urban Health*. 2008;85(3):402–410.

35. Pearce F. *When the Rivers Run Dry: Water—The Defining Crisis of the Twenty-first Century*. Boston, Mass: Beacon Press; 2006.

36. State using ancient remedy to treat Lake Apopka. *The Gainesville Su*. Feb. 15, 2009:5B.

37. The National Climatic Data Center. NOAA Paleoclimatology Program. A paleo perspective on global warming. Available at: www.ncdc.noaa.gov/paleo/globalwarming/home.html. Accessed November 23, 2009.

38. Kasotia P. The health effects of global warming: developing countries are the most vulnerable. *UN Chronicle* Online Edition. Available at: www.un.org/pubs/chronicle/2007/issue2/0207p48.htm. Accessed May 23, 2009.

39. Shannon MW, Best D, Binns HJ, et al. Global climate change and children's health. *Pediatrics*. 2007;120(5):1149–1152.

40. Moore TG. Health and amenity effects of global warming. Revised May 1996. Hoover Institution, Stanford University. Available at: www.stanford.edu/~moore/health.html. Accessed May 23, 2010.

41. Peters DH, Bloom G, Rahman M. Research for future health systems. *Global Forum Update on Research for Health*. 2006;3:133–137.

42. Manton KG, Stallard E, Corder L. Changes in the age dependence of mortality and disability: Cohort and other determinants. *Demography*. 1997;34:135–157.

43. World Health Organization. The world health report 2004. Preventing chronic diseases: A vital investment. Available at: www.who.int/whr/2004/chapter1/en/index1.html. Accessed May 23, 2010.

44. Scully JL. Disability and genetics in the era of genomic medicine. *Nat Rev Genet*. 2008;9:797–802.

45. Zhao G, Ford ES, Ahluwalia IB, Li C, Mokdad AH. Prevalence and trends of receipt of cancer screenings among us women with diagnosed diabetes. *J Gen Intern Med*. 2008;24(2):270–275.

46. Borden KA, Cutter SL. Spatial patterns of natural hazards mortality in the United States. *Int J Health Geogr*. 2008;7(1):64–76.

47. Council on School Health, Murray RD, Gereige RS, et al. Disaster planning for schools. *Pediatrics*. 2008;122(4):895–901.

48. Institute of Medicine. About the IOM. Available at: www.iom.edu/en/About-IOM.aspx. Accessed November 6, 2009.

49. Institute of Medicine. *The Future of the Public's Health in the 21st Century*. Washington, D.C.: National Academies Press; 2004.

50. Hyder AA, Bloom G, Leach M, et al. Exploring health systems research and its influence on policy processes in low income countries. *BMC Public Health*. 2007;7:309–320.

51. World Health Organization. About WHO. Available at: www.who.int/about/en/. Accessed November 6, 2009.

52. World Health Organization. Health and the Millennium Development Goals. 2005. Available at: www.who.int/hdp/publications/mdg_en.pdf. Accessed May 23, 2010.

53. World Health Organization. *A Safer Future: Global Public Health Security in the 21st Century.* Nonserial Publication. World Health Organization; 2007.

54. Murray CJL, Lopez AD. Mortality by cause for eight regions of the world: Global burden of disease study. *Lancet.* 1997;349:1269–1276.

55. Lopez AD, Mathers CD, Ezzati M, Jamison DT, Murray CJL. Global and regional burden of disease and risk factors, 2001: Systematic analysis of population health data. *Lancet.* 2006;364:1747–1757.

56. Mathers CD, Fat DM, Inoue M, Rao C, Lopez AD. Counting the dead and what they died from: An assessment of the global status of cause of death data. *Bull World Health Organ.* 2005;83(3):171–177.

57. Bishai DM, Shah NM, Walker DG, Brieger WR, Peters DH. Social franchising to improve quality and access in private health care in developing countries. *Harvard Health Policy Review.* 2008;9(1):184–197.

58. Syed SB, Hyder AA, Bloom G, et al. Exploring evidence-policy linkages in health research plans: A case study from six countries. *Health Res Policy Syst.* 2008;6:4–13.

59. Draper DA, Hurley RE, Lauer J. Public health workforce shortages imperil nation, Research Brief No. 4. Center for Studying Health System Change. 2008. Available at: www.hscchange.org/CONTENT/979/.

60. Association of Schools of Public Health. ASPH Policy Brief Confronting the Public Health Workforce Crisis. Executive Summary. Washington, D.C.: ASPH, 2008.

61. Calhoun JG, Ramiah K, Weist EM, Shortell SM. Development of a core competency model for the master of public health degree. *Am J Public Health.* 2008;98:1598–1607.

62. Centers for Disease Control. WISQARS leading causes of death reports, 1999–2006. Available at: http://webapp.cdc.gov/sasweb/ncipc/leadcaus10.html. Accessed November 6, 2009.

63. Pratt LA, Brody DJ. Depression in the United States Household Population, 2005–2006. NCHS data brief No. 7. National Center for Health Statistics. September, 2008. Available at: www.cdc.gov/nchs/data/databriefs/db07.pdf. Accessed November 6, 2009.

64. World Health Organization. Depression. Available at: www.who.int/mental_health/management/depression/definition/en/. Accessed November 6, 2009.

65. Gostin LO. (2003) Tradition, profession, and values in public health. In: Jennings B, Kahn J, Mastroianni A, Parker LS, eds. *Ethics and Public Health: Model Curriculum.* ASPH; 2003:13–20. Available at: www.asph.org/document.cfm?page=723. Accessed May 23, 2010.

66. Jennings B. Introduction: A strategy for discussing ethical issues in public health. In: Jennings B, Kahn J, Mastroianni A, Parker LS, eds. *Ethics and Public Health: Model Curriculum.* ASPH; 2003:1–12. Available at: www.asph.org/document.cfm?page=723. Accessed May 23, 2010.

GLOSSARY

Numbers in parentheses following a glossary term indicate the chapters in which the word, phrase, or acronym was listed as a key term.

A

abstract (5)
> In a research article, a brief summary of the entire article, typically comprising a sentence or two from each section of the work to provide readers a brief overview of the design and findings of the study.

acceptability (15)
> One of the dimensions of access in the framework by Penchansky and Thomas, it is the relationship of clients' attitudes about personal and practice characteristics of providers to the actual characteristics of existing providers, as well as provider attitudes about acceptable personal characteristics of clients.

accessibility (15)
> One of the dimensions of access in the framework by Penchansky and Thomas, it is the relationship between the location of supply and the location of clients, taking into account client transportation resources and travel time, distance, and cost.

accommodation (15)
> One of the dimensions of access in the framework by Penchansky and Thomas, it is the relationship between the manner in which the supply resources are organized to accept clients; the clients' ability to accommodate to these factors; and the clients' perception of their appropriateness.

acid fast (13)
A property of microorganisms, usually bacteria, such that, even after staining and subsequent rinsing with acid, the stain remains in the organism's cell wall.

acquired immune deficiency syndrome (AIDS) (8)
The late clinical stage of HIV infection that is classified based on $CD4^+$ cell counts and is associated with opportunistic infections and specific types of cancers.

action stage (11)
A stage from the stages of change or transtheoretical model in which the individual has changed a behavior for less than 6 months.

active surveillance (3)
Seeking out individuals who are newly exposed or diagnosed by contacting health care providers or by searching medical records.

activity pattern (10)
The sequence and duration of activities performed by a person during a specified period of time that are relevant to exposures.

additive (10)
In toxicology, the response of a target organism to multiple agents that produce biological effects independently of one another: effects are simply added together.

adjusted odds ratio (6)
To statistically modify an odds ratio, most often to account for confounding variables.

adjusted rate (4)
A rate that has been statistically modified to account for some characteristic(s) of the population, such as age or gender.

administrative information systems (15)
Systems used to assist in managing financial and administrative data within an organization, including billing, resource management, budgeting, and cost control.

adverse events (3)
Negative side effects associated with a drug or treatment.

affordability (15)
One of the dimensions of access in the framework by Penchansky and Thomas, it is the relationship of prices of services and providers' insurance

or deposit requirements to the clients' income, ability to pay, and existing health insurance.

airborne transmission (8)
A method of transmitting infectious agents in which the source releases the microbe into the air, usually by breathing, coughing, or spitting, and the host comes in contact with it.

alpha particles (9)
Energetic, positively charged particles consisting of two protons and two neutrons.

American Medical Association (AMA) (14)
Founded in 1847, a leading professional organization for physicians. It played a major role in state-level legislation for physician licensing and founded the Council on Medical Education to accredit medical schools.

analytic epidemiology (4, 5)
The branch of epidemiology that seeks to quantify the relationship between exposure (risk factor) and outcome.

Andersen framework (15)
The dominant theoretical approach to evaluating health care access, developed by Ronald Andersen in 1968. The framework views access as a function of three categories of variables: (1) predisposing factors, (2) enabling factors, and (3) an individual's need for health care.

antagonism (10)
In toxicology, the interaction of two or more agents that results in lesser effects than could be anticipated if each agent was considered individually.

apothecaries (14)
People who created and dispensed curative remedies.

appraisal support (11)
A type of social support, providing constructive and useful feedback and affirmations for self-evaluation.

assessment (2, 4)
One of the three core functions of public health, it includes gathering information about a health problem in order to create a clear picture of the situation that needs to be addressed, its potential causes, and which groups of people are most affected.

assurance (2)

One of the three core functions of public health, it includes making certain that public money and resources are being used responsibly to carry out policies and monitoring the success of public health programs so they can be changed or discontinued as deemed appropriate.

asthma (9)

A chronic respiratory disease commonly diagnosed among children that is characterized by frequent episodic wheezing, shortness of breath, tightening of the chest, and coughing.

attack rate (8)

The number of people who become ill after being exposed to a substance (cases) out of the number of susceptible people.

attenuate (5, 13)

Weaken. In epidemiology, to reduce the strength of a measure. In infectious disease, to make a bacteria or virus less virulent.

audit trail (12)

Documenting how and when analytic decisions were made in a research study.

availability (15)

One of the dimensions of access in the framework by Penchansky and Thomas, it is the relationship of the volume and type of existing services or resources to the clients' volume and types of needs.

axial coding (12)

Reviewing data for the purpose of more richly coding on a particular theme. See also coding.

B

background (5)

In a research article, the opening section that includes an overview of the problem, the current state of knowledge on the topic, and the rationale for the current research. Also called the introduction.

barriers to care (14)

Factors that limit a person's access to or use of health services.

baseline (6)

A value or measurement made at the beginning of a research study or during a pretreatment visit.

BCG vaccine (13)

A vaccine for tuberculosis named after the French scientists (Bacille, Calmette, and Guerin) who first produced the vaccine from an attenuated strain of *Mycobacterium tuberculosis*.

Belmont Report (1)

A framework for the ethical design and conduct of research involving human subjects, created by the National Commission for the Protection of Human Subjects of Biomedical and Behavioral Research in 1976; it distinguishes research from practice, outlines three basic ethical principles (respect for persons, beneficence, and justice), and lists specific requirements to meet the ethical principles (informed consent, assessment of risks and benefits, and fair selection of subjects).

beneficence (17)

Facilitating good; one of the three core principles of public health ethics. In the Belmont Report, beneficence refers to the obligation to do no harm to human subjects and to maximize benefits and minimize harm in research.

beta particles (9)

Fast-moving electrons emitted from the nucleus during radioactive decay.

bias (5, 6)

A systematic difference between the results of a study and the true measure.

biologically plausible (5)

The concept that an exposure-outcome relationship makes sense, with or without a specific biological mechanism.

biomarker (10)

Any chemical that can be measured in the body or in bodily fluids and that reveals information about exposure to that chemical or another biochemically related one.

biomonitoring (9)

Collecting biological samples from individuals to assess chemical exposures.

biostatistics (1)

A branch of statistics that is devoted to understanding health and health outcomes and that provides the analytic tools to assess and interpret public health data and complex studies.

bivariate (6)

Data description that focuses on two measurements at a time.

blinding (5)
Preventing an individual from knowing the exposure status of a research participant.

Blue Cross (14)
Developed as a nonprofit insurance plan for hospital services (a prepaid hospital services plan) in 1929.

Blue Shield (14)
Developed as a nonprofit insurance plan for non-hospital medical services in 1939.

bundled payments (15)
Paying hospitals and physicians a combined fee for all the care associated with a given patient episode.

C

Calmette, Albert (13)
A French physician, microbiologist, and immunologist who developed the BCG vaccine for tuberculosis in the early twentieth century with his colleague Camille Guerin.

Canada Health Act (2)
Legislation passed in 1980 that established a comprehensive single-payer health care system and guaranteed access to medical care for all Canadians regardless of ability to pay, age, or health status.

cancer (9)
A broad term used to describe the rapid growth of abnormal cells beyond their typical boundaries that have the potential to spread (metastasize) from one organ or cell type to another.

capitation (14, 15)
A payment method used by managed care plans in which a provider is given a fixed amount of money, paid in advance, per patient per month for the delivery of health care services, regardless of actual services provided.

carbon monoxide (9)
A compound created during incomplete combustion processes that can bind to hemoglobin and cause hypoxia.

cardiovascular diseases (16)
A group of diseases that affect the heart and vascular system and includes high blood pressure, coronary heart disease (including myocardial infarction and angina pectoris), heart failure, and stroke.

case (5, 8)
A person with the disease or outcome of interest. In infectious disease, a person who has clinical signs of an infection.

case definition (3)
A thorough description of quantifiable and objective clinical symptoms, diagnostic criteria, or exposure classification used to identify someone as having an exposure or outcome.

case-control study (5)
An observational study in which participants are sampled based on the outcome; a group of people with the outcome and a group of people without the outcome are selected, and their past exposures are assessed and compared.

causal inference (5)
The process of determining whether an exposure causes an outcome in an observational study based on the available evidence for temporal sequence, strength of association, consistency, biological plausibility, and dose-response.

Census (3)
An accounting of all citizens, done every ten years in the United States.

census tracts (16)
Small, relatively permanent statistical subdivisions of a county of 1,500 to 8,000 people each.

Centers for Disease Control and Prevention (CDC) (2)
One of the agencies within the Department of Health and Human Services that works to protect health and promote quality of life through the prevention and control of disease, injury, and disability.

Centers for Medicare & Medicaid Services (2, 15)
The agency within the U.S. Department of Health and Human Services responsible for overseeing and administering Medicare, Medicaid, and the Children's Health Insurance Program.

chain of infection (8)
The steps in the spread of an infectious disease; includes a source of the infection, a host for the infection, and a method for carrying the infection from the source to the host.

Children's Health Insurance Program (CHIP) (14)
A program designed to provide health coverage to uninsured children and pregnant women in families with incomes too high to qualify for most state

Medicaid programs and too low to afford private insurance coverage. Created in 1997 under Title XXI of the Social Security Act, CHIP is subject to federal guidelines, but states have flexibility in establishing eligibility requirements and covered benefits.

climate change (17)

Changes in the earth's temperature and weather patterns.

clinical information systems (15)

A computerized data system used to manage administrative, financial, and treatment-related information within a health care facility.

clinical phase (7)

A phase of the drug approval process in which a drug is tested on humans (there are three clinical phases in the United States).

coding (12)

In qualitative data analysis, reading the data, identifying major themes, and assigning labels to and defining categories that emerge.

cognitive dissonance (10)

In social psychology, the uncomfortable feeling that results from holding conflicting information or theories in our mind. According to this psychological model, we resolve the dissonance by rejecting the information that causes the most inconsistencies.

cohort (6)

A group of individuals with the same exposure status.

cohort study (5)

An observational study in which the incidence of the outcome is compared in an exposed group of people and an unexposed group of people; subject participants are sampled based on exposure.

collapse therapy (13)

Prior to the use of medications for the treatment of tuberculosis, it was believed that collapsing the portions of the lung affected by tuberculosis would eventually cure the disease.

commercial insurer (14)

A company that sells life and casualty insurance.

communicability (3)

The ease with which a health outcome (disease) spreads within a population; one of the criteria used to determine whether surveillance will be conducted on a health outcome.

community (11)

A group within which individuals feel a sense of belonging. Communities can be defined in a number of ways, such as geographic location, shared interests, shared identities, and ability to harness collective power.

community assets (11)

Strengths and resourses available to, and within, a community.

community coalitions (11)

Broad groups that bring together individuals, groups, and organizations around a particular issue.

community competence (11)

A community's ability to engage in problem solving by collectively identifying common needs; by establishing agreed-upon goals, priorities, and strategies for meeting these needs; and by undertaking necessary action.

community focus (12)

Used in ethnography when an entire community is the focus of the research.

community immunity (8)

The concept that not all members of a population need to be immunized against an infectious disease because being a member of a group (community) that is largely immune to an agent reduces the chance that a susceptible member of the group will contact an infected member. Also called herd immunity.

community level (2)

Level of the social-ecological framework in which the target of change is the community (neighborhood, school, workplace) and the focus is on changing a policy or the group perception or norms.

community needs (11)

Concrete or abstract strengths and resources that are not currently available or realized in a community. Needs reflect the reality of how things are versus how they should be for individuals, groups, and communities.

community organizer (11)

An individual who challenges individuals, groups, and communities to act on behalf of their common interests.

community organizing (11)

The process of helping communities to identify common interests and problems and to collectively set goals and strategies to overcome identified problems.

community trial (5)
A type of experimental study design in which the unit of analysis is the group rather than the individual.

community-based participatory research (11)
An approach to conducting research that emphasizes the engagement of community partners in all phases of the research (and intervention or programming) process.

comparative effectiveness research (7, 15)
Evaluating the impact of different treatment options on a particular set of patients to identify the most effective strategy.

comparative safety study (7)
A study in which the safety of two treatment options is compared.

complete-case analysis (6)
The practice of including only individuals who have valid data points for all measures in an analysis.

complexity (of a social network) (11)
Description of a social network pertaining to the variety of functions the network serves the individual.

component vaccine (8)
A vaccine that is made up of only the parts of the microbe to which the immune system will react.

concepts (11)
The primary structures or building blocks of theory.

conclusion (5)
In a research article, the final section in which the authors explain the implications of their findings.

confidence interval (6)
A random interval, computed based on the random sample, which has a 95 percent probability of including the population odds ratio.

confounder (4, 5, 6)
A variable other than the exposure of interest that may confuse or change the relationship between the exposure of interest and the outcome of interest.

confounding bias (4, 5, 6)

Confounding occurs when some factor other than the exposure of interest obscures or confuses the relationship between the exposure and outcome of interest.

confounding by indication (6, 7)

Confounding bias that occurs when individuals' exposure status is a result of an underlying need (indication) for exposure; for example, individuals who have a severe form of disease may be prescribed a different form of medication than individuals with less severe forms and therefore a direct comparison of the outcomes of the two groups would be confounded.

confounding by severity (7)

Confounding bias that occurs when a patient will preferably use a medication due to a certain risk that is a direct risk factor for the outcome. In this scenario, the confounder is the severity of the disease the drug is supposed to treat.

confounding by time (7)

Confounding bias that occurs when disease progression (or the treatment effect) over time results in preferential drug use.

congruence (12)

The way in which what the researcher asks, where he or she asks it, and how he or she works toward an answer all fit together.

consciousness raising (11)

One of the behavior change strategies of the stages of change or transtheoretical model; it involves learning new information that supports the need and motivation for behavior change.

consistency (5)

The consideration of whether the results of the current study are the same or different from previous studies on the topic.

constructs (11)

Key concepts that are named and defined for use in a particular theory.

contact investigation (13)

The process in which the contacts to an infectious case are screened for infection and disease and offered treatment if they are found to be infected.

contact rate (10)

The rate at which an exposed organism comes into contact with the media where a contaminant is present. This may be the inhalation rate, the amount and frequency a certain food is ingested, etc.

contact tracing (8)

In infectious disease outbreak investigations, the practice of identifying all persons with whom an infected individual has come into contact and may have exposed to the disease.

contact transmission (8)

The specific method of getting the infection from the source to the host; may be direct or indirect.

contemplation stage (11)

A stage of the stages of change or transtheoretical model in which an individual intends to change behavior in the next six months.

continuous quality improvement (15)

An approach to organizational management that emphasizes providing high-quality, efficient, and scientifically sound processes.

continuous source (8)

A type of infectious disease outbreak scenario in which there is a single source of ongoing exposure that is infecting people.

control (subject) (5)

In a research study, an individual who does not have the outcome or disease of interest.

control group (6)

The collection of individuals in an experimental study who are not exposed or who receive a placebo.

convenience sampling (12)

A sample derived by talking with whomever is available and willing to participate in the research study.

conventional insurance (14)

An insurance plan that pays a portion of the health care costs after a deductible is met. These plans cover care provided by any providers and hospitals and requires that either the provider or patient file a claim to receive reimbursement for care provided. (Also called indemnity insurance.)

copayment (14)

The amount of money an individual with insurance coverage must pay at the time of health service delivery.

core functions (2)

The central activities of a field; in public health, the core functions are assessment, policy development, and assurance.

correlation (5)

A measure of the degree to which two variables are associated.

cost (3)

The financial or human (morbidity, mortality, productivity) loss associated with a health outcome or exposure; one of the criteria used to determine whether surveillance will be conducted on a health outcome.

count (4)

The number of individuals experiencing an event or exposure of interest.

counterconditioning (11)

One of the behavior change strategies of the stages of change or transtheoretical model; it involves identifying healthier alternative behaviors for unhealthy behaviors.

criteria air pollutants (9)

Six compounds (particulate matter, sulfur dioxide, nitrogen oxide, ozone, carbon monoxide, and lead) named in the Clean Air Act for which the EPA has acceptable levels and which it monitors regularly.

critical collaborative ethnography (12)

Includes participatory, action-based, indigenous, and collaborative ethnographic practices that focus on resistance, social change, and political action.

critical consciousness (11)

The community's awareness of the underlying or root causes of the way things are. Often, critical consciousness involves or leads to action for social change.

cross-sectional study (5)

A type of observational study in which exposure and outcome information are collected at the same point in time.

crude odds ratio (6)

An odds ratio calculated directly from a 2×2 table without accounting for any confounding variables.

crude rate (4)
A rate calculated directly from surveillance or other data without adjusting for demographic or other variables.

cues to action (11)
A construct of Health Belief Model. The individual's exposure to internal or external prompts or reminders to change their health behavior.

cultural barriers (15)
Factors that inhibit people who need medical attention from seeking it, or once they obtain care, from following recommended posttreatment guidelines.

D

data (6)
Pieces of information used in a study.

deductible (14)
The portion or amount that an insured individual must pay first before the insurance company will begin to pay for services.

deductive reasoning (12)
Moving from cause to effect (general to specific).

density (of a social network) (11)
Description of a social network that pertains to how well members of the network know each other and interact.

Department of Health and Human Services (HHS) (2, 14)
The primary federal department responsible for health and health care in the United States. It comprises the Office of the Secretary and eleven agencies, including the Centers for Disease Control and Prevention, Food and Drug Administration, and National Institutes of Health.

Department of Veteran Affairs (VA) (2)
The agency responsible for providing military veterans with a wide range of benefits, including health care as a single-payer health system, in which the government acts as the financer and provider of health services for the covered population.

dependent variable (5)
The outcome in an epidemiological study.

descriptive (6)

Using numerical and graphical techniques to describe a sample.

descriptive epidemiology (4, 8)

Classifying a health event or exposure based on person, place, and time variables.

detection bias (16)

Documenting a higher rate of disease among a group because of increased awareness among that group or higher perceived susceptibility within the population.

diagnosis-related group (15)

A way to classify hospital patients based on clinical information, including the principal diagnosis (why the patient was admitted), complications and comorbidities (other secondary diagnoses), surgical procedures, and demographic factors.

dichotomize (5, 6)

To classify people or responses into two groups.

differential misclassification (5)

Inaccurately classifying study participants and doing so differently based on their exposure or outcome status.

diffusion of innovations (17)

The spreading of both the prevalence of new products and behaviors and instructions on how to perform them.

direct transmission (8, 9)

Occurs when the source touches the host and transmits infection.

directly observed therapy (13)

The standard of care for patients with active tuberculosis in which patients are given anti-TB medications and are observed taking every dose, usually by health department staff or other medical personnel.

disability-adjusted life expectancy (DALE) (17)

The number of years an individual in a population is expected to live adjusted for disability.

disability-adjusted life years (10, 15)

A measure of the years of life lost due to premature mortality and the years of productive life lost due to disability.

disability-free life expectancy (DFLE) (17)

The number of years an individual in a population is expected to live without disability.

discrimination (16)

The differential actions toward others that are a result of racism.

discussion (5)

In a research study, the section that includes the data interpretation. It may cite other studies that have found similar or different results and suggest reasons for these differences, include a synopsis of the study's strengths and weaknesses, describe the meaning of the work in the larger context of the field, and suggest future areas of study.

Donabedian's quality model (15)

A conceptual framework that helps define and measure quality in health care organizations by focusing on three domains: structure, process, and outcomes.

dose (10)

The amount of a chemical agent that crosses the boundary of an exposed individual.

dose response (5, 9)

The pattern that exists between exposure and outcome along a gradient; a variation in the level of outcome that occurs in response to a variation in the level of exposure.

dose-response assessment (10)

The process of finding out (quantitatively) how potent an agent is.

double-blind study (5)

An experimental study in which neither the subject nor the researcher knows to which exposure group the subject has been randomized.

Dracunculiasis (8)

A disease caused by a parasite, *Dracunculiasis medinensis*, which can invade the intestinal wall and migrate to the body's extremities. The disease is contracted when a person drinks stagnant water contaminated with the larvae of the parasite or walks unprotected in infected waterways. Also called Guinea worm disease.

dramatic relief (11)

One of the behavior change strategies of the stages of change or transtheoretical model. Involves provoking and highlighting negative emotions associated with unhealthy behavior.

drug utilization study (7)

A study that evaluates factors associated with the use of a specific medication, including time, place, or population.

E

ecological fallacy (5)

Inappropriately using results from a population-level (group-level) study to make an inference at the individual level.

ecological study (5)

A type of observational epidemiological study in which the unit of analysis is the population (group) rather than the individual.

effectiveness study (7)

A study designed to quantify the real-life drug effect.

emotional support (11)

A type of social support in which a person offers expressions of empathy, love, and caring.

Employee Retirement and Income Security Act of 1974 (ERISA) (14)

Legislation that exempted employers from minimum benefit mandates under state law and provided the advantage for employers to design benefit packages tailored to their employee population.

employer-based health insurance (14)

Group health insurance coverage provided through, and often paid for in part by, an employer.

empowerment (11)

A process through which individuals develop the belief in their ability to make a difference in their own lives and in the lives of others.

enabling factors (15)

A component of the Andersen model of health care access; includes the availability of providers in a community, an individual's insurance coverage, and existence of a regular source of care.

endemic (1, 4, 8, 9)

A disease that is typically present in a given population. The term may also denote the rate at which a disease is expected to occur.

environment (9)

The external world, including personal, occupational, social, and physical environments.

environmental epidemiology (9)

The study of the effect on human health of physical, biological, and chemical factors in the external environment, broadly conceived.

environmental health (1, 9)

The study of the relationship between the environment (broadly defined; may include the physical or social environment) and health and the impact of various exposures on health.

environmental justice (9)

Equitably distributing the risks associated with an environmental toxicant across a community.

Environmental Protection Agency (EPA) (2)

The agency is responsible for developing and enforcing environmental regulations for such areas as clean air and water; giving grants to fund state environmental programs, nonprofits, and educational institutions; conducting research on environmental issues; teaching the public about the environment; and sponsoring partnerships in the United States.

environmental reevaluation (11)

One of the behavior change strategies of the stages of change or transtheoretical model; it involves acknowledging the negative impact of unhealthy behavior on important others.

epidemic (1, 4, 8, 9)

A disease that occurs at a higher than expected frequency or rate within a population.

epidemic curve (8)

A graph of the number of infections per unit of time that can be used to identify the type of outbreak and possible mechanisms of spread.

epidemiology (1, 4)

The study of the distribution and determinants of health, outcomes, and disease in a population. Literally, the study of that which is upon the people.

equity of access (15)

A measure of the even and fair distribution of health care use.

eradication (8)

Completely eliminating an infectious disease. To date, only smallpox has been eradicated.

ethical analysis (17)

A set of steps, developed by Bruce Jennings, to use when trying to clarify and resolve an ethical problem.

ethics, public health

See public health ethics.

ethnographic data collection (12)

The process of collecting information by observing and participating in various activities and interviewing participants within the target group or community.

ethnography (12)

A qualitative method that uses observations, interviews, and other existing data such as reports, photos, and diaries as a means of exploring cultural groups or problems embedded in sociocultural groups or networks.

etiology (1, 4)

The biological basis or cause of a disease.

exclusion criteria (5)

Factors or characteristics (for example, age or existing health conditions) that make a person ineligible to participate in a research study or clinical trial.

experimental study (5)

A study in which a researcher assigns participants to an exposure and follows them over time to assess the incidence of the outcome of interest.

exposure (4, 5, 10)

In general, the independent variable under investigation in a study. In environmental studies, the extent of contact between a hazardous agent and an individual or population.

exposure assessment (10)

The process of estimating (quantitatively) the amount of contact between an agent and a target individual or population.

exposure science (10)

The discipline that studies how individuals and populations come into contact with hazardous agents, including a quantification of that contact.

extrapulmonary disease (13)
Tuberculosis disease that is found anywhere outside of the lungs.

extremely drug resistant (13)
By international consensus, it is multi-drug resistant TB, resistance to isonia-zid and rifampin, plus resistance to two important classes of second line drugs, the quinolones and the second line aminoglycosides and/or the related drug capreomycin.

F

fecal-oral route of transmission (8)
A method of an infectious agent (bacterium or virus) spreading through the ingestion of the fecal matter of infected individuals.

fee-for-service (15)
A payment system in which health care providers are paid a fee for each service provided.

fetal alcohol spectrum disorders (9)
A collection of disorders present at birth that result from ingesting alcohol during pregnancy; symptoms include a spectrum of physical malformations and developmental disability.

field notes (12)
Informal notes taken by a qualitative researcher during interviews and observations to document impressions about the various qualitative data-gathering experiences.

fieldwork (12)
In an ethnographic study, the act of collecting data at the location or in the community or institution where the action under study is taking place (rather than from an academic setting, for example).

financial barriers (15)
Factors that restrict access to health care either by patients' inability to pay for needed medical services or by discouraging physicians and hospitals from treating patients who have low income.

five-number summary (6)
A list of the quintiles of a distribution, typically accompanying a histogram.

focused ethnography (12)
A method that focuses on gathering data to answer specific questions about certain problems rather than focusing on an entire community or cultural group.

Food and Drug Administration (FDA) (2)
An agency within the U.S. Department of Health and Human Services that is responsible for ensuring a safe food, cosmetic, and medicine supply for the United States.

frameworks (11)
Conceptualizations that draw on several theories or theoretical constructs to understand a health issue.

Framingham Heart Study (5)
A large, ongoing cohort study based in Framingham, Massachusetts, that began in 1948 and has followed three generations of Framingham residents to assess risk and protective factors for cardiovascular disease and related conditions.

frequency (3, 6)
The numbers of people within certain categories. Also, how often a health event occurs in a population; one of the criteria used to determine whether surveillance will be conducted on a health outcome.

Future Health Systems (17)
A research consortium that is working with six low- and middle-income countries to better understand specific health system factors that contribute to a significant health problem within each country.

futures research (17)
Using a variety of methodological tools such as trend analysis and extrapolation to project what is likely to occur.

G

gamma rays (9)
Packets of electronic energy (photons) that are the most energetic in the electromagnetic spectrum.

genomics (17)
The study of genes and their function; examining molecular mechanisms and the relationship of genes and the environment.

geographic dispersion (of a social network) (11)
Description of social network pertaining to the physical distance members are from each other.

gibbous deformity (13)
A hunchback deformity of the spine caused by collapse of one or more of the vertebral bones of the spine.

grounded theory (12)

A process through which researchers work up from the data to develop explanations for or theories about the phenomena observed or the narratives participants provide; thus explanations are grounded in the data.

group-level data (5)

Summary exposure and outcome information for an entire population (rather than information from each individual member of the population).

Guerin, Camille (13)

A French veterinarian, microbiologist, and immunologist who developed the BCG vaccine for tuberculosis in the early twentieth century with his colleague Albert Calmette.

H

hazard (10)

A source of potential adverse health effect. Also, a substance's potency or ability to cause harm. Hazards may be chemical agents (asbestos or benzene), physical (ionizing radiation or sound pressure), or biological (the pathogens responsible for tuberculosis or malaria).

hazard identification (10)

The process of finding out (qualitatively) what hazards might exist.

hazard index (10)

The ratio of the chronic (lifetime) daily intake calculated from exposure assessment to the reference dose.

hazardous air pollutants (9)

Contaminants known to cause cancer or other serious health effects or environmental damage that are monitored by the EPA.

health (1)

According to the World Health Organization, "a state of complete physical, mental, and social well-being and not merely the absence of disease or infirmity."

Health and Human Services (HHS) (2)

See Department of Health and Human Services.

health belief model (11)

One of the most widely used public health theories for explaining an individual's likelihood of performing a health behavior. Developed by Godfrey Hochbaum.

health communications campaign (11)
> A strategy that employs different types of media to disseminate one or more health-promoting messages to a defined audience.

health disparities (1, 16)
> Disproportionate disease burden or adverse health outcomes experienced by disadvantaged social groups when compared with more advantaged social groups.

health information exchange (15)
> The use of information and computer technology in health care settings to facilitate and promote communication and the flow of information between providers.

health information technology (15)
> The use of information and computer technology in health care settings for information storage and for communication.

health insurance (14)
> Provides a mechanism for shifting the risk from an individual to a group by pooling resources, and all members of the insured group share actual losses.

Health Maintenance Act of 1973 (14)
> Provided start-up funds to establish new health maintenance organizations (HMOs) and added employer mandates to offer HMOs as an option if available in their community.

health maintenance organization (HMO) (14)
> A type of managed care plan that typically has tight controls on how enrollees access care, including using a primary care provider (PCP) and obtaining referrals from the PCP for specialty care.

health management and policy (1)
> A concentration within public health that is most concerned with issues of health care access and the policies at various levels of an organization or government and how these policies impact health outcomes.

health policy (14)
> Authoritative decisions made in the legislative, executive, or judicial branches of government that are intended to direct or influence the actions, behaviors, or decisions of others regarding health or the pursuit of health.

health savings account (14)
A medical savings account that is paired with a high-deductible health plan and is used to pay for health care expenses until the high deductible is met. Individuals or their employers can make tax-free contributions.

health services research (15)
The multidisciplinary field of scientific investigation that studies how social factors, financing systems, organizational structures and processes, health technologies, and personal behaviors affect access to health care, the quality and cost of health care, and ultimately our health and well-being.

Healthy People (16)
The health blueprint for the United States created by the Centers for Disease Control and Prevention in collaboration with scientific experts and public participants every ten years that sets specific, measurable targets for health and health behaviors.

healthy worker effect (5)
The concept that people who are in the workforce are typically healthier than people who are not in the workforce and also are advantaged in other ways (socially, economically) because of employment.

helping relationships (11)
One of the behavior change strategies of the stages of change or transtheoretical model; it involves seeking social support for behavior change.

herd immunity (8)
The concept that not all members of a population need to be immunized against an infectious disease because being a member of a group (herd) that is largely immune to an agent reduces the chance that a susceptible member of the group will contact an infected member. Also called community immunity.

Hill-Burton Act (14)
Legislation passed in 1947 that provided funding for hospital and other health care facility construction.

histogram (6)
A graphical method of displaying the distribution of measurements within a sample in which each bar represents the frequency of sampled participants within each range of the measurements.

homogeneity (of a social network) (11)
Description of social network pertaining to the similarity of network members.

hormesis (10)

A pattern of toxicological response to a chemical or physical agent for which an optimum level of exposure exists, whereas both too little and too much exposure cause adverse health effects.

host (8)

Any being that is capable of being infected with the organism that carries the disease.

Human Immunodeficiency Virus (HIV) (8)

A retrovirus that spreads from person to person by exposure to infected blood or body fluids, most frequently through sexual contact, needle sharing, or birth.

human subjects (1)

Individuals involved in the research study.

hypothesis (4, 8)

A testable theory; a statement of the investigator's expectation of the relationship between exposure and outcome.

hypothetical population (6)

A theoretical population about which one makes inferences based on samples.

I

inactivated vaccine (8)

A vaccine that contains a disease-causing organism that is not live (infectious), but enough of the organism is present in the vaccine to elicit an immune response.

inapparent infection (8)

Laboratory results that indicate infection despite the absence of symptoms.

incidence or incidence rate (4, 5, 13)

The amount or rate of new cases of a disease or health outcome in a population among members of the population who are at risk for the disease or health outcome (the population at risk).

inclusion criteria (5)

Factors or characteristics (for example age or the lack of existing health conditions) that must be present for a person to be eligible to participate in a research study or clinical trial.

incubation period (8)

The length of time between exposure to an infectious agent and the onset of symptoms.

indemnity insurance (14)

An insurance plan that pays a portion of the health care costs after a deductible is met. These plans cover care provided by any providers and hospitals and requires that either the provider or patient file a claim to receive reimbursement for care provided. (Also called conventional insurance.)

Independent Ethics Committee (IEC) (1)

A group established by an academic institution or other organization to review research proposals in order to assure the ethical conduct of research studies involving human subjects. (Also called an Institutional Review Board.)

independent variable (5)

The exposure of interest in epidemiological studies.

indirect transmission (9)

A mechanism by which an infectious agent is transferred when the source touches an object that then comes into contact with the host.

individual level (2, 11)

Level of the social-ecological framework in which the target of change is the individual and the focus is on changing personal characteristics.

inductive reasoning (12)

Moving from effect to cause (specific to general).

inequality (16)

Like disparity, refers to populations being unequal on a particular measure of health, with disadvantaged populations faring worse than more advantaged populations.

inequity (16)

The ethical considerations underlying health disparities and social justice.

infant mortality rate (4)

The number of individuals who die between birth and one year of age, usually expressed per 1,000 live births. The infant mortality rate is one of the vital statistics measures often used to describe the adequacy of a nation's health care system.

inferential (6)

Using a random sample to draw conclusions, or make inferences about, an entire population.

infiltrate (13)

A nonspecific term describing an area of inflammation seen on a chest X-ray, usually indicating an infection of the lung, including tuberculosis.

informational support (11)

A type of social support in which a person provides advice, suggestions, and information to help solve problems.

initiator (10)

An agent capable of initiating the chain of events that leads to the development of a cancer, typically by producing mutations in the DNA of a cell that activates or shuts down the expression of genes that regulate the cell's replication. Examples include ionizing radiation or chemicals such as nitrosamines.

inoculation (8)

The process of transferring material or fluids from an infected person to a noninfected person to elicit an immune response. Also called variolation (used for smallpox).

Institute of Medicine (IOM) (1, 17)

An advisory body to the United States that uses expert panels to create reports on topics of current interest in the health and medical field; it is part of the National Academy of Sciences and was founded in 1970.

Institutional Review Board (IRB) (1, 5)

A group established by an academic institution or other organization to review research proposals in order to ensure the ethical conduct of research studies involving human subjects. (Also called an Independent Ethics Committee.)

instrumental support (11)

A type of social support in which a person offers tangible aid and services that provide assistance to meet needs.

intensity (of a social network) (11)

Description of social network pertaining to the emotional closeness of network members.

intervention (11)

A program or initiative developed with the goal of producing behavior changes or improved health status.

intervention trial (5)

A randomized controlled trial that tests the impact of drugs or other efforts to reduce the severity of a disease in individuals who are at high risk of the outcome (secondary prevention).

interview guide (12)

A series of broad, general questions that address a specific research question meant to guide the research interview and to make sure that all participants are given the opportunity to answer the same questions.

interviewer bias (6)

A type of bias introduced because of differences in the way the individuals collecting data (interviewers) assess or report responses.

intramuscular (vaccine) (8)

A vaccine injected into the muscle.

intranasal (vaccine) (8)

A vaccine delivered through the nose.

introduction (5)

In a research article, the opening section that includes an overview of the problem, the current state of knowledge on the topic, and the rationale for the current research. Also called the background.

investigational new drug (IND) application (7)

The formal request for authorization to use an investigational drug in humans.

ionizing radiation (9)

Energy in the form of waves or particles that has enough force to remove electrons from atoms.

isolation (1)

The practice of separating people who are infected with an agent and exhibit signs of disease from people who are not infected.

J

judgment sampling (12)

See purposive sampling.

justice (17)

Fairness. In the Belmont Report, justice refers to the fair distribution of risks and benefits associated with research.

K

Kefauver-Harris Amendment (7)

Legislation that amended the Food, Drug, and Cosmetic Act and strengthened the requirements for premarketing safety studies and asked for proof of efficacy before a drug can be marketed in the United States.

Koch, Robert (13)

A German physician considered by many to be the father of bacteriology. Among his contributions to the field was his discovery of the organism responsible for causing tuberculosis.

Koch's postulates (8)

The process of connecting microbes and infectious disease; Robert Koch hypothesized that if a microbe was responsible for a certain disease, it should be possible to isolate the microbe from the diseased individual, grow it in the laboratory, then use it to infect a healthy individual with the same disease, and reisolate the microbe from the newly infected individual.

L

latent tuberculosis infection (13)

The presence of the organism that causes tuberculosis somewhere in the body in a dormant state. People with latent tuberculosis infection are not sick, have no symptoms, and their chest X-ray is almost always normal.

LD$_{50}$ (10)

The amount of a substance that kills 50 percent of a test population.

lead (9)

A water-soluble metal that can cause neurological damage, especially in young (developing) children.

linkages (11)

How theoretical constructs are related to each other.

live attenuated vaccine (8)

A vaccine that contains a live (infectious) microbe that has been altered in the laboratory to allow the immune system to recognize it as foreign but to prevent it from causing the disease during vaccination.

live vaccine (8)

A vaccine that contains a live (infectious) microbe that is similar enough to the disease-causing microbe that it allows the body to later recognize the disease microbe as foreign but not cause disease in the person vaccinated.

local health department (2)

Often organized at the county level, most provide a wide range of services, including health screenings, immunizations, community outreach and education, epidemiology and disease surveillance, vital statistics, maternal and child health services, food safety and restaurant regulation, tuberculosis testing, infectious disease control, and some primary health care services.

locality development (11)

A community organizing strategy that involves achieving group consensus about common concerns and collaborating in problem solving (also called community development).

logistic regression (model) (5, 6)

An analytic tool used in epidemiology to calculate an adjusted odds ratio.

long form (of Census) (3)

An additional questionnaire used with the United States Census 2000 to collect information about health and living conditions from one in six households.

longitudinal study (5)

A study that follows people over time; another name for a cohort study.

lost to follow-up (5)

Study participants who do not complete the research study.

lowest observed adverse effect level (LOAEL) (9, 10)

The smallest dose of a stressor or agent that statistically and biologically causes an alteration of the morphology, functional capacity, growth, development, or life span of organism.

lowest observed effect level (LOEL) (10)

The lowest dose of an agent observed to cause any effect during a toxicological experiment.

M

maintenance stage (11)

A stage of change from the stages of change or transtheoretical model in which an individual has changed a behavior for more than 6 months.

managed care plan (14)

A health insurance plan that uses a contracted network of providers to deliver care to their enrollees and incorporate processes for the management of patients. The plans negotiate reduced payment rates with providers in order to control costs. This is the predominant type of health insurance in the United States.

marker (16)

An indicator or predictor, often used when the desired target is difficult to measure directly.

matched case-control study (5)

A case-control study in which a control (person without the outcome) is chosen for each case (person with the outcome) who is similar on one or more demographic, health, or other variables.

material resources (16)

Economically based assets such as access to goods and services.

maximum (6)

The 100th percentile in a five-number summary.

maximum concentration level (MCL)

The highest allowable concentration of a substance or contaminant permissible by the National Primary Drinking Water Standards.

mean (6)

Average.

measure of effect (5)

A numeric representation of the amount by which an exposure increases or decreases the risk of an outcome, typically expressed as a relative risk or odds ratio in epidemiological studies. Similar to measure of excess risk, although the term *effect* indicates a causal relationship exists between exposure and outcome.

measure of excess risk (5)

A numeric representation of the amount by which an exposure increases or decreases the risk of an outcome, typically expressed as a relative risk or odds ratio in epidemiological studies. Similar to measure of effect, although this term does not indicate a causal relationship exists between exposure and outcome.

measurement error (6)

A type of error that occurs when a recorded measure is not completely correct.

median (6)

The value above which 50 percent of the population falls and below which 50 percent of the population falls; the 50th percentile in a five-number summary.

Medicaid (14)

A program created under Title XIX of the Social Security Amendment of 1965 designed to provide assistance to states to cover the medical expenses of individuals (especially women and their children) who are low income.

medical home (14)

A physician's office or other source of medical care that provides acute and preventive care, manages chronic illnesses, coordinates specialty care, and provides around-the-clock on-call assistance.

Medicare (14)

A health insurance program for Americans age sixty-five and older regardless of their income created under Title XVIII of the Social Security Amendment of 1965.

methods (5)

In a research article, a detailed description of the steps taken in the current study, often including the data source(s), a description of how study participants were selected, and details about the measures and analyses used in the study.

methyl mercury (9)

A lipid-soluble form of the metal mercury that can accumulate in predatory fish and result in neurological damage in humans who consume contaminated fish.

microbe (8)

A minute living organism.

midwives (14)

Practitioners who attend and assist with births.

miliary tuberculosis (13)

A form of tuberculosis in which the organism has spread throughout the body and is usually evident by small nodules that are too numerous to count, measuring between 1 to 4 millimeters in size.

Millennium Development goals (17)

Eight goals established and tracked by the World Health Organization and supported by 189 countries. Goals relate to poverty, hunger, education, health, and the environment.

Millennium Project (17)

A broad group of researchers, business leaders, policy makers, and others who work to understand the state of the future; they use trends from the past twenty years to predict the next ten years.

minimum (6)

The 0th percentile in a five-number summary.

Minority Health and Health Disparities Research and Education Act (16)

Legislation passed in 2000 that authorizes many programs and initiatives to address particular disparities.

misclassification (5)

Assigning a research subject to the wrong category (for example, classifying someone as exposed when he or she actually was not exposed).

missing data (6)

Information that is not available in a study, for example because data were not collected or were lost or because participants did not answer certain questions.

mission, public health (1)

Fulfilling society's interest in assuring conditions in which people can be healthy.

mixed methods (12)

Research that uses both quantitative and qualitative methods.

models (11)

Conceptualizations that draw on several theories or theoretical constructs to understand a health issue.

morbidity (1, 11)

The existence of any form of disease, or the degree to which a health condition affects a patient.

mortality (1)

Death, often expressed as a mortality rate per 100,000 population, the details of which are captured as part of vital statistics collection from the death certificate.

MTB complex (13)

The group of organisms that are genetically closely related that cause similar tuberculosis disease in humans. It includes the following sub-species: *Mycobacterium tuberculosis*, *Mycobacterium bovis*, *Mycobacterium africanum*, *Mycobacterium canetti*, and *Mycobacterium microti*.

multi-drug resistant (13)
Tuberculosis that is resistant to the most effective tuberculosis drugs currently in use, rifampin and isoniazid.

multifactorial (4)
Caused by many different variables or factors.

multivariate (6)
Data description that focuses on many measurements at a time.

***Mycobacterium tuberculosis* (13)**
The organism that causes tuberculosis. It is a bacillus from a group of bacteria known as the mycobacteria, known for their thick cell walls.

N

naled (9)
An organophosphate pesticide.

narrative (12)
The stories that participants tell in a qualitative research project.

National Institutes of Health (NIH) (2)
An agency under the U.S. Department of Health and Human Services that provides leadership in setting research priorities for the nation, funds research efforts at private and public institutions, is actively involved in the publication and dissemination of research findings, and supports the training of experts in medical sciences.

naturalistic research (12)
Research that is not conducted in a laboratory but is conducted in the real world of the lives and experiences of the people, patients, clients, or populations being studied.

neural tube defects (5)
A class of disabilities present at birth that relate to improper closure of the spinal column during development and includes spina bifida and anencephaly.

new drug application (NDA) (7)
The vehicle through which drug sponsors formally propose that the FDA approve a new drug for sale and marketing in the United States.

nitrate (9)

A naturally occurring oxidation product of nitrite that can methylate hemoglobin and cause blue baby syndrome in infants.

nitrogen oxide (9)

A compound that can cause respiratory problems, especially in children.

no observed adverse effect level (NOAEL) (9, 10)

The highest dose at which there is no statistically or biologically observed alteration of the morphology, functional capacity, growth, development, or life span of organism.

no observed effect level (NOEL) (10)

The highest dose of an agent that caused no observable effect in exposed laboratory animals during a toxicological experiment.

noncompliant (5)

Study participants who do adhere to the exposure instructions of a trial.

nonionizing radiation (9)

One of the two major types of radiation, it has the ability to move atoms but not to chemically change (ionize) them; weaker than ionizing radiation.

nonmaleficence (17)

Not harming; one of the core principles of public health ethics.

Nuremberg Code (1)

An outline of assurances (ten tenets) that must be in place in order to conduct human subjects research; it resulted from the Nuremberg trials of 1946–1947 in which German physicians and their associates were tried, and many convicted, for killing or disabling thousands of people in Nazi concentration camps during World War II.

O

obesity (9, 17)

Having a body mass index (BMI) greater than or equal to 30 (kg/m^2).

observational study (5)

A class of epidemiological studies in which subjects are not assigned to any exposure group, but are instead observed based on their naturally occurring (by choice or by environment) exposures to determine whether these factors influence their chances of having a particular health outcome.

odds ratio (OR) (5, 6)

A measure of excess risk or effect calculated in case-control studies. (Also, the measure obtained for any analysis using logistic regression.)

Office of the Surgeon General (OSG) (2)

Part of the Office of Public Health and Science that oversees the Commissioned Corps of the U.S. Public Health Service. The surgeon general is the country's chief health educator and provides Americans with the latest scientific information on how to improve their health and reduce the risk of illness and injury.

open coding (12)

An approach to coding data with no preconceived ideas about what will be found.

open-ended interviews (12)

A method of collecting information through one-on-one interviews that may be informal conversations, may use an interview guide of general topics to be covered, or may be statements requiring the participants to fill in the blanks.

organization and community level (11)

Level of the social-ecological framework where the target of change is the social environment, and the focus is on changing community norms, values, attitudes, and power structures.

outbreak (8)

A scenario in which the number of actual cases of an infectious disease is higher than the number of expected cases.

outcome (4, 5, 15)

The endpoint of interest in a study or the dependent variable.

outcome measures (15)

Used along with utilization measures to assess health care access; death rates, disease incidence, complications due to treatment, disability, and patient satisfaction are often used to measure access to care.

outliers (12, 15)

Data or participants who do not fit the typical patterns or hypothesized model.

out-of-pocket payments (14)

Payments made by individuals (rather than insurance companies or government programs) for health services.

ozone (9)

A photochemical oxidant that reacts with volatile organic compounds in the atmosphere to produce smog.

P

pandemic (1, 4, 9)

A global epidemic.

participation (11)

The engagement of community members, leaders, and structures in community organizing and research efforts, such as problem identification, priority setting, and research and intervention development, implementation, and evaluation.

participatory action research (12)

An example of critical collaborative ethnography in which researchers conduct field research but community participants are collaborators in the design, data collection, and data analysis process.

particulate matter (9)

Small compounds and particles suspended in the air that can be inhaled and create negative health effects.

passive surveillance (3)

A method of collecting data that allows individuals to report to a central agency or system without being contacted directly for the purpose of data collection.

pathway of exposure (10)

The series of processes that lead from a source of environmental contaminants to an exposed individual. These may include emissions, transport, chemical or biological degradation, bioaccumulation, etc.

pay-for-performance (15)

A payment system in which providers are rewarded for meeting pre-established performance measures for quality and efficiency, such as following clinical practice guidelines or adopting the use of electronic medical records.

peer debriefing (12)

A process by which other researchers provide feedback on the data collection and analysis to the researcher conducting the study.

perceived barriers (11)

A construct of health belief model that indicates an individual's belief that changing a health behavior will be difficult or cause them discomfort.

perceived benefits (11)

A construct of health belief model that indicates an individual's belief that changing a health behavior will reduce their risk of developing a disease or another adverse outcome.

perceived control (11)

A construct included in theory of planned behavior. It asserts that an individual's intent to perform a health behavior depends, in part, on how confident the individual feels that he or she has control over performing the behavior.

perceived severity (11)

A construct of health belief model that indicates an individual's belief that developing a disease (or other issue) would be serious.

perceived susceptibility (11)

A construct of health belief model that indicates an individual's belief that a health behavior will put them at risk for something to which they are averse (such as developing a disease).

perceived threat (11)

A construct of health belief model. It is a combination of how susceptible to developing a disease a person feels (or other adverse issue) and how severely that person believes the disease would impact him or her.

percentile (6)

A numbered point or range of values with an equal number of observations below which a certain percent of observations or members of a population occur.

person (8)

Part of descriptive epidemiology; includes detailing the demographics or other personal characteristics relevant to an outbreak investigation.

personal health record (15)

A complete medical history managed by an individual to facilitate health care delivery, typically in an electronic format.

person-time (4, 5)

A measure of the amount of time during which a person is at risk of developing the outcome of interest.

person-years (5)

The amount of time (in years) a person contributes to the denominator in a cohort study; person-time expressed in years.

pharmacodynamics (7)

The science of how drugs act through receptors or other mechanisms in the body.

pharmacoepidemiology (7)

The application of epidemiological reasoning, methods, and knowledge to the study of the uses and effects of drugs in human populations.

pharmacokinetics (7)

The science of how drugs are absorbed, distributed, metabolized, and excreted by the body.

phenomenological (12)

A research approach aimed at capturing the lived experience of the individuals or groups about whom we have questions.

photovoice (12)

A participatory action research strategy by which people create and discuss photographs as a means of catalyzing personal and community change.

physical environment (9)

The objects that surround us and the places we construct (the built environment).

place (8)

Part of descriptive epidemiology; may make use of a map to determine the geographical area in which an outbreak is occurring or describe the type of place, for example, a day care center or classrooms in a school.

placebo (5)

An inactive substance that looks like the treatment.

point source (8)

A type of infectious disease outbreak scenario in which there is a single source of exposure that occurred at a single point in time.

point-of-service plans (14)

A hybrid between HMO and PPO plans that includes a network of providers and requires members to be assigned to a primary care physician. They offer limited coverage to members who choose to go out of network for medical care, and out-of-network services require a deductible and a higher copayment than in-network services.

policy development (2)
One of the three core functions of public health, it is the process of formulating the best strategy to approach a public health problem and implementing the new program or law.

policy formation (14)
The first of three phases in policy making, it involves identifying a problem, setting a policy agenda, and developing legislation with input and negotiation by all of the interested parties.

policy implementation (14)
The second of three phases in policy making, it involves developing rules and regulations to guide the implementation and operationalization of the policy.

policy modification (14)
The third of three phases in policy making, it evaluates the consequences of legislation to see if it meets the original intent, or if circumstances change, what modifications are needed to more effectively address the problem.

poliovirus (8)
A virus that causes poliomyelitis, a disease with no symptoms (inapparent infection) in approximately 95 percent of those infected but can cause flaccid paralysis in about 1 percent of infected people.

polychlorinated biphenyls (PCBs) (9)
A class of compounds used as coolants and lubricants that accumulate in fish, meat, and dairy products and cause a variety of negative health outcomes in humans, including cancer.

polymorphism (9)
A genetic change or mutation at a specific place in the genotype. Also, the existence of more than one phenotype within a population that is regularly present and persists.

population (1, 2, 5)
A group of individuals who share a common set of characteristics, such as place of residence or demographic traits.

population at risk (4)
The members of a population who have a nonzero chance of acquiring or developing the health outcome of interest.

population health (2)

Assessing or discussing health in the context of groups rather than individuals.

population odds ratio (6)

The odds ratio we would compute if we had randomized the entire population to two intervention groups in an experimental study.

postmarketing (7)

Studies conducted once a drug is FDA approved and publicly available.

postmarketing surveillance (5)

Monitoring the health effects of a drug after it has been approved by the appropriate agency and is available to the general public (on the market).

power (statistical) (5)

The ability to reject the null hypothesis when the null hypothesis is false; the probability of avoiding type 2 error.

precautionary principle (10)

The idea that even in the absence of full certainty about the extent and mechanisms of potential threats, actions should be taken to prevent serious and irrevocable damage.

preclinical phase (7)

A phase of the U.S. drug approval process in which efficacy and safety are established in animal models.

precontemplation stage (11)

A stage of the stages of change or transtheoretical model in which an individual has no intention to change a behavior within the next 6 months.

predisposing factors (15)

A component of the Andersen model of health care access; includes personal resources, education, race, and age.

preexisting image (12)

Family pictures, newspaper photographs, photographs of rituals, archival materials, and photoblogs.

preferred provider organization (PPO) (14)

A type of managed care plan that is more loosely organized than a health maintenance organization (HMO) and has different levels of cost-sharing with enrollees who visit providers outside their health plan's contracted network.

premarketing (7)

A study that occurred before a drug was approved by the FDA and allowed to be marketed to the general public.

premium (14)

A fixed periodic cost (for a health insurance plan).

prepaid hospital services plan (14)

A payment system developed in 1929 designed to provide a regular source of income for hospitals and provide some protection for consumers against large medical bills.

preparation stage (11)

A stage of the stages of change or transtheoretical model in which an individual intends to change a behavior within the next month and has taken steps to do so.

prevalence (4)

The amount or frequency of a health outcome that exists in a population at a certain point or over a certain period of time.

preventability (3)

Whether it is possible to eliminate the spread of a disease or to limit its impact; one of the criteria used to determine whether surveillance will be conducted on a health outcome.

prevention (1, 2)

One of the hallmarks of public health, a concept that involves taking action to assure that a negative event or exposure does not occur or that the impact of a negative event or exposure is minimized. (See also primary, secondary, and tertiary prevention.)

prevention trial (5)

A randomized controlled trial that targets primary prevention, for example, testing the efficacy (ability to produce an effect) of a vaccine in healthy individuals.

preventive effect (6)

The amount by which an intervention reduces the odds of an outcome.

primary care provider (14)

A designated physician who serves as the typical source of health care and provides a referral for specialized care in a health maintenance organization (HMO) or other managed care plan.

primary prevention (2, 5)
One of the three levels of prevention; involves preventing a health outcome or negative exposure from occurring.

private financing (14)
Payment for health care services comes from private health insurance companies or individuals.

probability (6)
A proportion that quantifies chance on a scale from 0 to 1, with 0 indicating no chance and 1 indicating certainty.

probability sample (6)
A sample in which the chance of selecting any given subset of the population is known.

problem focus (12)
Used in ethnography to describe a study that focuses on a specific problem rather than studying the community as a whole.

prodromal stage (8)
The early phase of symptoms of infection, often including nonspecific symptoms such as headache, fever, body aches, and malaise.

promoter (10)
An agent capable of stimulating a cell already primed by an initiator to replicate out of control. Examples include DDT or some components of cigarette smoke.

propagated (8)
An infection that is spread from person to person.

proportion (4)
A quantitative measure; the count of health events divided by the population from which those events arose.

prospective (5)
Into the future.

prospective payment system (15)
A payment system in which hospitals are paid a predetermined rate for each Medicare admission.

protective factor (4)
Any personal attribute, environmental exposure, or other feature of a person or his or her environment that decreases the likelihood that a negative health outcome will occur.

public financing (14)

Health care services that are paid for by local, state, or federal government sources such as Medicare or Medicaid.

public health (1)

A multidisciplinary field that seeks to improve or maintain the health of a population through prevention and social justice while acting according to the values and norms of the population and within a social-ecological framework.

public health competencies (17)

Skills and knowledge that someone trained in public health should be able to demonstrate.

public health ethics (17)

The principles and values that help guide actions designed to promote health and prevent injury and disease in the population.

public interest (3)

The importance of a particular health issue to the general population; one of the criteria used to determine whether surveillance will be conducted on a health outcome.

pulmonary tuberculosis (13)

Tuberculosis disease that affects the lung. Over 85 percent of tuberculosis cases affect the lung.

purposive sampling (12)

Participants are selected based on the likelihood that they are informed and able to provide information about the particular research topic.

***p* value (6)**

The probability that the sample statistic will be as far or farther away from the hypothesized value on repeated sampling.

Q

qualitative research or qualitative studies (5, 12)

A holistic approach to answering research questions that is derived from the recognition that human lives are complex and that in-depth understanding is not described by numbers. The focus of this research is on the human experience: the context of human behavior, or in other words, what people do and how and why they do it. Qualitative research may also be called interpretive research.

quality-adjusted life years (15)
A measure of health care outcomes that adjusts gains (or losses) in years of life after a health care intervention and considers the quality of life during those years.

quantitative data (4)
Information that can be represented by numbers; for example, data that come from surveys that require respondents to choose from specified answer choices.

quantitative study designs (5)
A class of research studies including observational and experimental studies in which the data collected can be represented numerically.

quarantine (1)
The practice of separating people who have been exposed to an infectious agent but are asymptomatic from other people who are not infected.

R

racism (16)
The system of structuring opportunity and assigning value based on the social interpretation of phenotype (race).

radiation (9)
Energy that travels in the form of waves or high-speed particles.

randomized controlled trial (RCT) (5)
A type of experimental study in which participants are assigned at random to an exposure group or a control group.

rate (4)
A measure of disease frequency that includes time in the denominator.

recall bias (5, 6)
The type of bias that results when people with a different exposure or outcome status remember past events or exposures differently.

reciprocal determinism (11)
The interdependent relationship between the person, his or her behavior, and the environment.

reciprocity (of a social network) (11)
Description of social network pertaining to if and how support is both given and received.

reference dose (RfD) (9, 10)
The maximum dose of a chemical deemed safe for a human population, as used for U.S. EPA regulations. This level is derived from the NOEL or NOAEL reported by toxicological experiments on animals, with the use of appropriate safety factors.

referral sampling (12)
Selecting study participants by identifying key individuals to interview and asking them to recommend others. Also called snowball sampling.

registries (3)
Data systems that collect information from people with a specific type of disease or health outcome in a central repository.

reinforcement management (11)
One of the behavior change strategies of the stages of change or transtheoretical model; it involves increasing rewards for healthy behavior and decreasing rewards for unhealthy behavior.

relationship level (2, 11)
Level of the social-ecological framework in which the target of change is social influences and the focus is on changing the nature of social relationships.

relative risk (RR) (5)
A measure of excess risk or effect calculated in cohort studies or other epidemiological studies in which incidence can be measured.

representative sample (3, 6)
A selection of individuals that reflect the individuals (by demographic or other factors) in the underlying population of interest.

research design (12)
A plan or proposal to conduct research that should involve a philosophical point of view, strategies of inquiry, and specific methods for data collection and analysis.

researcher-produced images (12)
Photographs taken by the researcher to describe communities or groups, as in documentaries.

residual confounding (6)
Confounding that remains after some adjustments to data have been made.

resistant (13)

When an organism does not respond as expected after exposure to antibiotics that are known to be effective against it in the laboratory, it is said to be resistant.

response rate (5)

The percent of people sampled to participate in a survey who complete the survey.

results (5)

In a research article, the section describing the findings of the study, which often includes tables and figures that provide data from the analyses.

retrospective (5)

In the past.

risk (6, 10)

Probability; in environmental health, the probability that a certain undesirable (health) effect will take place, given a level of exposure to a specified toxic agent.

risk assessment (10)

The process of identifying threats to public health and estimating the likelihood of their occurrence.

risk characterization (10)

The final step of a risk assessment in which information from the hazard identification, dose-response assessment, and exposure assessment stages are integrated.

risk factor (4)

Any personal attribute, environmental exposure, or other feature of a person or his or her environment that increases the likelihood that a negative health outcome will occur.

Rochester Radiation Cohorts (5)

A series of studies that began in the mid-1950s designed to determine whether adverse effects, specifically cancer, are related to medical irradiation.

route of exposure (9, 10)

The way in which a chemical or biological agent can cross the boundary of an organism. These are most typically inhalation, ingestion, dermal absorption, and puncture.

S

safe haven laws (17)
Laws that allow children to be left at an organization such as a fire or police station without the threat of prosecution for parents or caregivers.

sampling (12)
Choosing research participants according to certain criteria.

sampling distribution (6)
The distribution of the statistic for repeated samples.

sampling variability (6)
The spread of the distribution of the statistic for repeated samples, that is, the spread of its sampling distribution.

sanitarium (13)
A health facility for long-term health care, usually referring to the long-term care associated with tuberculosis treatment prior to the widespread use of anti-tuberculosis medications.

scrofula (13)
Refers to tuberculosis-associated lymphadenitis, usually in the neck. Scrofula can be disfiguring because many of the lymph nodes affected by tuberculosis ulcerate and leave draining lesions and scars.

secondary prevention (2, 5)
One of the three levels of prevention; involves detecting disease while it is still in its early stages and reducing its progression and effects.

selection bias (6)
Bias that results when the sampled participants are not a representative probability sample of the population of interest.

selective pressure (13)
In reference to microorganisms, it is the exposure to conditions, usually antibiotics, that kill off susceptible organisms but allows those with characteristics resistant to those conditions to survive, reproduce, and eventually replace the other organisms that demonstrated susceptibility to the condition (antibiotics).

self-insurance (14)
Paying for health benefits directly instead of offering commercial health insurance (common among large employers).

self-efficacy (11)

A construct included in several health behavior theories (such as health belief model, social cognitive theory, stages of change). It pertains to an individual's belief that he or she can successfully perform as needed, such as in making a health behavior change.

self-liberation (11)

One of the behavior change strategies of the stages of change or transtheoretical model; it involves the individual making a commitment to change a health behavior.

self-reevaluation (11)

One of the behavior change strategies of the stages of change or transtheoretical model; it involves the individual seeing behavior change as important to his or her self-identify.

sensitivity (5)

A measure of accuracy; in a research study, the ability to correctly identify people who have the outcome (labeling cases as cases).

sensitivity analysis (6)

A method of external bias adjustment in which data pertaining to the bias are fabricated and the analysis is repeated.

severe acute respiratory syndrome (SARS) (8)

A novel coronavirus disease that appeared in 2002 and resulted in a pandemic.

severity (3)

Seriousness, often measured in terms of morbidity or mortality; one of the criteria used to determine whether surveillance will be conducted on a health outcome.

simple random sample (6)

The simplest form of a probability sample; one in which any subset of size n has an equal chance of being selected from a population of size N.

single-blind study (5)

An experimental study in which the subject does not know to which exposure group he has been randomized.

size (of social network) (11)

Description of social network pertaining to the number of members in the network.

smallpox (8)

A disease caused by variola virus transmitted through respiratory secretions and contact with the virus that results in fever, malaise, and pustules. Successfully eradicated in 1980.

snowball sampling (12)

Selecting study participants by locating some key individuals to interview and then asking them to recommend others who might be willing to participate. Also called referral sampling.

social action (11)

A community organizing strategy that uses public demonstration and sometimes adversarial methods to bring attention to issues (also called systems advocacy).

social and behavioral science (1, 11)

An area of public health focused on understanding, predicting, and influencing health behaviors of individuals, groups, and populations.

social cognitive theory (11)

An interpersonal-level theory developed by Albert Bandura that asserts that behavior is influenced by vicarious experiences and that learning and behavior change involves an interdependent relationship between the person, his or her behavior, and the environment.

social construct (16)

A classification that is culturally defined rather than biologically defined.

social constructivist (12)

A philosophical point of view that assumes meanings are constructed by human beings as they engage with the world. It also assumes that people engage with their world and make sense of it based on their historical and social perspectives that come from their culture.

social-ecological model or social-ecological framework (1, 2, 11, 16, 17)

Conceptual framework that acknowledges the complicated relationships that exist between individuals and their environments. It helps to organize the numerous factors that influence health and health behaviors into defined categories or levels.

social environment (11)

The individuals and groups one encounters or with whom one interacts.

social franchising (17)

A system in which small provider groups organize into units under a contract that provides business support, training, and quality monitoring.

social justice (1, 11)

The idea that all individuals in a population should have access to the same programs and services, regardless of social condition or standing.

social liberation (11)

One of the behavior change strategies of the stages of change or transtheoretical model. Involves the recognition that social changes are being made to better support healthy behaviors.

social network (11)

The web of relationships a person has with others that can serve diverse functions, such as providing employment opportunities, connections to others, and various types of social support.

social planning (11)

A community organizing strategy. Involves solving social problems through coordination of social services, program development, and planning for adequate resource allocation (also called policy change).

social resources (16)

Assets associated with relationships with others, such as social networks or social support.

social support (11)

Intentional aid and assistance that is received through social interactions. It includes four types of support: emotional, instrumental, informational, and appraisal.

societal level (2, 11)

Level of the social-ecological framework in which the target of change is local, state, and national laws and policies, and the focus is on changing government regulations and other regulatory processes, procedures, or laws to protect health.

socioeconomic position (16)

A term that encompasses social and economic factors that influence the positions that individuals in groups hold within a society.

source of infection (8)

The person, animal, or insect that carries an organism from one to another or an inanimate source such as food or the environment that causes infection.

Spatial Hazard Event and Loss Database for the United States (SHELDUS) (17)

One of the most comprehensive data banks for tracking natural disasters, encompassing eighteen different types of hazards by county.

specificity (5)

A measure of accuracy; in a research study, the ability to correctly classify people without the outcome as not having the outcome (labeling controls as controls).

spina bifida (5)

A type of neural tube defect characterized by incomplete closure of the spinal column; it can be visible or hidden and may cause a range of disability, including impaired bowel and bladder function and lower extremity paralysis.

sporadic (9)

Occurring occasionally (used to describe infectious diseases).

stage of (cancer) diagnosis (16)

A measure of how advanced cancer is at the time of diagnosis.

stages of change (11)

A theory developed by DiClemente and Prochaska that asserts that behavior change is not a one-time event but rather is a process that involves movement through five stages (precontemplation, contemplation, preparation, action, and maintenance) and that individuals use specific strategies to achieve change. (See also transtheoretical model).

stakeholders (10, 14, 17)

All the people, individually or as groups and institutions, that have a legitimate interest in a particular issue or proposed plan.

standard population (4)

A population for which the age and sex distribution is known.

state health department (2)

Typically, an umbrella agency under which local health departments exist and operate, and such departments are funded by a combination of state and federal dollars.

statistic (6)

A quantity computable from the data collected on the sample.

statistically significant (6)
A measure for which the *p* value is less than a specified threshold (often 0.05 or 5 percent), indicating the null hypothesis can be rejected.

stimulus control (11)
One of the behavior change strategies of the stages of change or transtheoretical model. Involves increasing cues for healthy behaviors and decreasing cues for unhealthy behaviors.

stratify (4)
Dividing data into categories for comparison.

strength of association (5)
The size of a measure of excess risk/measure of effect.

stroke belt (3)
A term applied to the southeastern United States because of a higher prevalence of stroke and other cardiovascular diseases and also many of the risk factors for these outcomes (obesity, high blood pressure, etc.) in the region.

structural barriers (15)
Impediments to medical care directly related to the number, type, concentration, location, or organizational configuration of health care providers.

subjective norm (11)
A construct included in theory of reasoned action and theory of planned behavior that asserts that an individual's intention to perform a health behavior is, in part, dependent on the importance he or she places on what important others think he or she should do.

subject-produced images (12)
Photographs or videotapes created by research participants that capture aspects of their world to allow the researchers an insider view.

sulfur dioxide (9)
A compound that results when fuel combustion reacts with water vapor to produce sulfuric acid and sulfates that irritate the respiratory tract.

surveillance (3)
A system for collecting, analyzing, and interpreting data on a continuous basis for planning and evaluating public health activities.

synergism (10)
In toxicology, the interaction of two or more agents that results in greater effects than could be anticipated if each agent was considered individually.

systematic differences (15)
Regular, measured differences.

T

telescoping (5)
Reporting more distant events as being closer to the present and during the exposure window of interest.

temporal sequence (5)
The order in which events occurred; specifically, whether the exposure occurred before the outcome in an epidemiological study.

teratogen (9)
A substance capable of causing birth defects.

tertiary prevention (2, 5)
One of the three levels of prevention; involves reducing complications and mortality associated with a health condition that is already present by providing medical care or rehabilitation services.

theory (11)
Conceptualization that systematically organizes numerous factors that influence health and health behavior into manageable groupings (constructs) and illustrates the relationships among these factors and constructs.

theory of planned behavior (11)
An extended version of theory of reasoned action that takes into account circumstances in which an individual's behavior is influenced by factors that are out of his or her control.

theory of reasoned action (11)
A widely used public health theory that asserts that health behavior is determined by the individual's readiness or intention to perform a specific health behavior.

therapeutic trial (5)
A randomized controlled trial designed to improve health outcomes once an individual has a disease (tertiary prevention).

threshold (10)
The exposure level or dose of an agent above which toxicity or adverse health effects can occur and below which toxicity or adverse health effects are unlikely.

time (8)

Part of descriptive epidemiology; details the start and end points of an out-break and any related information about duration.

time trends (5)

The pattern of change in a health measure (exposure or outcome) over time.

total exposure (10)

The sum of all exposures received by an individual through all pathways and routes of exposure.

toxicants (9)

Chemicals that have an adverse effect on living organisms.

toxin (9)

A toxicant from a biological source.

traditional ethnography (12)

Research typically done in a single setting, such as a village or a community that is unfamiliar to the researcher and involves observations, interviews, and participation in various activities.

transtheoretical model (11)

A theory developed by DiClemente and Prochaska that asserts that behavior change is not a one-time event, but rather is a process that involves move-ment through five stages (precontemplation, contemplation, preparation, action, and maintenance), and that individuals use specific strategies to achieve change (also see stages of change).

treatment group (6)

The collection of individuals in an experimental study who are exposed.

trend (4)

The movement of a measure in one direction over time.

tuberculin skin test (13)

A diagnostic test that determines an individual's response to proteins isolated from tuberculosis injected into the skin. A positive test is indicated by an area of induration at the site of injection that develops forty-eight to seventy-two hours after the injection.

tuberculosis (TB) (8, 13)

An infectious disease caused by the organism *Mycobacterium tuberculosis* that has a propensity to affect the lungs and is carried by about one-third of the world's population.

two-by-two (2×2) **table (5)**
A table with two rows, one for the exposed and one for the unexposed subjects, and two columns, one for those with the outcome and one for those without the outcome, that is used in observational studies to calculate a crude relative risk or odds ratio.

U

unintended effect (17)
Change brought about by an action that was not planned for.

unit of analysis (5)
The level at which information is collected and then analyzed, often individual or population (group).

univariate (6)
Data description that focuses on one measurement at a time.

universal health care (14)
Health care coverage for all citizens and other eligible residents in a country or governmental region that provides, at a minimum, basic health care services such as primary care and hospital services

usual care (5)
The standard level of health care or health services in a population.

utilization measure (15)
A quantifiable way to assess use of health care services; includes visits to medical providers and number of medical procedures, hospitalizations, and emergency department visits.

V

vaccination (8)
The process prevents infectious diseases by taking advantage of the body's ability to recognize and attack foreign materials inside it and to create a memory of the method of attack, thereby recognizing the foreign object again in the future.

validity (6)
A lack of bias in data or results.

value-based purchasing (15)
A process that ties provider reimbursement rates to quality of care provided.

variable (6, 11)

A value, category, or construct being measured.

variolation (8)

The process of transferring material or fluids from an infected person to a noninfected person to elicit an immune response, especially with smallpox. Also called inoculation.

vector (8)

Animals or insects known to carry (infectious) organisms.

vicarious experience (11)

Observing the behaviors of others and the outcomes of their behaviors.

vital statistics (3)

Primarily legal certifications such as birth and death certificates used as a source of public health data.

W

World Health Organization (WHO) (1, 7)

The body within the United Nations that coordinates health-related activities (surveillance, planning, policy suggestions, and technical support) on a global scale.

Y

years of potential life lost (15)

The number of years of potential life lost by each death occurring before a predetermined end point, such as age sixty-five or seventy years.

INDEX